Contemporary Issues in Peripheral Vascular Disease

Books Available in Cardiovascular Clinics Series

Contemporary Issues in Peripheral Vascular Disease

John A. Spittell, Jr., M.D. / Editor

Professor Emeritus of Medicine
Mayo Medical School
Consultant, Division of Cardiovascular Diseases and Internal Medicine
Mayo Clinic
Rochester, Minnesota

CARDIOVASCULAR CLINICS
Albert N. Brest, M.D. / Editor-in-Chief

James C. Wilson Professor of Medicine
Jefferson Medical College
Philadelphia, Pennsylvania

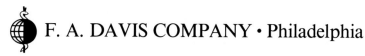 F. A. DAVIS COMPANY · Philadelphia

Printed in the United States of America
Last digit indicates print number: 10 9 8 7 6 5 4 3 2 1

acquisitions editor: Robert H. Craven
production editor: Gail Shapiro

As new scientific information becomes available through basic and clinical research, recommended treatments and drug therapies undergo changes. The author(s) and publisher have done everything possible to make this book accurate, up to date, and in accord with accepted standards at the time of publication. The authors, editors, and publisher are not responsible for errors or omissions or for consequences from application of the book, and make no warranty, expressed or implied, in regard to the contents of the book. Any practice described in this book should be applied by the reader in accordance with professional standards of care used in regard to the unique circumstances that may apply in each situation. The reader is advised always to check product information (package inserts) for changes and new information regarding dose and contraindications before administering any drug. Caution is especially urged when using new or infrequently ordered drugs.

Library of Congress Cataloging in Publication Data

Cardiovascular clinics. 22/3
   Philadelphia, F. A. Davis, 1969–
      v. ill. 27 cm.
     Editor: v. 1- A. N. Brest.
     Key title: Cardiovascular clinics, ISSN 0069-0384
     1. Cardiovascular system—Diseases—Collected works   I. Brest,
Albert N., ed.
     [DNLM: W1 CA77N]
RC681.A1C27   6.6.1   70-6558
ISBN 0-8036-80880   MARC-S

Preface

Disorders of the peripheral circulation are, if anything, increasing in frequency with the increasing age of our population. Aneurysmal disease and venous thromboembolism continue to be significant causes of mortality and morbidity because their recognition and diagnosis remain difficult and all too infrequent. Unfortunately, too, peripheral vascular disorders continue to be inadequately addressed in many, if not most, medical school curricula and residency training programs. At the same time, advances in basic knowledge, diagnostic methodology, and therapeutic options have piqued the interest of clinicians in peripheral vascular disease.

Inasmuch as it has been eight years since an issue of Cardiovascular Clinics has been devoted to peripheral vascular disease, it is the purpose of this issue to focus on the new developments and their application to the up-to-date management of peripheral arterial disease and venous thromboembolic disease and their complications.

John A. Spittell, Jr.

Editor's Commentary

An earlier (1983) edition of CARDIOVASCULAR CLINICS dealt with Clinical Vascular Disease and covered a wide array of arterial and venous diseases involving various peripheral and systemic vascular beds. In addition, special topics such as the Vasculitides, lymphedema, and differential diagnosis of leg ulcers were covered. Much of the material in that issue remains clinically vital, and the reader of this volume may wish to refer to the earlier book. No attempt was made in the present volume to simply repeat the earlier material, but instead it was our goal to contemporize the information where needed, and again to include additional special topics such as arteriovenous communications, penetrating aortic ulcer, and endothelium-derived factors and peripheral vascular disease. I am once again indebted to my friend, John A. Spittell, Jr., M.D., for his guidance in the development of this volume; and both of us are indebted to the contributors for their exemplary efforts.

Albert N. Brest, M.D.
Editor-in-Chief

Contributors

John P. Cooke, M.D., Ph.D.
Assistant Professor of Medicine
Director, Section of Vascular Medicine
Division of Cardiovascular Medicine
Stanford University School of Medicine
Stanford, California

Edward Genton, M.D.
Department of Cardiology
Ochsner Clinic
Cardiology Section
New Orleans, Louisiana

Peter Gloviczki, M.D.
Mayo Clinic
Rochester, Minnesota

Robert Graor, M.D.
Cleveland Clinic Foundation
Cleveland, Ohio

Bruce H. Gray, D.O.
Cleveland Clinic Foundation
Cleveland, Ohio

Larry H. Hollier, M.D.
Chairman, Department of Surgery
Clinical Professor of Surgery
Louisiana State University Medical Center and Tulane University Medical Center
New Orleans, Louisiana

John W. Joyce, M.D.
Associate Professor of Medicine
Mayo Medical School
Division of Cardiovascular Diseases and Internal Medicine
Mayo Clinic
Rochester, Minnesota

Francis J. Kazmier, M.D.
Division of Vascular Medicine
Ochsner Clinic
New Orleans, Louisiana

Irene Meissner, M.D.
Consultant, Department of Neurology
Mayo Clinic
Assistant Professor of Neurology
Mayo Medical School
Rochester, Minnesota

Steven W. Merrell, M.D.
Mayo Clinic
Rochester, Minnesota

Wayne L. Miller, M.D., Ph.D.
Assistant Professor of Medicine
Senior Associate Consultant
Cardiovascular Diseases and Internal Medicine
Mayo Clinic
Rochester, Minnesota

Bahram Mokri, M.D.
Vice Chairman, Department of Neurology
Mayo Clinic
Associate Professor of Neurology
Mayo Medical School
Rochester, Minnesota

William M. Moore, Jr., M.D.
Fellow in Vascular Surgery
Ochsner Clinic
New Orleans, Louisiana

Philip J. Osmundson, M.D.
Consultant, Cardiovascular Division
Mayo Clinic
Associate Professor of Medicine
Mayo Medical School
Rochester, Minnesota

Edward C. Rosenow, III, M.D.
Arthur M. and Gladys D. Gray Professor of Medicine
Division of Thoracic Diseases and Internal Medicine
Mayo Clinic
Rochester, Minnesota

Thom W. Rooke, M.D., F.A.C.C.
Assistant Professor of Medicine
Director of Vascular Disease Center
Mayo Clinic
Rochester, Minnesota

Jay H. Ryu, M.D.
Assistant Professor of Medicine
Division of Thoracic Diseases and Internal Medicine
Mayo Clinic
Rochester, Minnesota

Roger F. J. Shepherd, M.B., B.Ch.
Consultant, Cardiovascular Diseases and Internal Medicine
Mayo Clinic
Rochester, Minnesota

John A. Spittell, Jr., M.D.
Professor, Mayo Medical School
Consultant, Cardiovascular Diseases
Mayo Clinic
Rochester, Minnesota

Robert G. Tancredi, M.D.
Consultant, Division of Cardiovascular Diseases
Mayo Clinic
Rochester, Minnesota

Jess R. Young, M.D.
Chairman, Department of Vascular Medicine
Cleveland Clinic Foundation
Cleveland, Ohio

Contents

PART 1

Etiologic and Diagnostic Considerations

CHAPTER 1

Endothelium-Derived Factors and Peripheral Vascular Disease

John P. Cooke, M.D., Ph.D.

Twenty-five years ago, Nobel laureate Lord Florey challenged the conventional paradigm of the endothelium as merely a nonthrombogenic barrier when he stated that "endothelial cells (are) . . . more than a sheet of nucleated cellophane."[1] In the intervening time it has become quite clear that the endothelium plays a major role in control of vasomotor tone and structure, blood fluidity, lipid metabolism, and angiogenesis. The normal endothelium synthesizes an astounding variety of proteins and maintains a delicate balance between growth inhibitory and growth-promoting factors, vasoconstrictors and vasodilators, as well as antithrombotic and hemostatic mechanisms. Disturbances of the delicate balance between opposing endothelial influences are associated with a number of vasculopathies, characterized by vasospasm, thrombosis, or abnormal vessel growth.

NORMAL ENDOTHELIAL FUNCTION

EFFECTS ON COAGULATION

The endothelium plays a major role in modulating blood fluidity. It synthesizes and releases activators and inhibitors of fibrinolysis.[2-4] Prostacyclin produced by the endothelium inhibits platelet reactivity, but its action is opposed by another endothelial product, thromboxane A_2; in addition, the endothelium produces von Willebrand's factor, which is necessary for platelet–vessel wall interactions.[5-7] The endothelium also synthesizes membrane-associated molecules such as thrombomodulin and heparan sulfate, which contribute to its antithrombogenic properties[8,9]; conversely, it also generates adhesive molecules that bind platelets or leukocytes to the endothelium.[10,11] This diversity of endothelial synthetic functions allows this tissue to maintain blood fluidity under normal circumstances but provides mechanisms for hemostasis in the event of vessel injury.

EFFECTS ON VASCULAR GROWTH AND STRUCTURE

In the same manner, dynamic equilibrium exists between growth promoters and inhibitors released from the endothelium. The endothelium is capable of manufacturing platelet-derived growth factor, insulin-like growth factor, fibroblast-growth factor, and other cytokines and growth-promoting factors.[12-14] The effects of these growth-promoting paracrine substances are balanced by endothelial products that suppress smooth muscle proliferation, such as transforming growth factor.[15] It is now known that many of the vasoactive agents produced by the endothelium also affect proliferation of vascular smooth muscle. Endothelium-derived prostanoids and other relaxing factors inhibit proliferation of vascular smooth muscle, whereas endothelin and angiotensin II promote growth.[16-20] The ability of endothelial products to alter the growth state of vascular smooth muscle cells likely has important physiologic consequences. Remodeling the vessel wall is an ongoing process in response to changes in hemodynamic forces as well as neurohumoral stimuli. For example, when blood flow increases through a conduit vessel, it dilates and then returns to its basal dimensions when flow normalizes.[21] If the increase in blood flow persists for a prolonged period (as in the case of a conduit vessel supplying an arteriovenous malformation), the increase in luminal diameter becomes permanent as the vessel remodels.[21,22] The endothelium is necessary for both phenomena to occur. Transient increases in blood flow trigger the release of prostacyclin and endothelium-derived relaxing factor, the latter vasodilator being primarily responsible for flow-mediated vasodilation.[23-25] It is not known what role these or other endothelial products play in the structural alterations induced by prolonged changes in blood flow. The mechanism by which the endothelium senses changes in flow also remains undetermined but may involve activation of ionic channels in the luminal aspect of the cell membrane.[26,27] The endothelium also responds to changes in transluminal pressure by releasing a vasoconstrictor substance, possibly a prostanoid.[28] In this way, the endothelium may contribute to autoregulation of vessel diameter in response to fluxes in the blood pressure.

EFFECTS ON VASCULAR TONE

Because of its intimate apposition to the vascular smooth muscle, the endothelium plays a major role in vascular tone. The endothelium is a rich source of converting enzyme, which metabolizes angiotensin I to the active vasoconstrictor, angiotensin II; the same enzyme inactivates the vasodilator bradykinin.[29] It also acts as a metabolic barrier to serotonin and catecholamines. These substances are taken up avidly by the endothelium and inactivated by monoamine oxidase.[29] In addition to its metabolic activity the endothelium provides a braking influence on the action of vasoconstrictors by releasing endogenous vasodilators. For example, in the absence of the endothelium, serotonin, histamine, and acetylcholine and other endogenous vasoconstrictors will activate the vascular smooth muscle.[30-34] In contrast, in the presence of the endothelium, receptors on its surface bind these agonists and modulate their action by stimulating the release of endothelial vasodilators such as prostacyclin and endothelium-derived relaxing factor (Fig. 1–1).[30-34] Endothelium-derived relaxing factor (EDRF) is now known to be nitric oxide or a nitric oxide–containing substance.[35-38] It is an extremely potent vasodilator that likely plays a major role in the regulation of vessel tone. Its chemical

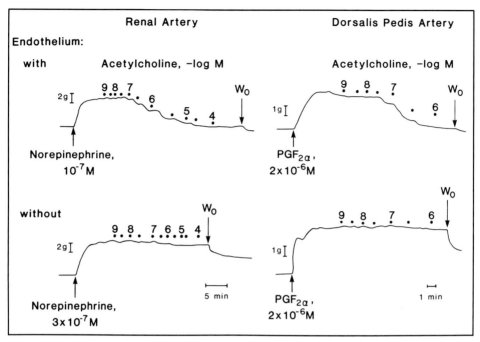

Figure 1–1. Tracings of original polygraph recordings of vasomotion in a human renal artery *(left panel)* and a dorsalis pedis artery *(right panel)*. Arterial rings with *(above)* and without endothelium *(below)* were contracted with norepinephrine or prostaglandin F_{2a}(PGF$_{2a}$). During the contraction, increasing concentrations of acetylcholine were added to the solutions bathing these vessels. In the presence of endothelium, human arteries relax in response to acetylcholine. This relaxation is due to the release of EDRF. In the absence of endothelium *(below)* no relaxations are observed. (From Luscher et al,[34] with permission.)

properties and mechanism of action resemble that of the class of drugs known as nitrovasodilators, and this substance can be thought of as an endogenous form of nitroglycerin. It is derived from the metabolism of arginine; specifically, it is the terminal guanidino nitrogen atoms of this amino acid that are oxidized to nitric oxide.[38] Synthesis of EDRF can be abrogated by specific inhibitors; intravenous injection of these inhibitors into animals causes a substantial rise in blood pressure (in the range of 30 mm Hg).[39] Intrabrachial arterial infusion of these inhibitors also causes dramatic and sustained increases in forearm vascular resistance in humans. This agent is not only a potent vasodilator but it also inhibits platelet aggregation[41–43] (Fig. 1–2). Its action on platelets is similar to that of other nitrates in that it appears to be mediated by a cyclic guanosine monophosphate (GMP)–dependent pathway. Of great interest is the recent finding that nitrovasodilators and the cyclic GMP analogues that mimic their action are also antimitogenic agents.[16] Therefore, this particular endothelial product appears to be an antiplatelet and growth inhibitory substance as well as a potent vasodilator.

ENDOTHELIAL DYSFUNCTION AND PERIPHERAL VASCULAR DISEASE

Because of its multifold actions to modulate vessel tone and growth and to regulate interactions of the vessel wall with blood constituents, dysfunction of the

DOSE–DEPENDENT INHIBITION OF PLATELET AGGREGATION BY ASPIRIN–TREATED ENDOTHELIAL CELLS

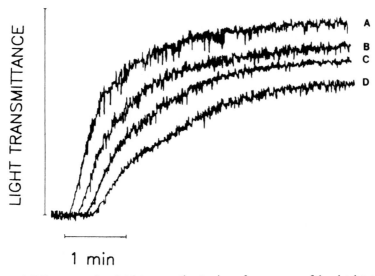

1 min

Figure 1–2. Representative platelet aggregation tracings after exposure of the platelets to increasing concentrations of endothelial cells in vitro (A = 0, B = 4.4×10^5, C = 8.8×10^5, and D = 1.3×10^6 endothelial cells added to the platelet-rich plasma in the aggregometer). Exposure of the platelets in vitro to increasing concentrations of the endothelial cells reduces the rate as well as the extent of platelet aggregation. This phenomenon was associated with an increase in cyclic GMP within the platelets. (From Stamler et al,[42] with permission.)

endothelium may be responsible for or contribute to a variety of vasculopathies. Atherosclerosis, restenosis, hypertension, and other disorders characterized by thrombosis, vasoconstriction, and/or abnormal vascular structure are associated with endothelial dysfunction. To focus the discussion, endothelial dysfunction in these disease states will be examined largely in terms of disturbances in the synthesis and release of one endothelial product, EDRF.

ATHEROSCLEROSIS: A RESPONSE TO ENDOTHELIAL INJURY

MECHANISMS OF ENDOTHELIAL INJURY

The most common cause of peripheral arterial occlusive disease is athcrosclerosis. This is a complex process that is thought to be initiated by a "response to injury" of the endothelium.[44] The specific injuries that precipitate atherogenesis are not known, although risk factors have been identified. One of these is serum cholesterol, specifically the low-density lipoprotein (LDL) fraction. Elevated levels of LDL cholesterol perturb the cell membrane, alter permeability and secretion, and may possibly induce the expression of intercellular adhesion molecules, cytokines, and growth factors.[45–47] One or more of these abnormalities may be responsible for the observation that within several days of a high-cholesterol diet, monocytes adhere to the endothelium, particularly at intercellular junctions.[44,48] They migrate into the subendothelium where they begin to accumulate lipid and become foam cells. This is the earliest event in the formation of the fatty streak. These activated macrophages release mitogens and chemoattractants that recruit additional macrophages as well as vascular smooth muscle cells into the lesion. Migration and proliferation of vascular smooth muscle cells into the lesion gradually transform it into a fibrous plaque. Platelets play a major role in the development of these lesions; injury to or dysfunction of the endothelium permits platelets to adhere to the vessel wall, releasing epidermal growth factor, platelet-derived growth factor, and other mitogens and cytokines that may induce smooth muscle migration and proliferation.[44]

The specific endothelial injuries that initiate atherogenesis are not known. However, one of the earliest known endothelial dysfunctions induced by hypercholesterolemia is a reduction in the release of EDRF. It is widely recognized that hypercholesterolemia alters vascular reactivity in animal models and in humans; this appears to be due primarily to a reduced release of EDRF, although some investigators have reported changes in sensitivity of the vascular smooth muscle to vasoconstrictors.[49–52] In hypercholesterolemic primates, swine, and rabbits, endothelium-dependent relaxation is attenuated; in parallel fashion, contractions to a wide range of vasoconstrictors are augmented owing to the imbalance caused by a reduction of EDRF release.[49–51] This disturbance of vasodilator function occurs long before any of the morphologic changes of atherosclerosis. Porcine coronary arteries from animals fed a cholesterol-rich diet for 8 weeks exhibit little or no morphologic changes; however, endothelium-dependent relaxations are reduced.[53] Indeed, endothelium-dependent relaxations in normal vessels can be dramatically reduced within minutes after in vitro exposure to LDL cholesterol.[54,55] It is likely that a reduced release of EDRF (nitric oxide) is one of the earliest vascular abnormalities in hypercholesterolemia and may play an important role in the initiation of atherogenesis. A reduction in the release of EDRF would enhance vasoconstriction, promote platelet–vessel wall interactions, and disrupt the balance between growth inhibitory and promoting influences on the vascular smooth muscle. Moreover, there is indirect evidence that EDRF may also inhibit macrophage migration into the vessel wall;[56] a reduction in EDRF release might also favor monocyte adhesion and migration. All of these events would tend to promote atherogenesis.

RESTORATION OF ENDOTHELIAL FUNCTION

Aggressive treatment of hypercholesterolemia improves vascular function and structure. There is abundant evidence in animal models that treatment of hypercholesterolemia inhibits atherogenesis and can cause lesions to regress and vasomotor function to normalize. Iliac arteries from primates fed a cholesterol-rich diet exhibit morphologic changes of atherosclerosis and reduced endothelium-dependent vasodilation.[57] After the animals have been switched to a low-cholesterol diet, there is a gradual regression of the atherosclerotic lesions associated with a normalization of endothelial function. Abnormal endothelial function and atherogenesis also may be prevented by treatment of hypercholesterolemic animals with HMG CoA reductase inhibitors; the same beneficial effect is observed in hypercholesterolemic animals treated with fish oil.[58,59]

The beneficial effect of dietary changes and antilipid agents is clearly due to a reduction in the levels of LDL cholesterol; in contrast, the salutory effects of fish oil cannot be ascribed solely to changes in serum cholesterol because its effects on serum lipids are modest and variable.[59-61] However, the effects of fish oil on prostanoid synthesis are notable. The omega-3 unsaturated fatty acids in fish oil compete with arachidonic acid for metabolism by cyclo-oxygenase.[61,62] Normally arachidonic acid is converted into prostacyclin (PGI_2), which has vasodilator, antiplatelet, and antimitogenic activity; or thromboxane (TxA_2), a potent vasoconstrictor, platelet activator, and chemoattractant. Eicosopentaenoic acid in fish oil replaces arachidonic acid as the substrate for prostanoid synthesis. It is converted into an active form of prostacyclin (PGI_3), but an inactive form of thromboxane (TxA_3). Thus, eicosopentaenoic acid creates a favorable imbalance in prostanoid metabolism, which favors vasodilation, inhibition of platelet aggregation, and suppression of smooth muscle growth. Fish oil also increases the release of EDRF.[59] These effects of fish oil may be responsible for the reduced incidence of coronary artery disease in Greenland Eskimos, inasmuch as this group consumes large quantities of marine lipid.[63,64]

Aggressive medical therapy may improve vascular function and structure in humans. Indeed, a number of angiographic studies have revealed that aggressive antilipid therapy may induce plaque regression.[65,66] Preliminary evidence suggests that treatment also may improve vascular function. As an example, it is known that patients with atherosclerosis of coronary or peripheral vessels exhibit enhanced vasoconstriction and/or attenuated vasodilation of these vessels.[67,68] Initial studies suggest that the administration of fish oil may normalize coronary vasomotion in these patients.[69,70]

Recently, we have investigated the utility of L-arginine to improve vascular function. As previously mentioned, L-arginine is the precursor for EDRF. We hypothesized that the reduced release of EDRF in hypercholesterolemic subjects was due to reduced intracellular availability or metabolism of arginine, and further

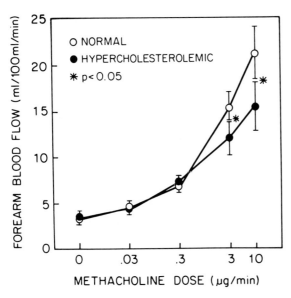

Figure 1-3. Forearm blood flow response to intra-arterial methacholine in normal *(open circles)* and hypercholesterolemic *(closed circles)* subjects without clinical evidence of atherosclerosis. The response to methacholine was significantly reduced in the hypercholesterolemic subjects, suggesting an endothelial vasodilator dysfunction. (From the Journal of Clinical Investigation 86:228–234, 1990, by copyright permission of the American Society of Clinical Investigation.)

proposed that administration of the EDRF precursor could restore normal vaso-motion. This hypothesis has been confirmed in animal studies. Increases in hind limb blood flow in response to intra-arterial acetylcholine are reduced in hypercholesterolemic rabbits; normal responses were restored after an intravenous infusion of L-arginine.[71] Endothelium-dependent responses of arteries isolated from these animals and studied in vitro were also improved by L-arginine.[72,73] In young hypercholesterolemic subjects without clinical evidence of atherosclerosis, forearm blood flow in response to intra-arterial methacholine (which stimulates the release of EDRF) is reduced[74] (Fig. 1–3). Preliminary studies suggest that vasomotion in these subjects may be normalized after intravenous infusion of L-arginine.[75]

In summary, hypercholesterolemia induces an endothelial dysfunction that initiates atherogenesis. The specific endothelial injury that precipitates atherogenesis remains undetermined. However, it is clear that atherogenesis may be reversed, even at later stages of the disease. A number of ongoing studies will determine the role of aggressive antilipid therapy, calcium entry antagonists, or other agents to induce regression of atherosclerotic disease. We will need to determine the nature of the endothelial dysfunction that initiates atherogenesis so that new therapies can be directed at the mechanisms of the disease.

RESTENOSIS AND MYOINTIMAL HYPERPLASIA

PATHOLOGY OF RESTENOSIS

When atherosclerotic arterial occlusive disease of the peripheral vessels progresses to the point that symptoms begin to interfere with the patient's lifestyle or when the viability of the extremity becomes threatened, interventional techniques are indicated, such as catheter balloon angioplasty or atherectomy, endarterectomy, or venous bypass grafting. Acute failure of these procedures is due generally to thrombosis precipitated by gross endothelial denudation exposing the thrombogenic constituents of the subendothelial space. Hemorrhage into the vessel wall due to plaque rupture or dissection also contributes to early closure.

Long-term success of these procedures is limited by a different disorder known as myointimal hyperplasia (Fig. 1–4). This process is characterized by migration of vascular smooth cells from the media to the intima where they proliferate and transform into secretory cells, synthesizing extracellular matrix that contributes to the bulk of the lesion.[76–78] It appears that this process is precipitated by endothelial denudation, platelet–vessel wall interactions, and the release of growth factors. Inflammatory cells also contribute, releasing cytokines (such as interleukin-1) and other paracrine substances that stimulate migration and proliferation. The injured vascular smooth muscle cells also appear to release growth factors and chemotactic agents that participate in the proliferative process. This disorder causes symptomatic restenosis in approximately 30% of patients within 6 months of balloon angioplasty or atherectomy and contributes to most late failures of bypass grafts.[76–78] The so-called transplant atherosclerosis that is now responsible for 40% of deaths following an initially successful heart transplantation histologically resembles myointimal hyperplasia.[79]

Although myointimal hyperplasia appears to be initiated by loss of the endothelium, it continues after the endothelium has regenerated. We and others have found that these regenerating endothelial cells are morphologically and functionally

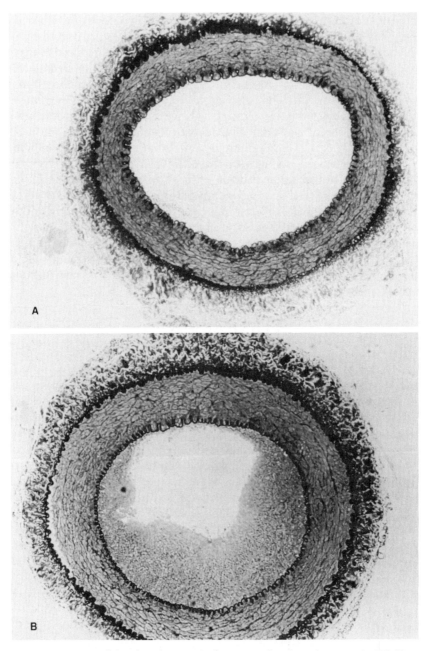

Figure 1–4. (*A*) Low-power light microphotograph of a cross section through a normal rabbit iliac artery. (*B*) Cross section through a rabbit iliac artery injured 4 weeks previously using a balloon catheter. Myointimal hyperplasia has significantly reduced the diameter of the vessel lumen. (From Weidinger et al,[81] with permission.)

abnormal, and may be contributing to the disease process.[80-81] Unlike normal endothelial cells, which are fusiform and aligned with flow, these cells are irregularly sized, cuboidal, and not aligned with flow (Fig. 1–5). Adherent platelets may be observed, usually in association with gaps at the interendothelial junctions.

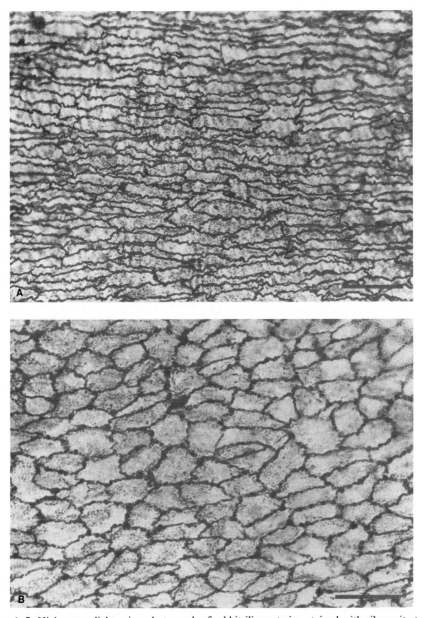

Figure 1-5. High-power light microphotograph of rabbit iliac arteries, stained with silver nitrate and examined en face to demonstrate endothelial morphology. (*A*) The normal endothelium from an uninjured rabbit iliac artery is composed of fusiform cells that are aligned with blood flow. (*B*) Four weeks after a balloon catheter injury, the endothelium has regenerated but the cells are polygonal, irregularly sized, and not aligned with blood flow. Magnification bars represent 40 μm. From Weidinger et al,[81] with permission.)

These abnormal cells produce less EDRF, and this deficiency may contribute to ongoing platelet-vessel interactions and vascular smooth muscle proliferation. This in indicated by the observation that the intimal thickness is related to the severity of endothelial dysfunction.[81]

THERAPEUTIC STRATEGIES

Medical therapy to limit restenosis has been disappointing. Antiplatelet therapy undoubtedly reduces the incidence of acute thrombosis after revascularization procedures but does not inhibit myointimal hyperplasia.[82] Heparin, warfarin sodium (Coumadin), calcium entry antagonists, and corticosteroids also have no beneficial effect on this lesion.[83-86] Trials with fish oils have been contradictory.[87-90] Considered in aggregate, these trials suggest there may be a modest reduction of restenosis with fish oil treatment, but this modest effect is attained with large quantities of the agent that are not well tolerated by many patients. Angiotensin converting enzyme inhibitors may have some promise. In an animal model of restenosis after balloon angioplasty, converting enzyme inhibition was associated with a 50% reduction in the size of the lesion when treatment was initiated prior to, and continued for several weeks after, the balloon injury.[91] The mechanism of this beneficial effect is not known but may be due to a local effect of these agents on the vessel wall. Specifically, it is now known that the blood vessel contains all the elements of the renin-angiotensin system and may generate angiotensin II locally.[92] Angiotensin II is not only a potent vasoconstrictor but promotes vascular smooth muscle growth by inducing the expression of proto-oncogenes and the synthesis of PDGF and other autocrine growth factors.[19,20] Preliminary evidence suggests that balloon injury activates the local renin-angiotensin system of the vessel wall, resulting in locally elevated concentrations of angiotensin II (V. J. Dzau*, personal communication). If activation of the local renin-angiotensin system in the injured vessel contributes to myointimal hyperplasia, this would explain the beneficial effect of converting enzyme inhibitors. Clinical trials of converting enzyme inhibitors to prevent myointimal hyperplasia are now in progress.

The implications of the dysfunction observed in regenerating endothelium may apply to other situations resulting in endothelial loss. At sites of arterial bifurcation, flow becomes turbulent. At these sites, there is increased endothelial cell turnover with focal areas of endothelial damage and denudation.[93,94] It is possible that the endothelium regenerating at these sites is also abnormal. Indeed, a recent study revealed evidence of endothelial vasodilator dysfunction at coronary artery branch points, even in patients with no angiographic evidence of coronary atherosclerosis.[95] This early endothelial dysfunction may explain the tendency for atheroma to form at arterial bifurcations.

HYPERTENSION, ENDOTHELIUM, AND ARTERIAL DISEASE

Hypertension is a known risk factor for the development of atherosclerotic arterial occlusive disease. In animal models, hypertension induces vasomotor abnormalities, including a reduction in endothelium-dependent relaxation, as well as the elaboration of a vasoconstrictor from the endothelium that appears to be a prostanoid.[96-100] It is not known whether these abnormalities play a major role in elevating vascular resistance or are merely epiphenomena of the hypertensive process. Antihypertensive treatment does normalize vascular response in these exper-

---

*V. J. Dzau, M.D., Chief, Division of Cardiovascular Medicine, Stanford University School of Medicine, Stanford, CA.

imental models,[101,102] suggesting the endothelial abnormalities may be secondary to the elevated blood pressure.

Two recent studies indicate that the observations made in animal models of hypertension apply to patients with essential hypertension.[103,104] In both of these studies forearm blood flow was measured in response to intra-arterial infusion of acetylcholine (which releases EDRF) and sodium nitroprusside (which causes vasodilation independent of the endothelium). In the patients with essential hypertension, the response to acetylcholine was blunted in comparison with the response of the normotensive subjects. By contrast, the endothelium-independent vasodilation to sodium nitroprusside was unaffected. It appears therefore that in hypertensive humans, the release of EDRF is attenuated. Whether this is a primary or secondary phenomenon is not known; however, the reduction in EDRF release certainly may contribute to the increase in vascular resistance. Moreover, it may be speculated that the reduction in EDRF release also may contribute to the proliferation of vascular smooth muscle observed in hypertension. This endothelial dysfunction also may promote increased platelet–vessel wall interactions, which may contribute to the acceleration of atherosclerosis in this population of patients.

SUMMARY

The endothelium plays a major role in modulating vascular tone, vascular growth, and interactions of the vessel wall with blood constituents. Therefore, abnormalities in endothelial function may play a primary or contributory role to a variety of vasculopathies that are characterized by thrombosis, excessive vasoconstriction, or vascular smooth muscle proliferation. Our increasing understanding of the complexity of endothelial functions will permit us to understand the mechanisms of vascular disease and to design new therapies directed at these mechanisms of disease.

REFERENCES

1. Florey, L: The endothelial cell. Br Med J 2:487, 1966.
2. Todd, AS: The histological localization of fibrinolytic activator. J Pathol Bacteriol 78:281, 1959.
3. Levin, EG and Loskutoff, DJ: Cultures bovine endothelial cells produce both urokinase and tissue-type plasminogen activators. J Cell Biol 94:631, 1982.
4. Levin, EG: Latent tissue plasminogen activator produced by human endothelial cells in culture: Evidence for enzyme-inhibitor complex. Proc Natl Acad Sci USA 80:6804, 1983.
5. Bunting, SR, Gryglewski, R, Moncada, S, et al: Arterial walls generate from prostaglandin endoperoxides a substance (prostaglandin X) which relaxes strips of mesenteric and coeliac arteries and inhibits platelet aggregation. Prostaglandins 12:897, 1976.
6. Jaffe, EA, Hoyer, LW, and Nachmann, RL: Synthesis of antihemophilic factor antigen by cultured human endothelial cells. J Clin Invest 52:2725, 1973.
7. Jaffe EA, Hoyer, LW, and Nachmann, RL: Synthesis of von Willebrand factor by cultured human endothelial cells. Proc Natl Acad Sci USA 71:1906, 1974.
8. Marcum, JA, McKenney, JB, and Rosenberg, RD: Acceleration of thrombin-antithrombin complex formation in rat hindquarters via heparin-like molecules bound to the endothelium. J Clin Invest 74:341, 1984.
9. Esmon, C and Owen, W: Identification of an endothelial cell cofactor for thrombin-catalyzed activation of protein C. Proc Natl Acad Sci USA 78:2249, 1981.
10. Streeter, PR, Berg, EL, Rouse, BTN, et al: A tissue-specific endothelial cell molecule involved in lymphocyte homing. Nature 331:41, 1988.
11. Tonnesen, MG: Neutrophil-endothelial cell interactions: Mechanisms of neutrophil adherence to vascular endothelium. J Invest Dermatol 93:53S, 1989.

12. Fox, PL and DiCorleto, PE: Regulation of production of a platelet-derived growth factor-like protein by cultured bovine aortic endothelial cells. J Cell Physiol 121:298, 1984.

13. Hansson, H-A, Jennische, E, and Skottner, A: Regenerating endothelial cells express insulin like growth factor-1 immunoreactivity after arterial injury. Cell Tissue Res 250:499, 1987.

14. Vlodavsky, I, Folkman, J, Sullivan, R, et al: Endothelial cell-derived basic fibroblast growth factor: Synthesis and deposition into subendothelial extracellular matrix. Proc Natl Acad Sci USA 84:2292, 1987.

15. Antonelli-Orlidge, A, Saunders, KB, Smith, S, et al: An activated form of transforming growth factor-beta is produced by cocultures of endothelial cells and pericytes. Proc Natl Acad Sci USA 86:4544.

16. Garg, UC and Hassid, A: Nitric oxide-generating vasodilators and 8-bromocyclic guanosine monophosphate inhibit mitogenesis and proliferation of cultured rat vascular smooth muscle cells. J Clin Invest 83:1774, 1989.

17. Loesberg, C, Wijk, RV, Zandbergen, J, et al: Cell cycle-dependent inhibition of human vascular smooth muscle cell proliferation by prostaglandin E1. Exp Cell Res 160:117, 1985.

18. Dubin, D, Pratt, RE, Cooke, JP, et al: Endothelin, a potent vasoconstrictor, is a vascular smooth muscle mitogen. J Vasc Med Biol 1:150, 1989.

19. Geisterfer, AAT, Peach, MJ, and Owens, GK: Angiotensin II induces hypertrophy, not hyperplasia, of cultured rat aortic smooth muscle cells. Circ Res 62:749–756, 1988.

20. Naftilan, AJ, Pratt, RE, and Dzau, VJ: Induction of platelet-derived growth factor A-chain and c-myc gene expressions by angiotensin II in cultured rat vascular smooth muscle cells. J Clin Invest 83:1419, 1989.

21. Holtz, J, Forstermann, U, Pohl, U, et al: Flow dependent, endothelium-mediated dilation of epicardial coronary arteries in conscious dogs: Effects of cyclo-oxygenase inhibition. J Cardiovasc Pharmacol 6:1161, 1984.

22. Langille, BL and O'Donnell, F: Reductions in arterial diameter produced by chronic decreases in blood flow are endothelium-dependent. Science 231:405, 1986.

23. Frangos, VA, Eskin, SG, McIntire, LV, et al: Flow effects on prostacyclin production by cultured human endothelial cells. Science 227:1477, 1985.

24. Kaiser, L, Hull, SS, and Sparks, HV: Methylene blue and ETYA block flow-dependent dilation in canine femoral artery. Am J Physiol 250:H974, 1986.

25. Cooke, JP, Osmundson, PJ, Creaser, MA, and Shepherd, JT: Sex differences in control of cutaneous blood flow. Circulation 82:1607–1615, 1990.

26. Olesen, S-P, Clapham, DE, and Davies, PF: Hemodynamic shear stress activates a K^+ current in vascular endothelial cells. Nature 331:168, 1988.

27. Cooke, JP, Rossitch, E, Jr, Andon, N, et al: Flow activates a specific endothelial potassium channel to release an endogenous nitrovasodilator. J Clin Invest (in press).

28. Harder, DR: Pressure-induced myogenic activation of cat cerebral arteries is dependent on intact endothelium. Circ Res 60:102, 1987.

29. Shepherd, JT and Vanhoutte, PM: The Human Cardiovascular System: Facts and Concepts. Raven Press, New York, 1979, p. 22.

30. Furchgott, RF, and Zawadzki, JV: The obligatory role of endothelial cells in the relaxation of arterial smooth muscle by acetylcholine. Nature 286:373, 1980.

31. DeMey, JG, and Vanhoutte, PM: Role of the intima in cholinergic and purinergic relaxation of isolated canine femoral arteries. J Physiol (London) 316:347, 1981.

32. Houston, DS, Shepherd, JT, and Vanhoutte, PM: Adenine nucleotides, serotonin, and endothelium-dependent relaxations to platelets. Am J Physiol 248:H389, 1985.

33. Vane, JR, Anggard, EE, and Botting, RM: Regulatory functions of the vascular endothelium. N Engl J Med 323:27, 1990.

34. Luscher, TF, Cooke, JP, Houston, BS, et al: Endothelium-dependent relaxation in human arteries. Mayo Clin Proc 62:601, 1987.

35. Ignarro, LJ, Byrns, RE, Buga, GM, et al: Endothelium-derived relaxing factor from pulmonary artery and vein possesses pharmacologic and chemical properties indentical to those of nitric oxide radical. Circ Res 61:866, 1987.

36. Palmer, RMJ, Ferrige, AG, and Moncada, S: Nitric oxide release accounts for the biological activity of endothelium-derived relaxing factor. Nature 327:524, 1987.

37. Furchgott, RF: Studies on relaxation of rabbit aorta by sodium nitrite: The basis for the proposal that the acid-activatable inhibitory factor from retractor penis is inorganic nitrite and the endothelium-derived relaxing factor is nitric oxide. In Vanhoutte, P. (ed): Mechanisms of Vasodilation. Raven Press, New York, 1988, p. 401.

38. Palmer, RMJ, Ashton, DS, and Moncada, S: Vascular endothelial cells synthesize nitric oxide from L-arginine. Nature 333:664, 1988.
39. Rees, DD, Palmer, RMJ, and Moncada, S: Role of endothelium-derived nitric oxide in the regulation of blood pressure. Proc Natl Acad Sci USA 86:3375, 1989.
40. Vallance, P, Collier, J, and Moncada, S: Effects of endothelium-derived nitric oxide on peripheral arteriolar tone in man. Lancet 2:997, 1989.
41. Furlong, G, Henderson, AH, Lewis, MJ, et al: Endothelium-derived relaxing factor inhibits in vitro platelet aggregation. Br J Pharmacol 92:181, 1987.
42. Stamler, JS, Mendelsohn, ME, Amarante, P, et al: N-acetylcysteine potentiates platelet inhibition by endothelium-derived relaxing factor. Circ Res 65:789, 1989.
43. Radomski, MW, Palmer, RMJ, and Moncada, S: Comparative pharmacology of endothelium-derived relaxing factor, nitric oxide and prostacyclin in platelets. Br J Pharmacol 92:181, 1987.
44. Ross R: The pathogenesis of atherosclerosis—An update. N Engl J Med 314:488, 1986.
45. Bjorkerud, S and Bondjers, G: Endothelial integrity and viability in the aorta of the normal rabbit and rat as evaluated with dye exclusion tests and interference contract microscopy. Atherosclerosis 15:285, 1972.
46. Dainiak, N, Warren, HB, Kreczko, S, et al: Acetylated lipoproteins impair erythroid growth factor release from endothelial cells. J Clin Invest 81:834, 1988.
47. Cybulsky, MI, and Gimbrone, MA, Jr: Endothelial cells express a monocyte adhesion molecule during atherogenesis (abstr). FASEB J 4(4):A1135, 1990.
48. Faggiotto, A, Ross, R, and Harker, L: Studies of hypercholesterolemia in the nonhuman primate. I. Changes that lead to fatty streak formation. Arteriosclerosis 4:323, 1984.
49. Henry, PD and Yokoyama, M: Supersensitivity of atherosclerotic rabbit aorta to ergonovine. Mediation by a serotonergic mechanism. J Clin Invest 66:306, 1980.
50. Verbeuren, TH, Jordaens, FH, Zonnekeyn, LL, et al: Effect of hypercholesterolemia on vascular reactivity in the rabbit. Circ Res 58:552, 1986.
51. Heistad, DD, Armstrong, MLI, Marcus, ML, et al: Augmented responses to vasoconstrictor stimuli in hypercholesterolemic and atherosclerotic monkeys. Circ Res 54:711, 1984.
52. Shimokawa, H, Kim, P, and Vanhoutte, PM: Endothelium-dependent relaxation to aggregating platelets in isolated basilar arteries of control and hypercholesterolemic pigs. Circ Res 63:604, 1988.
53. Cohen, RA, Zitnay, KM, Haudenschold, CC, et al: Loss of selective endothelial cell vasoactive functions in pig coronary arteries caused by hypercholesterolemia. Circ Res 63:903, 1988.
54. Andrews, HE, Bruckdorfer, KR, Dunn, RC, et al: Low-density lipoproteins inhibit endothelium-dependent relaxation in rabbit aorta. Nature 327:237, 1987.
55. Kugiyama, K, Kerns, SA, Morrisett, JD, et al: Impairment of endothelium-dependent arterial relaxation by lysolecithin in modified low-density lipoproteins. Nature 344:160, 1990.
56. Johnson, G, III, Tsao, PS, Mulloy, D, et al: Cardioprotective effects of acidified sodium nitrite in myocardial ischemia with reperfusion. J Pharmacol Exp Ther 252:35, 1990.
57. Harrison, DG, Armstrong, ML, Freiman, PC, et al: Restoration of endothelium-dependent relaxation by dietary treatment of atherosclerosis. J Clin Invest 80:1808, 1987.
58. Osborne, JA, Lento, PH, Siegfried, MR, et al: Cardiovascular effects of acute hypercholesterolemia in rabbits: Reversal with lovastatin treatment. J Clin Invest 83:465, 1989.
59. Shimokawa, H and Vanhoutte, PM: Dietary cod-liver oil improves endothelium-dependent responses in hypercholesterolemic and atherosclerotic porcine coronary arteries. Circulation 78:1421, 1988.
60. Philipson, BE, Rothrock, DW, Conner, WE, et al: Reduction of plasma lipids, lipoproteins, and apoproteins by dietary fish oils in patients with hypertriglyceridemia. N Engl J Med 312:1210, 1985.
61. Knapp, HR, Reilly, IAG, Alessandrini, P, et al: In vivio indices of platelet and vascular function during fish-oil administration in patients with atherosclerosis. N Engl J Med 314:937, 1986.
62. Needleman, P, Raz, A, Minkes, MS, et al: Triene prostaglandins: prostacyclin and thromboxane biosynthesis and unique biological properties. Proc Natl Acad Sci USA 176:944, 1979.
63. Nelson, AM: Diet therapy in coronary disease: Effect on mortality of high-protein, high-seafood, fat-controller diet. Geriatrics 27(12):103, 1972.
64. Kromhout D, Bosschieter, EB, and de Lezenne Coulander, C: The inverse relation between fish consumption and 20-year mortality from coronary heart disease. N Engl J Med 312:1205, 1985.
65. Blankenhorn, DH, Brooks, SH, Selzer, RH, et al: The rate of atherosclerosis change during treatment of hyperlipoproteinemia. Circulation 57:355, 1978.

66. Blankenhorn, DH, Nessim, SA, Johnson, RL, et al: Beneficial effects of combined cholestipolnia-cin therapy on coronary atherosclerosis and coronary venous bypass grafts. JAMA 257:3233, 1987.

67. Ludmer, PL, Selwyn, AP, Shook, TL, et al: Paradoxical vasoconstriction induced by acetylcholine in atherosclerotic coronary arteries. N Engl J Med 315:1046, 1986.

68. Cox, DA, Vita, J, Treasure, CB, et al: Atherosclerosis impairs flow-mediated dilation of coronary arteries in man. Circulation 80:458, 1989.

69. Vekshtein, VI, Teung, AC, Vita, JA, et al: Fish oil improves endothelium-dependent relaxation in patients with coronary artery disease. Circulation 80(Suppl II):434, 1989 (abstr).

70. Fleishhauer, FJ, Lee, TC, Nellessen, U, et al: Fish oil improves endothelium-dependent coronary vasodilation in cardiac transplant recipients. Circulation 82(Suppl III):457, 1990.

71. Girerd, XJ, Hirsch, AT, Cooke, JP, et al: L-Arginine augments endothelium-dependent vasodila-tion in cholesterol-fed rabbits. Circ Res 67:1301–1308, 1990.

72. Cooke, JP, Andon, NA, Girerd, XJ, et al: Arginine restores cholinergic relaxation of hypercholes-terolemic rabbit thoracic aorta. Circulation 83:1057–1062, 1991.

73. Rossitch, E, Jr, Alexander, E, III, Black, PM, et al: L-arginine normalizes endothelial function in cerebral vessels from hypercholesterolemic rabbits. J Clin Invest 87:1295–1299, 1991.

74. Creager, MA, Cooke, JP, Mendelsohn, ME, et al: Impaired vasodilation of forearm resistance ves-sels in hypercholesterolemic humans. J Clin Invest 86:228, 1990.

75. Creager, MA, Girerd, XJ, Gallagher, SJ, et al: L-arginine improves endothelium-dependent vaso-dilation in hypercholesterolemic humans. Circulation 82:346, 1990.

76. McBride, W, Lange, RA, and Hillis, LD: Restenosis after successful coronary angioplasty: Patho-physiology and prevention. N Engl J Med 318:1734, 1988.

77. Blackshear, JL, O'Callaghan, WG, and Califf, RM: Medical approaches to prevention of restenosis after coronary angioplasty. J Am Coll Cardiol 9:834, 1987.

78. Liu, MW, Roubin, GS, and King, SB: Restenosis after coronary angioplasty: Potential biologic determinants and role of intimal hyperplasia. Circulation 79:1374, 1989.

79. Gao, S-Z, Alderman, EL, Schroeder, JS, et al: Accelerated coronary vascular disease in the heart transplant patient: Coronary arteriographic findings. J Am Coll Cardiol 12:334, 1988.

80. Shimokawa H, Aarhus, LL, and Vanhoutte, PM: Porcine coronary arteries with regenerated endo-thelium have a reduced endothelium-dependent responsiveness to aggregating platelets and serotonin. Circ Res 61:256, 1987.

81. Weidinger, FF, McLenachan, JM, Cybulsky, M, et al: Persistent dysfunction of regenerated endo-thelium following balloon angioplasty of rabbit iliac artery. Circulation 81:1667, 1990.

82. Schwartz, L, Bourassa, MG, Lesperance, J, et al: Aspirin and dipyridamole in the prevention of restenosis after percutaneous transluminal coronary angioplasty. N Engl J Med 318:1714, 1988.

83. Ellis, SG, Roubin, GS, Wilentz, J, et al: Effect of 18- to 24-hour heparin administration for pre-vention of restenosis after uncomplicated coronary angioplasty. Am Heart J 177:777, 1989.

84. Thornton, MA, Gruentzig, AR, Hollman, J, et al: Coumadin and aspirin in prevention of recur-rence after transluminal coronary angioplasty: A randomized study. Circulation 69:721, 1984.

85. Whitworth, HB, Rougin, GS, Hollman, J, et al: Effect of nifedipine on recurrent stenosis after percutaneous transluminal coronary angioplasty. J Am Coll Cardiol 8:1271, 1986.

86. Pepine, CJ, Hirshfeld, JW, Macdonald, RG, et al: A controlled trial of corticosteroids to prevent restenosis after coronary angioplasty. Circulation 81:1753, 1990.

87. Dehmer, GJ, Popma, JJ, van den Berg, EK, et al: Reduction in the rate of early restenosis after coronary angioplasty by a diet supplemented with n-3 fatty acids. N Engl J Med 319:733, 1988.

88. Grigg, LE, Kay, TWH, Valentine, PA, et al: Determinants of restenosis and lack of effect of dietary supplementation with eicosapentaenoic acid on the incidence of coronary artery restenosis after angioplasty. J Am Coll Cardiol 13:665, 1989.

89. Milner, MR, Gallino, RA, Leffingwell, A, et al: Usefulness of fish oil supplements in preventing clinical evidence of restenosis after uncomplicated coronary angioplasty. Am Heart J 117:777, 1984.

90. Resi, JG, Sipperly, ME, McCabe, CH, et al: Randomized trial of fish oil for prevention of restenosis after coronary angioplasty. Lancet July 22, 1989, p. 177.

91. Powell, JS, Clozel, J-P, Muller, RKM, et al: Inhibitors of angiotensin-converting enzyme prevent myointimal proliferation after vascular injury. Science 245:186, 1989.

92. Kifor, I and Dzau, VJ: Endothelial renin angiotensin pathway: Evidence for intracellular synthesis and secretion of angiotensins. Circ Res 60:422, 1987.

93. Wright, HP: Mitosis patterns in aortic endothelium. Atherosclerosis 15:93, 1972.
94. Reidy, MA and Bowyer, DE: Scanning electron microscopy of arteries. The morphology of aortic endothelium in haemodynamically stressed areas associated with branches. Atherosclerosis 26:181, 1977.
95. McLenachan, JM Vita, J, Fish, RD, et al: Early evidence of endothelial vasodilator dysfunction at coronary branch points. Circulation 82:1169, 1990.
96. Konishi, M and Su, C: Role of endothelium in dilator responses of spontaneously hypertensive rat arteries. Hypertension 5:881, 1983.
97. Winquist, RJ, Bunting, PB, Baskin, EP, et al: Decreased endothelium-dependent relaxation in New Zealand genetic hypertensive rats. J Hypertens 2:536, 1984.
98. Luscher TF and Vanhoutte, PM: Endothelium-dependent contractions to acetylcholine in the aorta of the spontaneously hypertensive rat. Hypertension 8:344, 1986.
99. Luscher, TF, Raij, L, and Vanhoutte, PM: Endothelium-dependent responses in normotensive and hypertensive Dahl rats. Hypertension 9:157, 1987.
100. Lockette, WE, Otsuha, Y, and Carretero, OA: Endothelium-dependent relaxation in hypertension. Hypertension 8 (Suppl II):61, 1986.
101. Luscher, TF, Vanhoutte, PM, and Raij, L: Antihypertensive treatment normalizes decreased endothelium-dependent relaxations in rats with salt-induced hypertension. Hypertension 9 (Suppl III):193, 1987.
102. Schultz, PJ and Raij, L: Effects of antihypertensive agents on endothelium-dependent and endothelium-independent relaxations. Br J Clin Pharmacol 28 (Suppl 2):151S, 1989.
103. Panza, J, Quyyumi, AA, Brush, JE, et al: Abnormal endothelium-dependent vascular relaxation in patients with essential hypertension. N Engl J Med 323:22, 1990.
104. Linder, L, Kiowski, W, Buhler, FR, et al: Indirect evidence for release of endothelium-derived relaxing factor in human forearm circulation in vivo: Blunted response in essential hypertension. Circulation 81:1762, 1990.

CHAPTER 2

Primary Hypercoagulable State

Edward Genton, M.D.

Hypercoagulability is a frequently used term, which was first introduced more than a century ago by Virchow, but until now has escaped precise definition. Most often, hypercoagulability refers to proneness to thrombosis or a prethrombotic state.

The vast majority of prethrombotic states are "acquired" secondary to a variety of disease states, while a much smaller group are "primary" disorders of genetic origin.

Many clinical conditions or disease states predispose patients to thrombosis. Most of these are acquired conditions such as myeloproliferative disorders, malignancies, vasculidities, hormonal abnormalities, obstetric disorders, and so on. In these, there is no consistent causative factor, but there is often evidence of vascular damage, alteration in blood flow leading to stasis, or release into the circulation of a thrombogenic substance that may activate coagulation factors. Some patients with "acquired hypercoagulability," such as those with liver disorders, may develop deficiency in coagulation factors or thrombosis inhibitors.

Hypercoagulability associated with congenital defects in the coagulation system is well described and, of those conditions recognized to date, all are associated with deficient or deranged proteins. An understanding of the role these proteins play in the coagulation scheme and the mechanism by which the derangement leads to thrombosis is necessary to determine an approach to management.

MECHANISM OF HEMOSTASIS AND THROMBOSIS

The hemostatic plug or intravascular thrombus in most instances is the result of alteration in the vessel wall, stimulation of platelet reactivity, and activation of the coagulation system. Most events are initiated by vessel wall damage leading to disruption of endothelium and adherence of platelets to subendothelial structures that triggers the release reaction from granules in the cytoplasm of platelets and activation of the prostaglandin pathway in platelet membrane. This results in the release of adenosine diphosphate, serotonin, and so on, into the site of vessel wall damage, formation of thromboxane A_2, and formation of platelet aggregates. The coagulation system is stimulated by contact of factor XII with the damaged vessel wall leading to its activation and initiation of the cascade of proteolytic reactions, resulting in sequential activation of the coagulation zymogens to their active form, and most are serine proteases (Fig. 2–1). The extrinsic system is also stimulated by activation of factor VII by exposure to "tissue factor" released from damaged vessel wall. Sequential activation of the coagulation factors creates a multiplier system, with a small number of molecules in the early sequence leading to the formation of a large amount of the later activated substances, in particular, thrombin. For example, the amount of thrombin that could be formed from 10 mL of whole blood

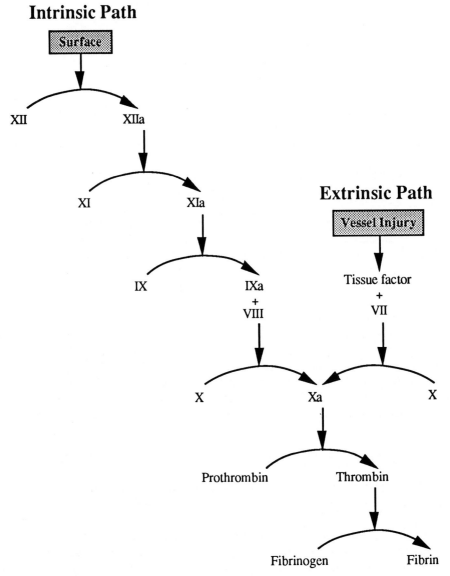

Figure 2–1. Diagram of intrinsic and extrinsic coagulation cascade showing sequential activation of zymogens.

would be a sufficient amount to convert all the fibrinogen in the circulation to fibrin.

The products from the activation of both intrinsic and extrinsic pathways lead to activation of factor X. From that point there is the final common pathway by which factor Xa converts prothrombin into thrombin, which degrades fibrinogen to fibrin and clot formation.

Regulatory mechanisms exist and are activated with the coagulation sequence, which limits propagation of hemostatic plug and prevents intravascular occlusion in most circumstances (Fig. 2–2). These mechanisms include the antithrombin III (AT III), protein C, and fibrinolytic pathways.[1-4] Antithrombin III binds serine proteases (including factors XII-A, XI-A, IX-A, X-A, and thrombin) by forming a stoichiometric 1:1 stable complex. This reaction of AT III with serine proteases is greatly enhanced by heparin or naturally occurring heparan-like proteoglycan substances that form a complex with, and cause an alteration in, the molecular configuration of the AT III molecule which enhances its inhibitory capability.

The protein C pathway includes protein C, protein S, and thrombomodulin. Protein C is synthesized in the liver and is present in plasma at a concentration of 2.7 to 5.0 mEq/mL. The T½ of the zymogen is 10 hours, and of the active form the T½ is 20 to 30 minutes. On exposure to thrombin, the protein is activated to a proteinase that degrades the activated form of factors V and VIII. In its active form protein C is cleared by binding to one of several plasma inhibitors including a specific inhibitor, alpha 1 antitrypsin, and plasmin activator inhibitor.

Protein S is a vitamin K–dependent protein synthesized in both the liver and probably also the endothelial cells with a level in plasma of 13 to 32 mEq/mL. Approximately 45% of the protein is unbound in plasma and the remainder bound reversibly with a protein in the complement system. The free proteins interact with endothelial cells and platelet surfaces where they potentiate the anticoagulant effect of activated protein C.

Thrombomodulin is an endothelial cell membrane protein that binds thrombin and modifies its specificity, thereby potentiating activation of protein C and decreasing the action of thrombin to convert fibrinogen to fibrin and activate factor

AT III + Heparin Proteoglycan Complex inhibits:

- thrombin
- Xa
- IXa

Protein C Pathway inhibits:

- thrombin
- VIIIa
- Va

Lipoprotein-Associated Coagulation Inhibitor inhibits:

- VII-tissue factor complex

Figure 2–2. Regulatory pathways that inhibit intravascular coagulation.

V. The thrombin bound to thrombomodulin is surrounded by protein C molecules and is unable to react with fibrinogen or with platelets. The protein C bound to protein S molecules proteolyzes factors Va and VIIIa, which inhibits thrombin formation.

The fibrinolytic system is comprised of plasminogen and plasminogen activators and inhibitors. The conversion of plasminogen to plasmin is triggered by plasminogen activators, which in the circulation is due principally to tissue plasminogen activator (TPA). Plasmin, in turn, degrades fibrin or fibrinogen to prevent the formation of intravascular occlusive lesions. TPA is released from various tissues, principally the endothelial cells, and has a high affinity for fibrin and adheres to fibrin strands as they form. Plasminogen also adheres to the fibrin and is converted to plasmin by TPA, which results in dissolution of fibrin strands at the site of thrombus formation while avoiding plasmin entering the circulation and degrading fibrinogen. Plasmin and plasminogen activators that enter the circulation are rapidly neutralized by inhibitors in plasma.

PRIMARY HYPERCOAGULABLE STATES

Several congenital conditions predispose to thrombosis and all involve quantitative or qualitative abnormalities in plasma coagulation proteins[1-4] (Fig. 2–3).

ANTITHROMBIN III DEFICIENCY

Antithrombin III deficiency, which was described in 1965, was the first congenital disorder leading to thrombosis to be identified. To date, more than 100 families have been reported with this inherited disorder. Numerous studies have indicated that inheritance is an autosomal dominant. Half of family members acquire the condition, and most affected patients who survive infancy are heterozygous with AT III functional levels of 40% to 60% of normal. Three types of the disorder have been characterized as based upon the measurement of AT III immunogically, by progressive serum protease inhibition in the absence of heparin, and by the

Primary Hypercoagulable States
Genetic Abnormalities Predisposing to Thrombosis

Deficiencies (Quantitative or Qualitative)

- **Coagulation**
  - **AT III**
  - **Protein C**
  - **Protein S**
  - **Fibrinogen**
- **Fibrinolytic**
  - **Plasminogen**
  - **Plasminogen activator**
  - **Plasminogen activator inhibitor (type I)**

Figure 2–3. Table of coagulation and fibrinolytic proteins that may produce hypercoagulability when deficient qualitatively or quantitatively.

cofactor activity of heparin to bind to the antithrombin III and catalyze the inhibition of serum proteases.[5] In the type I patients, all assays are abnormal. In the type II, the AT III level measured antigenically is normal, but the antithrombin and cofactor activities are decreased. And in type III, the antigen assay is normal, the antithrombin assay is normal, and only the heparin cofactor activity is decreased. The overall incidence of AT III deficiency varies widely from reports of estimates from 1:2000 to 1:20,000.

In patients with AT III deficiency, activated factor X is regularly found in plasma. However, thrombin is not evident, because as thrombin is formed, it rapidly binds to endothelial cell thrombomodulin receptors and is neutralized as previously described.

Patients with AT III deficiency have an increased incidence of thrombosis, with type I and type II deficiency being associated with thrombosis in about half of the patients. The type III deficiency patients apparently do not have clinical thrombosis unless they are homozygous.

Antithrombin III–deficient patients will develop clinical thrombotic events by age 55 in approximately 85% of cases. These events may occur at a young age but usually not until the late teens, and approximately 20% will have had an event prior to age 20.[5,6] The thrombotic episodes are characterized by occurring at a young age without apparent provocation and often involving unusual and multiple sites (e.g., renal mesenteric or cerebral veins). The thrombotic episodes tend to be recurrent, particularly during predisposing conditions such as pregnancies and surgical procedures. Overall, approximately 60% of patients will have their first episode in association with a recognized provocation and 40% appear to develop them spontaneously.

Most episodes involve the venous circulation in deep leg or mesenteric vessels, and pulmonary emboli are common.

PROTEIN C PATHWAY DEFICIENCY

Protein C and protein S deficiencies are also inherited as autosomal dominant. Patients recognized with this disorder usually are heterozygous with blood levels of the deficient protein approximately 30% to 50% of normal, inasmuch as homozygous patients are thought to die in the neonatal period, often with massive thrombotic events such as purpura fulminous.[6,7]

Protein C and protein S levels may be measured immunologically or functionally. Patients deficient in these factors present in a fashion similar to AT III with episodes of usually venous thrombosis that are recurrent, beginning from early adulthood and often without associated provocation. Arterial thrombosis before middle age is uncommon in these patients, making it difficult to be certain that these protein deficiencies increase significantly the incidence of arterial thrombotic events. Superficial thrombophlebitis appears to be more common in protein S and protein C deficiency than with AT III–deficient states.

It is curious that a significant percentage of patients with documented deficiency of protein C have no clinical episodes of thrombosis.

FIBRINOLYTIC SYSTEM DEFICIENCY

Congenital fibrinolytic mechanism defects predisposing to thrombosis have also been reported. Defects in the production or release of TPA or qualitative or quantitive abnormalities in plasminogen may occur. Several types of plasminogen activator inhibitor have been described and, if present in increased quantities, may increase patients' susceptibility to venous thrombotic events. Fibrinogen abnormalities may occur that lead to the formation of fibrin gels which are resistant to lysis by plasmin.[2,3]

MANAGEMENT

ANTITHROMBIN III DEFICIENCY

In most instances an acute thromboembolic episode responds to the "conventional approach" to treatment with heparin followed by oral anticoagulation to arrest the thrombotic process.[5] Heparin is relatively ineffective in these patients owing to the chronically reduced AT III level, which may be further decreased by depletion from combining with heparin. To confirm adequate heparin effect, the partial thromboplastin time should be monitored as is conventionally done. In the occasional patient in whom therapeutic prolongation of PTT is unachievable, the addition of AT III concentrates or fresh-frozen plasma to increase AT III levels may be required. Heparin therapy should overlap with the oral anticoagulant for several days before being discontinued.

PROPHYLAXIS IN THE ASYMPTOMATIC PATIENT

Theoretically, the patient with AT III deficiency is a candidate for lifelong prophylaxis. This is achievable with warfarin sodium (Coumadin), which works by reducing vitamin K–dependent clotting factors and possibly also by effecting an increase in AT III levels. Inasmuch as the incidence of thrombosis is low before the teenage years, it has not been established that routine prophylaxis of all patients is required. However, after patients reach their mid-teens, the incidence of thrombosis increases and it is reasonable to use prophylaxis unless contraindications exist.

Also, it is appropriate for all patients with AT III deficiency to receive prophylactic therapy during periods when they would be at high risk for developing a thrombotic event; these periods include prolonged bed rest, major surgery, long bone fracture, and especially pregnancy. In most such instances, oral anticoagulation with prothrombin times prolonged to 1.5:2 INR (international normalized ratio) is effective. The pregnant patient presents a particular challenge. Without treatment, the majority of patients would develop a thrombotic episode, but the drug treatment may produce significant morbidity and mortality in the fetus. The risk of warfarin embryopathy is most marked during weeks 6 through 12 of pregnancy. A reasonable approach to management of the patient during pregnancy is to discontinue warfarin and administer heparin subcutaneously to obtain moderate prolongation of PTT. This may be continued throughout the pregnancy, or warfarin may replace heparin if necessary, from the second trimester through term. At the time of delivery, anticoagulation should be discontinued and antithrombin III concentrate should be administered until anticoagulation could be resumed postpartum. Warfarin can be used safely in the breast-feeding mother.

Antithrombin III concentrate is commercially available. The preparation has had no recognized complication to date. The approach to intravenous administration is to infuse 0.67 units per kilogram for each 1% increase in the antithrombin III level desired in plasma or to administer 50 international units per kilogram over a 20-minute period, which should achieve an antithrombin III level in excess of 100%. The half-life of the concentrate is 18 to 26 hours, so that the preparation should be repeated at a dose of 35 to 40 units per kilogram every 24 hours. The level required to prevent thromboembolism is not precisely known, but levels above 75% of that for normal patients are probably desirable.

If fresh-frozen plasma is to be used as a substitute for AT III concentrate, 0.67 mL of plasma per kilogram is to be used for each 1% of increase desired in plasma level of AT III.

PROTEIN C AND PROTEIN S DEFICIENCY

Oral anticoagulants are the preferable treatment for protein C deficiency. However, especially during the early phases of warfarin therapy, the protein C level can be expected to drop below baseline level, thereby further increasing the risk of thrombosis. It is important therefore that heparin be given for 12 to 36 hours in conjunction with warfarin until the falls in factor X and prothrombin have occurred that are required for the antithrombotic effect.

In infants with homozygote protein C deficiency, conventional warfarin therapy has not been effective. Such patients require the administration of plasma or plasma fractions to establish adequate protein C levels to prevent the thrombotic episodes. With active thrombosis, heparin will arrest the process and then should be followed by conventional warfarin therapy.

DEFICIENCIES IN THE FIBRINOLYTIC PATHWAY

Because the abnormality in these patients is a failure of the fibrinolytic system to activate or of fibrin to lyse, the objective for therapy would be to prevent thrombosis formation. The response to antithrombotic prophylaxis is normal, and therapy with oral anticoagulants or heparin may be indicated during high-risk situations or in some patients chronically.

SCREENING PATIENTS FOR HYPERCOAGULABLE STATES

No precise guidelines are established to guide clinicians in screening for hypercoagulability. Clearly, all members of families with a documented deficiency should be screened to identify cases for prophylaxis during high-risk periods. No justification could be made for screening all patients with venous thrombotic events because the likelihood of finding abnormalities would be low and the cost would be high.

Emphasis has been placed on identifying clinical indicators that favor deficiency states. It is correct that primary hypercoagulability is often associated with strong family history, onset at a young age, recurrent episodes, and involvement of unusual sites. However, it has not been established that these features are often associated with deficiency states.

In a recently reported study[6] of patients with documented venous thrombosis, the prevalence of deficiency of AT III proteins C or S or abnormal plasminogen was 8.3% compared with 2.2% in control cases. Furthermore, the study examined the predictive value of history for familial, juvenile onset, or recurrent thrombosis for detecting a deficiency. The overall positive predictive value was 13%. In patients with all three features, the predictive value was 30%. Interestingly, more than a third of patients with protein deficiencies had none of the examined clinical features.

It may be concluded that routine screening of patients with venous thrombo-embolism is not indicated. With present information, screening should be reserved for cases with a combination of positive family history, recurrent episodes, young age at onset, and/or involvement of unusual sites.

REFERENCES

1. Rosenberg, RD and Bauer, KA: Thrombosis in inherited deficiencies of antithrombin protein C, and protein S. Hum Pathol 18:253, 1987.
2. Mooke, JL: Hypercoagulable states. Adv Intern Med 35:235, 1990.
3. Schafer, AI: The hypercoagulable states. Ann Intern Med 102:814, 1985.
4. Winter, JH, Fenech, A, Ridley, W, et al: Familial antithrombin III deficiency. Q J Med 204:373, 1982.
5. Hirsh, J, Provella, F, and Pini, M: Congenital antithrombin III deficiency incidence and clinical features. Am J Med 87(Suppl 3B):34S, 1989.
6. Heijboer, H, Brandjes, DPM, Buller, HR, et al: Deficiencies of coagulation inhibiting and fibrinolytic proteins in outpatients with deep vein thrombosis. N Engl J Med 323:1512, 1990.
7. Engesser L, Brockmans, AW, Briet, E, et al: Hereditary protein S deficiency: Clinical manifestations. Ann Intern Med 106:677, 1987.

CHAPTER 3

The Noninvasive Vascular Laboratory

Thom W. Rooke, M.D.

PRINCIPLES OF NONINVASIVE VASCULAR LABORATORY EVALUATION

Along with the history and physical examination, noninvasive vascular testing plays an important role in the assessment of peripheral circulatory disorders. The usual indications for performing noninvasive vascular testing can be divided into five broad categories.

DIAGNOSIS OF PERIPHERAL VASCULAR DISEASE

Occasionally, there may be doubt about the presence or absence of vascular disease, especially when the clinical examination is difficult (as it may be in patients with obesity, swollen limbs, orthopedic abnormalities, and so on) or when the history suggests an alternative, nonvascular diagnosis (for example, pseudoclaudication due to spinal stenosis mimicking true claudication). In these situations noninvasive testing may clarify a vascular diagnosis.

DOCUMENTATION AND QUANTIFICATION OF PERIPHERAL VASCULAR DISEASE

Although the diagnosis of peripheral vascular disease usually can be made on clinical grounds, it may be difficult occasionally to assess disease severity. Fortunately, noninvasive vascular testing can be used to both document the presence of peripheral vascular disease and objectively quantify its severity. Noninvasive testing therefore plays an important role not only in various aspects of patient management, but also as a means of satisfying the increasingly stringent demands for objective documentation of disease severity required of the physician by review groups and third party payers prior to treatment.

ASSESS DISEASE SIGNIFICANCE AND NEED FOR THERAPY

In some situations it is not enough simply to confirm the presence of peripheral vascular disease and determine its severity; sometimes the functional impact of disease on the patient must be assessed. For example, one patient with "severe" disease by laboratory assessment may be relatively symptom free, whereas another patient with objectively less disease may be more severely limited or affected. Specific noninvasive studies, including stress testing, can be used to assess the functional significance of disease and determine whether therapy is indicated.

FOLLOW PROGRESSION OR REGRESSION OF PERIPHERAL VASCULAR DISEASE OR RESPONSE TO THERAPY (SERIAL STUDIES)

A major strength of noninvasive testing is the ability to perform serial studies that can be used to determine disease trends, for example, whether disease is progressing or to what extent a particular therapy has been successful. Then appropriate treatments can be employed or altered as indicated.

LOCALIZATION AND CHARACTERIZATION OF VASCULAR LESIONS

Noninvasive vascular testing can be used to localize and characterize specific lesions; this ability is especially important when interventional therapies such as percutaneous transluminal angioplasty or revascularization surgery are being considered. The severity (percent stenosis) of a particular lesion, lesion length, presence of calcium, aneurysmal dilatation, and other factors can all be assessed.

To be clinically useful, noninvasive vascular tests must meet certain criteria. They should be *accurate* and *reproducible.* Both accuracy and reproducibility should be established each time a new test is introduced into a laboratory, and they must be checked periodically to ensure continued reliability. Tests should have *generalized applicability* in terms of the patients that can be studied (i.e., they should not be significantly limited by body habitus and should not require complex activities by patients who may have limited mobility or decreased level of consciousness, and so on). Patient *safety* and *comfort* are extremely important considerations. Tests must be *simple* and *quick,* and ideally they should be capable of being performed by a technician. Finally, tests need to be *inexpensive* so that their use can be employed liberally and cost effectively.

ANATOMIC VERSUS HEMODYNAMIC VERSUS FUNCTIONAL ASSESSMENTS

Noninvasive tests of peripheral vessels can be divided into three categories depending upon whether the information they provide is primarily anatomic, hemodynamic, or functional. Table 3–1 lists several common tests according to the type of information they provide.

Anatomic tests refer to those tests that give information about the location or appearance of a vascular lesion. Imaging studies, such as two-dimensional echocardiographic scanning, are classic examples of anatomic tests. Other tests, such as segmental pressures, are partly anatomic inasmuch as they help localize occlusive lesions to a particular region.

Hemodynamic tests provide information about blood flow and how it is affected by a specific vascular lesion. For example, Doppler changes in blood flow velocity occurring as the blood passes through a particular stenotic lesion (or for that matter, a drop in segmental limb pressure at certain level) provide information about the degree of hemodynamic impairment caused by the lesion.

Table 3–1. Anatomic versus
Hemodynamic/Functional Noninvasive
Vascular Laboratory Studies

Anatomic	Hemodynamic/Functional
Two-dimensional echo	Segmental pressures
Segmental pressures	Continuous wave Doppler
Continuous wave Doppler	Treadmill exercise
(CT scanning)*	Transcutaneous oximetry
(MRI scanning)*	Skin temperature
	Plethysmography
	Oculoplethysmography
	Laser Doppler
	MRI flow detection

*Noninvasive, but not usually found in a "vascular laboratory."

Functional tests are used to assess the significance of vascular disease. Consider the following: a patient presents complaining of somewhat atypical leg pain that occurs intermittently with walking, but may also occasionally occur at rest. A stenosis is identified in a lower limb artery by two-dimensional echocardiogram imaging and appears to limit the vessel lumen by about 50% (anatomic information). A Doppler (or segmental pressure) study documents a pressure drop across this lesion (hemodynamic information). Does this lesion explain the patient's leg pain? Despite having good information about the anatomic and hemodynamic characteristics of the lesion, uncertainty remains because the functional significance of the lesion to the patient remains undetermined. Additional testing, such as walking a patient on a treadmill, correlating symptoms with walking distance, and determining the change in distal limb pressures following exercise, would all help to clarify the functional significance of the lesion(s).

SPECIFIC NONINVASIVE TESTS

There are literally hundreds, if not thousands, of noninvasive vascular tests that have been developed, employed, and promoted over the years by various groups or individuals. Many of these tests represent truly novel approaches to circulatory assessment, whereas others may be little more than slight variations on a particular technique. The following tests are representative of those that, in this author's opinion, are accepted as standard noninvasive vascular laboratory techniques, or that show promise for the future. The list is obviously not all-inclusive.

For purposes of discussion, specific tests can be most easily considered if they are divided into those that primarily assess arteries, veins, or the microcirculation.

ARTERIAL STUDIES

Continuous Wave Doppler

The continuous wave Doppler is one of the most commonly used devices for studying arteries and veins. In its simplest form, it consists of a hand-held unit with a stethoscope earpiece attachment (Fig. 3–1) that allows direct interpretation of the Doppler velocity signal. Models with attached loudspeakers (for multiple listeners)

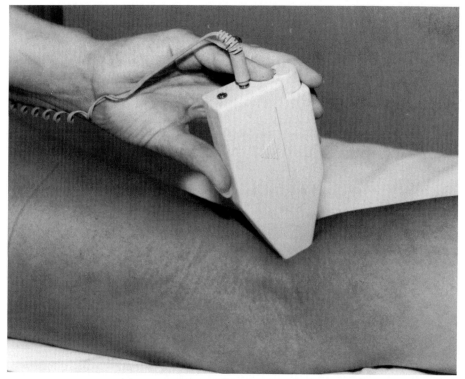

Figure 3–1. Hand-held continuous wave Doppler. This device can be used to assess flow in arteries or veins.

are also available, as are more complex units with bidirectional capabilities and real-time hard copy printouts. The principles of Doppler technology are beyond the scope of this work but have been reviewed elsewhere.[1–3]

Continuous wave Dopplers have two principal applications in the arterial examination: (1) as detectors of blood motion, they can be used along with inflatable cuffs to determine segmental pressures (see following section), or (2) the Doppler velocity signal can be analyzed to determine whether the underlying arterial flow is normal or abnormal. Figure 3–2 shows typical normal and abnormal Doppler signals from the femoral artery. Normal signals have a characteristic biphasic or triphasic pattern, which includes a component of rapid forward flow during systole followed by flow reversal (due to recoil from elastic arteries) during diastole. If one examines the arterial signal obtained distal to a significant stenosis, the velocity of forward flow during systole is attenuated, flow reversal during diastole is lost, and there may be forward diastolic flow. The limb can be interrogated at multiple levels and over different vessels, thus identifying sites of significant stenoses. Continuous wave Doppler can therefore be used to diagnose the presence of arterial occlusive disease, help gauge its severity, and to a certain extent localize the blockages.

The continuous wave Doppler is simple to use, portable, cheap, and readily applicable on virtually any patient (alone or more often in conjunction with other tests). Its major drawbacks include the fact that results are somewhat operator dependent, a relatively poor ability to quantify disease severity, and an inability to accurately study collateral blood flow.

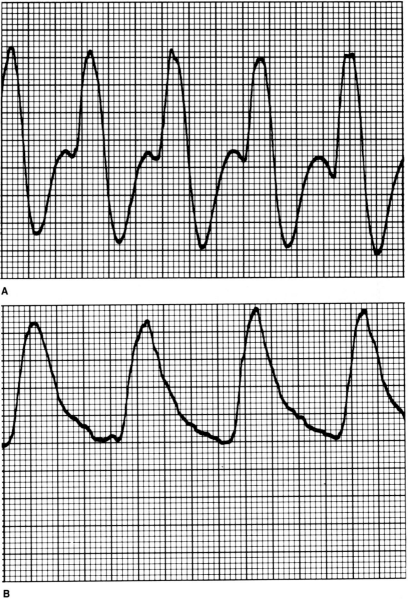

Figure 3–2. (*A*) Normal common femoral bidirectional Doppler velocity tracing. (*B*) Bidirectional Doppler velocity tracing from common femoral artery distal to a hemodynamically significant iliac artery stenosis.

Segmental Pressure

Segmental pressure measurements are used to (1) diagnose and document the presence of arterial occlusive disease, (2) assess disease severity, and (3) localize arterial obstructions to specific limb segments. The technique employs the use of a blood pressure cuff (or multiple cuffs) that can be sequentially inflated at different positions along the limb (Fig. 3–3). The arterial blood pressure in a given limb segment is determined by inflating the cuff around that segment to a pressure suf-

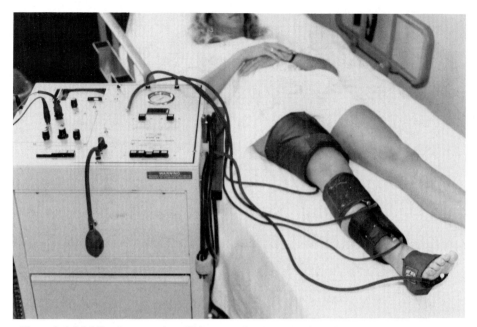

Figure 3–3. Multilevel pneumatic cuff placement for determination of segmental blood pressures.

ficient to occlude blood flow, then slowly deflating the cuff until arterial blood flow is detected distal to the cuff. A continuous wave Doppler is usually used for the purpose of detecting blood flow. In this manner the blood pressure at multiple limb levels can be determined.[4-6] In order to correct for variations between individuals in systemic arterial pressure, the segmental pressures are often divided by the brachial pressure to create an index; the ankle/brachial index (ABI) is a commonly used measurement of arterial sufficiency.

In our laboratory we usually assume the following relationship between resting, supine ABI and disease severity: greater than 0.9—normal, 0.8 to 0.9—mild, 0.5 to 0.8—moderate, and less than 0.5—"severe." In some patients, particularly those with relatively mild claudication, the ABI may be normal at rest but reduced following exercise. This effect occurs because the arterial obstruction(s) acts to limit blood flow during exercise; that is, at rest the vascular resistance of the leg is relatively high and the flow through a stenotic lesion may be sufficient to maintain a normal distal pressure, whereas after exercise the vascular resistance is lower and blood flow through the stenosis is no longer sufficient to keep distal pressure from falling. Thus, exercise may bring out occult arterial occlusive disease.[7] We use a standard protocol in our laboratory consisting of treadmill exercise with electrocardiographic monitoring for 5 min at 2 mph up a 10% grade. Patients are instructed to complete the test or stop if symptoms limit them. Determination of preexercise and postexercise ABIs along with symptom development enables an accurate assessment of functional disease severity.

Of all the arterial studies performed in the vascular laboratory, segmental pressure measurement is among the quickest, cheapest, easiest, most accurate, and most reproducible.[8] It has three major drawbacks: (1) arteries that have been rendered noncompressible by calcium deposition (a condition that is particularly common in diabetics) cannot be occluded by inflation of the blood pressure cuff and therefore pressure cannot be determined; (2) the level of obstruction can only be determined at and below the midthigh; and (3) the effect of nonpulsatile flow (as may occur through small collateral vessels) cannot be easily determined.

Inflow (Venous Occlusion) Plethysmography

Most plethysmographic techniques for measuring limb blood flow share two components: (1) a proximally placed pneumatic occlusion cuff that can be rapidly inflated to a pressure that is above venous but below arterial (during the brief period of cuff inflation, blood will become trapped in the limb); and (2) a method for determining the amount of blood trapped in the limb during the period of occlusion. This usually involves a plethysmograph of some type. Plethysmographs for this purpose may utilize electrical impedance, mercury-in-Silastic strain gauges, air or fluid displacement, or other methods to determine the change in limb size caused by transient venous occlusion.[9]

To perform a plethysmographic flow measurement, the limb is placed in a neutral, relaxed position and the venous occlusion cuff is rapidly inflated. Blood that flows into the limb becomes trapped, causing the limb to expand. The rate at which expansion occurs is measured by the plethysmograph, from which an estimate of arterial inflow can be made, usually in units of milliliters of blood per minute per 100 mL tissue. Success with this technique requires that the periods of venous occlusion be kept short, and only the initial rates of limb expansion should be used for flow calculations because a significant rise in venous pressure will oppose arterial inflow and cause low flow values.[10]

The strengths of venous occlusion plethysmography include its reasonable accuracy (for most situations) and its ability to be used repetitively and serially. Its drawbacks include the need for careful limb positioning and patient cooperation, the potential for artifacts, the requirement for blood flow to be in a steady state, and the inability to determine blood flow in a particular tissue (e.g., skin, muscle, and bone).

Oculoplethysmography

Oculoplethysmography (OPG) measures ocular arterial pressure, which in turn can be used as an index of cerebral perfusion pressure.[11,12] The technique involves the application of cups to both eyes (after application of a local anesthetic) through which a vacuum can be applied. This vacuum (up to 500 mm Hg) distorts the globe, raises intraocular pressure, and eliminates ocular pulsations. The vacuum is then slowly released and pulsations return when globe pressure falls below blood pressure; this allows systolic pressure in the eye to be determined. Because both eyes are studied simultaneously, they can be directly compared with one another as well as with the brachial blood pressure. A difference between eyes of 5 mm Hg is usually considered significant.[13]

The strength of OPG is that it is essentially a functional test of intracranial perfusion. Because of the circle of Willis, there is a tremendous potential for collateral flow in the cerebral circulation. If collateralization is well developed, a high-grade or even total arterial obstruction in the internal carotid system may have little or no effect on ocular (and presumably ipsilateral cerebral perfusion) pressure. In contrast, patients with ipsilateral carotid disease and poor collateralization may have markedly decreased OPGs. In comparison with some other methods, OPG can appear relatively insensitive at identifying carotid stenosis or occlusion, because collateral flow may render the readings normal; however, if the goal is to assess the functional adequacy of perfusion, it remains an outstanding and highly useful test.

Duplex Scanning

Combining two-dimensional real-time ultrasound imaging with continuous or pulsatile wave Doppler is referred to as duplex scanning. The technology involved in duplex scanning is sophisticated and constantly improving; its details are beyond the scope of this work (see Ref. 14 for reviews). Recent advances such as color flow imaging have further increased both the complexity and utility of duplex scanning. The two-dimensional ultrasound component of duplex scanning allows a real-time image of the blood vessels to be obtained, thus providing *anatomic* information about the vasculature. The Doppler and color flow components enable the velocity (and therefore the pressure gradient) across specific lesions to be determined, which gives *hemodynamic* information (see later section on continuous wave Doppler). When applicable, duplex scanning provides the most detailed noninvasive information possible about the anatomic and hemodynamic status of the arteries.

Duplex scanning has found widespread applicability in several areas including assessment of extracranial carotid disease; identification, measurement, and surveillance of aortic, popliteal, or other aneurysms; detection of arteriovenous fistulas; and assessment of specific upper and lower extremity arterial lesions. It also plays a more limited role in the evaluation of renal or mesenteric arterial occlusive disease, although improvements in equipment may lead to an expansion of this role. Numerous studies have shown good correlation between duplex scanning and arteriography.[15-18] Duplex scanning appears to be accurate enough to screen for lower extremity lesions suitable for angioplasty; in some centers this has reduced the need for preangioplasty angiograms.[19] The ability to study plaque morphology in detail (e.g., plaque thickness, surface character, and degree of calcification) suggests that duplex scanning may be increasingly important in research on atherosclerosis development and progression.[20] Finally, largely through the efforts of echocardiologists, the use of duplex scanning via a transesophageal approach has proved to be extremely precise in the diagnosis of aortic dissection.

The strengths of duplex scanning lie in its high degree of anatomic accuracy (relative to arteriography) and its ability to yield simultaneous hemodynamic information. It has, however, several definite drawbacks. Duplex scanning equipment is expensive and the studies can be quite time consuming to perform. In addition, scanning requires a skilled technical operator to obtain the study and an expert in ultrasound interpretation to analyze it. These drawbacks significantly limit its utility as a general screening tool. Unfortunately, once a laboratory has committed to the purchase of duplex equipment, it may be forced, for financial reasons, to utilize the equipment in ways that are not cost effective.

Magnetic Resonance Arterial Blood Flowimetry

Nuclear magnetic resonance (NMR) technology is showing promise as a noninvasive method for measuring limb blood flow. Recent adaptations and equipment have resulted in (relatively) simple-to-use, relatively low-priced NMR devices designed specifically for studying limb blood flow; the fact that these devices may be located in certain vascular laboratories represents a departure from the traditional association between NMR and disciplines such as radiology. The device works on the principle that magnetized blood (produced by surrounding the leg with a magnetic field) will generate a flow signal as it passes through a detector coil. Preliminary results on reproducibility and correlation with other flow-measuring techniques appear promising at this time.[21,22] The ultimate utility of NMR scanning as a vascular tool remains to be determined.

VENOUS STUDIES

Continuous Wave Doppler

The continuous wave Doppler (described in the preceding section on arterial studies) is also useful for examining the venous circulation in the upper or lower extremities.[23–25] The goals of the continuous wave Doppler examination are to identify the presence of venous obstruction or incompetence, qualitatively assess the severity of the venous disease, and roughly localize these abnormalities to a particular segment of the limb. In performing a continuous wave Doppler venous examination, the venous flow signal is obtained at several sites (in the lower limb these would routinely be the common femoral, superficial femoral, popliteal, and posterior tibial veins), and six specific characteristics of venous flow are determined and/or graded:

Patency—Can a venous signal be obtained? If so, the vein is patent.

Spontaneous flow—Does flow occur spontaneously, or are special maneuvers needed to make it occur? The presence of spontaneous flow reduces the chance of a venous occlusion near the listening site.

Phasicity—Is the flow phasic with respiration (i.e., decreased during inspiration and increased with expiration)? If so, venous occlusion proximal to the listening site is unlikely.

Augmentation—Does venous flow increase appropriately when the limb is manually compressed distal to the Doppler interrogation site? If the augmentation is less than expected, it suggests the presence of venous obstruction between the sites of compression and interrogation.

Competency—Does manual compression proximal to the interrogation site (or the Valsalva maneuver) cause a reversal in venous flow? If so, the valves between the sites of compression and interrogation are incompetent.

Pulsatility—Is the venous flow pulsatile? If so, it may reflect congestive heart failure, tricuspid regurgitation, arterial venous fistula, or other abnormalities. Pulsatility can occasionally be seen as a normal variant.

Most of the aforementioned variables, can, if desired, be graded on an arbitrary scale. In our laboratory we use mild, moderate, and severe to describe abnormalities in each of these areas.

The strengths of the venous continuous wave Doppler examination are its quickness, simplicity, and low cost. Unfortunately, it is subject to numerous artifacts and produces a significant number of false positives and negatives. For example, it is often impossible to determine if one is studying the appropriate deep vein or an unseen, nearby superficial vein. It is best therefore to use continuous wave Doppler for screening purposes and/or in conjunction with other tests.

Impedance Plethysmography

Impedance plethysmography (IPG) is a technique for detecting proximal, lower extremity deep venous obstruction (DVT). The device consists of two components: (1) a venous occlusion cuff that is placed around the thigh and (2) a set of electrodes (one proximal and one distal) that encircle the calf. A fixed voltage is placed between the electrodes and the amount of electrical current that subsequently flows from one electrode to the other is dependent upon the electrical impedance of the limb. In turn, the impedance is dependent upon the fluid volume contained within the limb. When the thigh cuff is inflated (to a level above venous but below arterial pressure), blood flows into the leg and becomes trapped. As the volume of the leg expands, its electrical impedance changes. This change in impedance is recorded by the IPG. After a period of venous filling has been achieved, the cuff is suddenly released and blood flows out of the leg. The rate of flow (and reduction in limb volume) is reflected by the rate of change in electrical impedance and current.

The presence of a proximal lower extremity deep venous thrombosis causes several changes in the IPG measurements. First, because a degree of venous hypertension is usually present due to the outflow obstruction, inflation of the venous occlusion cuff may not cause much additional blood trapping, and thus electrical impedance may change little. Second, when the venous occlusion cuff is released, the rate of outflow from the leg (and therefore the rate of change of electrical impedance) will be decreased due to the persisting outflow obstruction caused by the venous thrombosis. The presence of these abnormalities in a patient with appropriate clinical findings is strongly suggestive of DVT.

For the detection of acute, proximal (at or above the popliteal vein) deep venous thrombosis, the accuracy of IPG testing appears in many series to be quite good (sensitivity = 93%, specificity = 94%).[26] Its utility is further enhanced by the fact that a negative study predicts a low rate of subsequent pulmonary embolism; the test therefore has significant prognostic value.[27] Given the known difficulty with using clinical indicators to diagnose deep venous thrombosis, the value of a screening IPG is well recognized.

The strengths of IPG include its low cost, prognostic value, reasonable accuracy, and ability for use in serial studies. However, its potential shortcomings are numerous and include

> *Significant false-positive rate*—Anything that causes venous obstruction or venous hypertension can mimic an acute DVT. This includes extrinsic venous compression, old chronic DVT, congestive heart failure, or tricuspid regurgitation.
>
> *Significant false-negative rate*—The test is not useful for identifying infrapopliteal DVT and will often miss this lesion. In addition, any DVT that is nonobstructing (or only partially obstructing) venous outflow may be missed.
>
> *Artifacts*—Reduced leg compliance (due to tense swelling from any cause), inability by the patient to assume or maintain the correct positioning dur-

ing the study, pain with cuff inflation, and so on, all decrease the utility of the test.

For these reasons IPG is usually performed as a screening study, often in conjunction with a venous continuous wave Doppler examination. When positive, findings may be confirmed with a duplex scan or venogram if clinically indicated.

Exercise Venous Plethysmography

Lower limb venous function can be tested by performing a plethysmographic evaluation of limb volume before, during, and after exercise. For example, a plethysmograph can be placed around the lower limb and the subject can be requested to perform a specific exercise (such as deep knee bends or walking). As the lower extremity "muscle pump" is activated, blood is pumped out of the legs and into the central venous pool of the abdomen and chest. The unidirectional valves in the veins aid this process; in addition, they prevent the reflux of blood back into the legs following the exercise period. In a normal individual, plethysmography will show a progressive drop in leg volume during exercise, followed by a period after exercise during which leg volume slowly returns to normal. In legs with impaired pumping (due to venous obstruction, valvular incompetence, or other causes), the exercise-induced fall in venous volume will be less than expected. In addition, when venous incompetence is present, the postexercise return in volume will be more rapid than expected (Fig. 3–4). This principle underlies the use of "exercise venous plethysmography" as a means of evaluating venous function, especially incompetence.

Numerous plethysmographic devices have been devised for this purpose. These may utilize fluid displacement, air displacement, mercury-in-Silastic strain

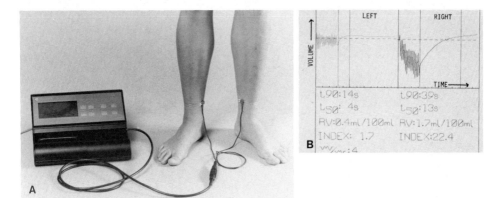

Figure 3–4. (*A*) Typical electrode placement for strain gauge exercise venous plethysmography. After a baseline measurement is obtained, the patient is exercised by performing deep knee bends, dorsal ankle flexions, or other maneuvers. (*B*) Recording during strain gauge plethysmography. On the right, there is a drop in ankle volume during the exercise period, followed by a slow period of volume recovery during the postexercise period. On the left, there is no decrease in volume during the exercise period. These findings suggest normal venous emptying and valvular competence on the right, and severe valvular incompetence and/or obstruction on the left. The machine automatically calculates the time required in seconds for 90% (T_{90}) and 50% (T_{50}) recovery of volume following exercise as well as the amount of blood displaced from the leg during exercise (refill volume, RV). The index, which reflects overall venous function, is obtained by multiplying the T_{50} by the refill volume.

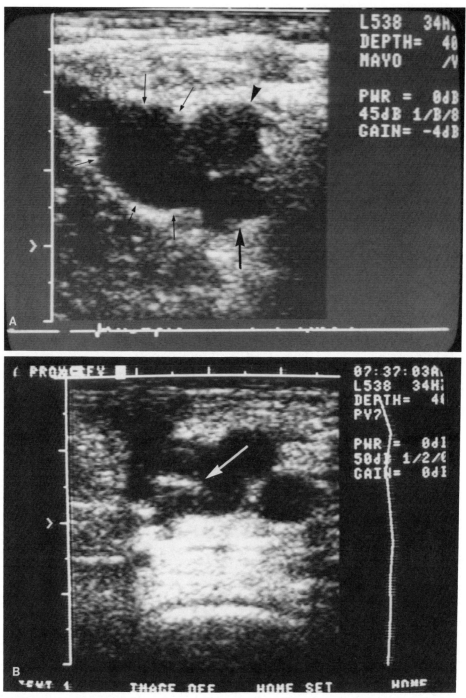

Figure 3–5. (*A*) Cross-sectional, two-dimensional, real-time ultrasound view of the common femoral vein (small arrows) and the superficial (large arrow) and deep femoral arteries (large arrow with stem) obtained at the level of the saphenofemoral junction in a normal individual. (*B*) Identical view obtained in a patient with deep venous thrombosis involving the common femoral vein. Note the hyperechoic mass (white arrow) within the common femoral vein.

gauges, or other modalities.[28-30] Although not strictly a true plethysmographic technique, photoplethysmography uses a cutaneous light-detecting sensor to pinpoint changes in skin blood volume, which can be used as an index of venous volume changes.[31]

The strengths of exercise venous plethysmography are that it is usually simple, quick, and easy to perform. In many cases, it represents the "gold standard" among techniques used for assessing the significance of venous incompetence or obstruction. Its major drawbacks include the fact that the patient must be cooperative and able to perform the required exercise(s). Also, some techniques (photoplethysmography in particular) are subject to a disquieting number of complicating factors and artifacts.[32]

Venous Duplex Scanning

Venous duplex scanning combines two-dimensional venous imaging with Doppler (or color flow) analysis of venous flow (see previous section on arterial imaging and venous continuous wave Doppler). The biggest application for venous duplex scanning is in the identification of DVT. For the detection of proximal DVT, several series now show sensitivities and specificities approaching 100%.[33-36] Criteria for diagnosing DVT with duplex scanning include (1) the presence of a noncompressible intravascular mass, (2) visualization of a partially obstructing thrombus, (3) lack of venous flow by color flow or Doppler, and (4) failure of flow to augment properly with appropriate maneuvers. Of these, the presence of venous noncompressibility is considered most diagnostic (Fig. 3–5). Duplex scanning also can be used to identify calf or superficial vein thrombosis, locate and assess veins prior to their harvesting for bypass procedures, determine venous incompetency, identify and visualize specific venous valves, and diagnose or rule out conditions that may mimic venous disease (such as ruptured Baker's cyst).[37] The biggest drawback for venous duplex analysis is the time and expense associated with its use; for this reason, it should be used selectively rather than for general screening.

MICROCIRCULATORY STUDIES

Temperature Measurement

Cutaneous temperature measurement can be used as an index of skin blood flow.[38,39] Cutaneous temperature has traditionally been measured using electronic thermistors that can be applied locally to obtain "spot" temperatures; however, recent advances have led to an increased role for thermographic techniques that measure temperature by quantifying infrared emission from skin. Regardless of the technique used, it is important to remember that skin temperature does not necessarily equate with cutaneous blood flow. For example, ambient temperature, the degree of arteriovenous shunting, vasomotor changes, skin thickness and composition, and numerous other real or theoretical factors can distort the relationship between skin blood flow and temperature. Typically, cutaneous temperature is studied in two ways: (1) *asymmetry* is sought between comparable sites on each limb—when present, a relative reduction in temperature usually reflects a relative reduction in blood flow; and (2) *skin rewarming time* can be determined following a standardized cold challenge such as 30 seconds of ice-water immersion. In the presence of normal, unobstructed arteries (as determined, for example, by digital pressure measurements), a delay in cutaneous warming (for example, of the hands or digits) suggests vasospasm.

The strengths of using skin temperature as an index of cutaneous blood flow are its simplicity and low cost. Weaknesses include the fact that decreased temperature is not necessarily a consequence of fixed vascular obstruction, because any factor that affects the vasomotor state (for example, drugs, medications, smoking, emotional state, or ambient temperature) will change blood flow and skin temperature.

Transcutaneous Oxygen Tension Measurement

Transcutaneous oxygen tension ($TcPo_2$) measurement represents a powerful new tool for the functional assessment of cutaneous blood flow.[40,41] The technique utilizes a Clark-type electrode that can be attached to the skin at virtually any body site by means of an airtight adhesive (Fig. 3–6). The electrode measures oxygen tension as O_2 diffuses from the superficial regions of the skin. Under conditions of high skin blood flow, $TcPo_2$ approaches arterial Po_2; when flow is high, the $TcPo_2$ will be relatively unaffected by small changes in blood flow. If flow is reduced to the point at which oxygen delivery to skin falls relative to the metabolic needs, the $TcPo_2$ will decrease. A similar drop in $TcPo_2$ will likewise occur if the metabolic rate is increased relative to the oxygen delivery. $TcPo_2$ therefore represents a functional assessment of the match between cutaneous O_2 delivery and O_2 demand, and it can be used to quantify the degree of ischemia in poorly perfused skin. In our noninvasive vascular laboratory, $TcPo_2$ is measured in a standard fashion according to the following protocol. In the case of a lower extremity study, the patient is put into the supine position, and two electrodes are attached to the dorsum of each foot approximately 1 to 2 cm apart. A reference electrode is similarly placed on the chest. The electrodes are equipped with heating elements that can control the elec-

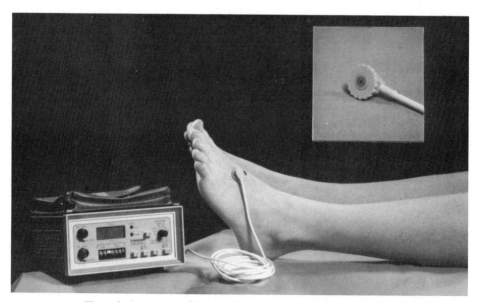

Figure 3–6. Apparatus for measuring transcutaneous oxygen tension.

Table 3–2. Interpretation of TcPo$_2$ Values (Lower Extremity)

	Resting TcPo$_2$ (mm Hg)	Resting RPI*	Change with Elevation	
			TcPo$_2$ (mm Hg)	RPI
Normal or mild impairment	>40	>0.6	<10	<0.2
Moderate impairment	>40	>0.6	>10	>0.2
Severe impairment	<40	<0.6	—	—

*Regional perfusion index, obtained by dividing distal TcPo$_2$'s by reference (chest) TcPo$_2$.

trode surface temperature; these elements are warmed to maintain a temperature of 45°C. This amount of heat has been previously shown to maximally vasodilate the small cutaneous vessels underlying the region beneath the electrode, thus producing a local zone of maximal vasodilation. This eliminates any vasomotor tone around the electrode and ensures that the skin blood flow (and TcPo$_2$) in the perielectrode region reflects true vessel patency and not vasoconstriction. The O$_2$ measurements are allowed to come to a steady value (typically requiring about 20 minutes) and then the feet are elevated to 30° for 3 minutes. This puts an additional stress on the leg circulation and may bring out or intensify TcPo$_2$ abnormalities not noted while supine. The TcPo$_2$ measurements are interpreted in terms of their absolute values as well as their values relative to the reference chest electrode (Table 3–2). The technique used in our laboratory can be modified to study most areas of the body. Different laboratories may use maneuvers other than leg elevation to identify abnormal TcPo$_2$ values; these include oxygen inhalation,[42,43] reactive hyperemia,[44] exercise,[45] and others. Regardless of which intervention is used, the reproducibility and accuracy of simple resting TcPo$_2$ measurement has proved to be excellent.

Although the potential applications of TcPo$_2$ measurement are almost limitless, we utilize it most often in four situations: (1) to assess the adequacy of skin blood flow in areas where the severity of the perfusion impairment is uncertain; (2) to measure success following revascularization[46]; (3) to predict the likelihood of ulcer or amputation site healing; and (4) to assess diabetic limbs, particularly when the vessels are noncompressible. In the case of ulcer or amputation site healing, data (unpublished) from our laboratory show that supine values greater than 40 mm Hg virtually always heal, whereas those less than 20 mm Hg do not. With regard to diabetics, there appears to be a cutaneous microvascular abnormality that coexists in addition to the arterial occlusive disease caused by atherosclerosis[47]; this abnormality further impairs TcPo$_2$ and may, in part, explain why skin healing is impaired in diabetics.

Laser Doppler Flowimetry

Laser Doppler flowimetry is an exciting new development for studying skin blood flow.[48–50] The device directs a low-power laser beam into the skin where it is reflected back from tissues that are either moving (blood) or stationary (other cutaneous structures). The light reflecting from a moving structure such as a blood cell undergoes a Doppler shift, whereas light striking a stationary tissue does not. The *amount* of light undergoing a Doppler shift is proportional to the volume of moving material (or blood) in the skin, and the *magnitude* of the shift is proportional to the blood velocity. By combining information about the volume and velocity of blood, the device can calculate and report skin blood flow in milliliters per minute per 100 mL of tissue.

Techniques for using laser Doppler flowimetry to assess skin blood flow are still being developed and tested. Heating electrodes can be used to warm the underlying skin and produce a state of maximum blood flow; overall vascular patency can therefore be assessed. A potentially important role for laser Doppler flowimetry is in the study of vasospasm and vasomotor changes, inasmuch as it is one of the few techniques that can accurately follow the instantaneous changes in skin blood flow produced by alterations in autonomic tone. Several problems remain with laser Doppler flowimetry at present, the most difficult being a relatively poor degree of reproducibility and a large number of factors that can produce flow artifacts.[51] However, it should be anticipated that these concerns will be resolved and that laser Doppler flowimetry will be used extensively in the future.

REFERENCES

1. Johnston, KW and Kassam, MS: Processing Doppler signals and analysis of peripheral arterial waveforms: Problems and solutions. In Bernstein, EF (ed): Noninvasive Diagnostic Techniques in Vascular Disease. CV Mosby, St. Louis, 1985, p 40.
2. Blackshear, WM, et al: Carotid artery velocity patterns in normal and stenotic vessels. Stroke 11:67, 1980.
3. Rittgers, SE, Thornhill, BM, and Barnes, RW: Quantitative analysis of carotid artery Doppler spectral waveforms—Diagnostic value of parameters. Ultrasound Med Biol 9:255, 1983.
4. Baker, JD and Dix, D: Variability of Doppler ankle pressures with arterial occlusive disease: An evaluation of ankle index and brachial-ankle pressure gradient. Surgery 89:134, 1981.
5. Carter, SA: Clinical measurement of systolic pressures in limbs with arterial occlusive disease. JAMA 207:1869, 1969.
6. Cutajar, CL, Marston, A, and Newcombe, JF: Valve of cuff occlusion pressures in assessment of pheripheral vascular disease. Br Med J 2:392, 1973.
7. Carter, SA: Response of ankle systolic pressure to leg exercise in mild or questionable arterial disease. N Engl J Med 287:578, 1972.
8. Osmundson, PJ, OFallon, WM, Clements, IP, et al: Reproducibility of noninvasive tests of peripheral occlusive arterial disease. J Vasc Surg 2:678, 1985.
9. Sumner, DS: Volume plethysmography in vascular disease: An overview. In Bernstein, EF (ed): Noninvasive Diagnostic Techniques in Vascular Disease. CV Mosby, St. Louis, 1985, p 97.
10. Hiatt, WR, Huang, SY, Regensteiner, JG, et al: Venous occlusion plethysmography reduces arterial diameter and flow velocity. J Appl Physiol 66:2239, 1989.
11. Gee, W, Mehigan, JT, and Wylie, EJ: Measurement of collateral cerebral hemispheric blood pressure by ocular pneumoplethysmography. Am J Surg 110:1516, 1975.
12. Gee, W, et al: Simultaneous bilateral determination of the systolic pressure of the ophthalmic arteries by ocular pneumoplethysmography. Invest Ophthalmol Vis Sci 15:86, 1977.
13. Eikelboom, BC, et al: Criteria for interpretation of ocular pneumoplethysmography (Gee). Arch Surg 118:1169, 1983.
14. Phillips, DJ and Strandness, DE, Jr: Duplex scanning: Practical aspects of instrument performance. In Bernstein, EF (ed): Noninvasive Diagnostic Techniques in Vascular Disease. CV Mosby, St. Louis, 1985, p 397.
15. Langlois, Y, et al: Evaluating caroid artery disease: The concordance between pulsed Doppler/spectrum analysis and arteriography. Ultrasound Med Biol 9:51, 1983.
16. Phillips, DJ, et al: Detection of peripheral vascular disease using the Duplex Scanner III. Ultrasound Med Biol 6:205, 1980.
17. Jager, KA, Phillips, DJ, Martin, RL, et al: Noninvasive mapping of lower limb arterial lesions. Ultrasound Med Biol 11:515, 1985.

18. Merritt, CR: Doppler color flow imaging. J Clin Ultrasound 15:591, 1987.
19. Cossman, DV, Ellison, JE, RVT, Wagner, WH, et al: Comparison of contrast arteriography to arterial mapping with color-flow duplex imaging in the lower extremities. J Vasc Surg 10:522, 1989.
20. Langsfeld, M, Gray-Weale, AC, and Lusby, RJ: The role of plaque morphology and diameter reduction in the development of new symptoms in asymptomatic carotid arteries. J Vasc Surg 9:548, 1989.
21. Salles-Cunha, SX, Halbach, RE, Battocletti, JH, et al: Noninvasive techniques in the evaluation of the peripheral circulation. J Clin Engineer 4:209, 1979.
22. Salles-Cunha, SX and Tolan, D: Evaluation of a magnetic resonance arterial blood flowmeter: Comparison with venous occlusion strain-gauge plethysmography. J Vasc Tech 155, 1989.
23. Kistner, RL: Diagnosis of chronic venous insufficiency. J Vasc Surg 3:185, 1986.
24. Comerota, AJ, White, JV, and Katz, ML: Diagnostic methods for deep vein thrombosis: Venous Doppler examination, phleborrheography, iodine-125 fibrinogen uptake, and phlebography. Am J Surg 150:14, 1985.
25. Baker, WH and Hayes, AC: The normal Doppler venous examination. Angiology 34:283, 1983.
26. Wheeler, HB and Anderson, FA, Jr: Can noninvasive tests be used as the basis for treatment of deep vein thrombosis? In Bernstein, EF (ed): Noninvasive Diagnostic Techniques in Vascular Disease. CV Mosby, St. Louis, 1985, p 805.
27. Wheeler, HB, et al: Suspected deep deep vein thrombosis: Management by impedance plethysmography. Arch Surg 117:1206, 1982.
28. Barnes, RW, et al: Noninvasive quantitation of venous reflux in the postphlebitic syndrome. Surg Gynecol Obstet 136:769, 1973.
29. Christopoulos, D, Nicolaides, AN, Cook, A, et al: Pathogenesis of venous ulceration in relation to the calf muscle pump function. Surgery 106:829, 1989.
30. Thulesius, O: Foot volumetry. In Bernstein, EF (ed): Noninvasive Diagnostic Techniques in Vascular Disease. CV Mosby, St. Louis, 1985, p 828.
31. Abramowitz, HB, et al: The use of photoplethysmography in the assessment of venous insufficiency: A comparison to venous pressure measurements. Surgery 86:434, 1979.
32. Rosfors, S: Venous photoplethysmography: Relationship between transducer position and regional distribution of venous insufficiency. J Vasc Surg 11:436, 1990.
33. Aitken, AG and Godden, DJ: Real-time ultrasound diagnosis of deep vein thrombosis: A comparison with venography. Clin Radiol 38:309, 1987.
34. Appelman, PT, DeJong, TE, and Lampmann, LE: Deep venous thrombosis of the leg: U.S. findings. Radiology 163:743, 1987.
35. Dauzat, MM, Laroche, JP, Charras, C, et al: Real-time B-mode ultrasonography for better specificity in the noninvasive diagnosis of deep venous thrombosis. J Ultrasound Med 5:625, 1986.
36. Lensing, AWA, Prandoni, P, Brandjes, D, et al: Detection of deep-vein thrombosis by real-time B-mode ultrasonography. N Engl J Med 320:342, 1989.
37. Rooke, TW and Martin, RP: Lower extremity venous imaging for the echocardiologist. J Am Soc Echo 3:158, 1990.
38. Stoner, HB, Taylor, L, and Marcuson, RW: The value of skin temperature measurements in forecasting the healing of a below-knee amputation for end-stage ischaemia of the leg in peripheral vascular disease. Eur J Vasc Surg 3:355, 1989.
39. Kurumatani, N, Iki, M, Hirata, K, et al: Usefulness of fingertip skin temperature for examining peripheral circulatory disturbances of vibrating tool operators. Scand J Work Environ Health 12:272, 1986.
40. Franzeck, UK, Talke, P, Bernstein, EF, et al.: Transcutaneous PO_2 measurements in health and peripheral arterial occlusive disease. Surgery 91:156, 1982.
41. Batay-Csorba, PA, Provan, JL, and Ameli, FM: Transcutaneous oxygen tension measurements in the detection of iliac and femoral arterial disease. Surg Gynecol Obstet 164:102, 1987.
42. Harward, TRS, Bernstein, EF, and Fronek, A: Oxygen inhalation–induced transcutaneous PO_2 changes as a predictor of amputation level. J Vasc Surg 2:220, 1985.
43. Mustapha, NM, Jain SK, Dudley, P, et al: The effect of oxygen inhalation and intravenous Naftidrofuryl on the transcutaneous partial oxygen pressure in ischaemic lower limbs. Prosthet Orthot Int 8:135, 1984.
44. Kram, HB, Appel, PL, White, RA, et al: Assessment of peripheral vascular disease by postocclusive transcutaneous oxygen recovery time. J Vasc Surg 1:628, 1984.
45. Byrne, P, Provan, JL, Ameli, FM, et al: The use of transcutaneous oxygen tension measurements in the diagnosis of peripheral vascular insufficiency. Ann Surg 200:159, 1984.

46. Osmundson, PJ, Rooke, TW, and Hallett, JW: Effect of arterial revascularization on transcutaneous oxygen tension of the ischemic extremity. Mayo Clin Proc 63:897, 1988.

47. Rooke, TW and Osmundson, PJ: The influence of age, sex, smoking, and diabetes on lower limb transcutaneous oxygen tension in patients with arterial occlusive disease. Arch Intern Med 150:129, 1990.

48. Oberg, PA, Tenland, T, and Nilsson, GE: Laser-Doppler flowmetry—A non-invasive and continuous method for blood flow evaluation in microvascular studies. Acta Medica Scandinavica Supplementum 687:17, 1984.

49. Sundberg, S: Acute effects and long-term variations in skin blood flow measured with laser Doppler flowmetry. Scand J Clin Lab Invest 44:341, 1984.

50. Rendell, M, Bergman, T, O'Donnell, G, et al: Microvascular blood flow, volume and velocity measured by laser Doppler techniques in IDDM. Diabetes 38:819, 1989.

51. Johnson, JM, Taylor, WF, Shepherd, AP, et al: Laser-Doppler measurement of skin blood flow: comparison with plethysmography. J Appl Physiol 56:798, 1984.

PART 2

Venous Disorders

CHAPTER 4

Acute Deep Venous Thrombosis

Roger F. J. Shepherd, M.B., B.Ch.

In the venous system, thrombosis may occur anywhere but most commonly involves the deep veins of the leg. In the calf this may remain asymptomatic as the clot often dissolves without sequela by natural fibrinolysis.[1] However, if the thrombotic process continues, it may become clinically significant. Up to 5% to 20% of calf vein thrombi will propagate proximally,[1-3] and if extension occurs into the popliteal or more proximal veins, the chance of pulmonary embolism increases from less than 5% to approximately 50%.[4-8]

With approximately 200,000 deaths annually, thromboembolic disease remains the third most common cause of death in the United States and is the most common preventable cause of hospital death.[3,9] Sudden death from pulmonary embolism is often unexpected, as it can occur in the presence of silent deep vein thrombosis.

Venous thrombosis also causes chronic debilitation from venous obstruction and incompetence, the so-called postphlebitic syndrome.[10] This presents at a variable length of time, which can be up to 5 to 10 years following the resolution of the acute episode of thrombosis, with recurrent leg edema, stasis changes, and, often, skin ulceration. Altogether it is estimated that up to 600,000 persons are hospitalized annually in the United States for thromboembolic disease.[7] Therefore, it is no surprise that more than 1000 articles have been written on this disease during the past 10 years, as this is a condition that all fields of medicine need to be able to diagnose and treat.

Noninvasive tests are commonly used in the diagnosis of deep venous thrombosis (DVT). Advances in technology have allowed a greater reliance to be placed on some of these tests, especially duplex ultrasound and impedance plethysmography, in making therapeutic decisions. Today the therapy for acute DVT is less empiric, and current recommendations can be based on objective clinical studies. In the era of diagnostic related groups affecting reimbursement, and increasing concerns of cost containment, the hospital stay may be shortened by earlier institution of warfarin anticoagulation. Newer thrombolytic agents have greater clot specificity with less potential for systemic lysis and hence the expectation of decreased risk of bleeding. In the future, Hirudin and low molecular weight heparin may show promise as potent antithrombotic agents. Embolectomy by catheter technique may have a renewed role in acute DVT. Advances in knowledge of the mechanisms of coagulation have furthered our understanding of deficiencies of natural coagulation inhibitors such as protein C, protein S, and antithrombin III and have identified the antiphospholipin antibody syndromes associated with thromboembolic events.

Of primary importance is the prevention of thrombosis, with recognition of high-risk groups and effective prophylaxis of thromboembolic disease.[7]

In this chapter discussion is limited to the diagnosis and treatment of acute DVT.

ORIGIN OF LEG VEIN THROMBI

A thrombus consists of red cells, platelets, and leukocytes bound by fibrin. The majority of thrombi are thought to form initially in the venous sinuses of the calf or in valve cusp pockets.[11-14] Once a thrombus forms, several events may occur: (1) the thrombus may propagate, (2) it may embolize, (3) it may be removed by fibrinolytic activity, or (4) it may undergo organization and become recanalized. An initial inflammatory response leads to fibroblast and capillary ingrowth, which helps to stabilize the thrombus. Organization occurs over weeks to months as the thrombus becomes incorporated into the vessel wall. Partial or complete recanalization may occur and the surface becomes covered by endothelium.[15]

Because the calf veins have multiple valves and sinuses, most DVT are believed to originate in the lower leg veins. This has been demonstrated in postoperative patients using ^{125}I leg scanning[1] and venography.[11] For example, a large venographic study showed that thrombosis in 92% of 535 limbs was limited to calf veins or was contiguous with more proximal veins. Only 8% had discontinuous or isolated proximal leg thrombosis.[16] Thrombosis can also occur at the site of local trauma.[17] Thrombosis of the left common iliac vein has been noted to be more frequent than that of the right, perhaps due to compression of the left common iliac vein by the overlying iliac artery.[18]

From a clinical viewpoint, the natural history and consequences of a lower extremity venous thrombosis are different depending on the site of the thrombus. Deep vein thrombosis traditionally is divided into calf and more proximal (popliteal, femoral, iliac) involvement. Because the tibial and peroneal veins in the calf are duplicated and run in parallel, a thrombosis confined to one of these is unlikely to cause significant obstruction to the outflow of blood. Small calf vein clots occur frequently, especially in postoperative patients, as shown by ^{125}I studies. Of those that are asymptomatic, half lyse spontaneously, and as a consequence these patients are unlikely to have deep vein incompetence.[1]

On the other hand, thrombi involving the more proximal veins are less likely to undergo spontaneous lysis, even with heparin therapy.[3,19,20] If recanalization occurs, it is often incomplete and does not reverse the valvular damage, which frequently leads to venous incompetence and subsequent venous hypertension. If there is no recanalization, collateral veins may help to relieve the obstruction. When patients with an acute DVT are followed by impedance plethysmography for the assessment of venous obstruction, a positive test returns to normal in 30% of patients at 3 weeks and 60% to 70% by 3 months, indicating relief of venous obstruction in approximately two-thirds of these patients either by recanalization or collateral veins.[2]

MECHANISM OF THROMBOSIS

Clotting is the normal physiologic response to injury. The formation of fibrin is crucial in forming a localized hemostatic plug to prevent loss of circulating blood volume, a process that involves complex biochemical interactions between coagulation factors, platelets, and the vessel wall. Normally a critical balance is maintained between those factors that lead to clot formation and those that inhibit it; however, in many disease states, abnormal clotting is a frequent complication.

Clotting begins with intimal damage and exposure of the vascular subendothelium to platelets and coagulation factors. Platelets aggregate and release vasoactive substances, including thromboxane A_2 and serotonin. The coagulation system is activated by intrinsic system exposure to the vessel subendothelium and extrinsic activation by tissue thromboplastin substances released from injured tissues. The coagulation process continues with sequential activation of coagulation factors leading to the formation of thrombin, which converts soluble fibrinogen into insoluble fibrin.[14] Whether this becomes clinically significant depends on the balance between the formation and removal of activated clotting factors and the formation and removal of fibrin. Normally the liver clears activated clotting factors from the circulation. Venous stasis may predispose to clotting because these activated factors along with platelet aggregates may accumulate. Hypercoagulable states such as those associated with cancer or inherited coagulopathies and those caused by vessel wall injury from surgery or local trauma are major predisposing factors for thrombosis. This is in accord with the triad postulated by Virchow more than a century ago of venous stasis, abnormality of clotting, and abnormality of the vein wall.

The vein wall not only provides a smooth nonadherent conduit for circulating blood, but also has an important role in the maintenance of the fluidity of the blood by inhibiting the coagulation system to prevent thrombosis as well as by initiating local fibrinolysis to remove any clot forming on the vessel wall. The endothelial cell surface contains a heparinlike substance that can bind circulating antithrombin III and contains thrombomodulin, which is an endothelial cell receptor for thrombin. The ability of thrombomodulin to activate protein C is increased 1000-fold by complexing with thrombin.[14,21] Substances are also synthesized in and released from the endothelial cells, and there is active interaction between these and elements in the blood. Key substances include the following:

1. *Prostacyclin (PGI$_2$)*. PGI$_2$, formed in both the endothelium and smooth muscle, has vasodilator properties and inhibits platelet aggregation.[22,23] Its production can be stimulated by thrombin, endoperoxidases from platelets, or contact with activated leukocytes.[24]

2. *Endothelium-derived relaxing factor(s) (EDRF)*. In 1980 a nonprostanoid substance formed in the endothelium was demonstrated, which acts synergistically with PGI$_2$ to inhibit platelet aggregation and is a more potent vasodilator.[25]

3. *Tissue plasminogen activator (t-PA)*. The endothelium produces t-PA, which acts locally on any developing thrombus by activating the fibrinolytic enzyme system.[26] In this system, plasminogen activators act on plasminogen, an inactive zymogen synthesized in the liver. Plasminogen binds to fibrin along with tissue plasminogen activator. This leads to the local formation of plasmin and degradation of fibrin. Free plasmin is rapidly com-

plexed and inactivated by α_2-antiplasmin. A plasminogen activator inhibitor is also formed in endothelial cells in addition to t-PA.[14,27]

Normally there is a small, continuous, basal release of PGI_2 and EDRF, which can be increased by various substances including those released from platelets, such as adenosine diphosphate, serotonin, and thromboxane A_2. Along with thrombin, these substances activate specific receptors on the endothelial cells to release EDRF.[22,28,29] Thrombin also stimulates the release of tissue plasminogen activator from cultured human endothelial cells.[30,31]

Naturally occurring plasma coagulation inhibitors include antithrombin III, protein C, and protein S. Antithrombin III is the predominant inhibitor of thrombin. By binding to heparin, it accelerates the rate of inactivation of thrombin. A small fraction also is bound to heparan sulfate proteoglycans synthesized by endothelial cells, where it can neutralize activated coagulation factors on the vessel wall and protect against thrombus formation.[32]

Protein C is an inactive zymogen activated by thrombin and enhanced by thrombomodulin. Active protein C acts as an inhibitor of coagulation by inactivating factor Va and VIIIa. Protein S acts in part as a cofactor for factor C. By promoting the binding of factor C to phospholipid, it enhances the rate of inactivation of factor Va. Further discussion can be found in a comprehensive review of venous thrombosis by Ogston.[14]

DIAGNOSIS

When a patient presents with the possibility of a DVT, a focused history is obtained. Predisposing risk factors such as prolonged immobilization during car or plane trips, use of estrogens, prior DVT, or family history of thrombosis should be elicited (Table 4–1).

On examination, prominent features include localized tenderness and edema. The calf may be locally or diffusely tender to palpation in infrapopliteal thrombosis. Tenderness directly over the superficial femoral and common femoral veins is a more specific finding for proximal DVT. Edema often first appears in the posterior malleolar area or in the most dependent part of the leg. In some patients there is a diffuse increase in tissue turgor of the calf, which is best assessed with the knee flexed. Some patients have painless edema, whereas other patients may manifest edema only after bed rest when the affected leg is dependent. Often DVT may be clinically silent with pulmonary embolism as the presenting symptom. An increased superficial venous pattern may be prominent and may not decrease with leg elevation owing to increased venous pressure. Distal cyanosis may indicate extensive blockage to venous return. In some patients, massive venous obstruction can progress to phlegmasia cerulea dolens. This condition usually results from proximal obstruction at the ileofemoral level with extensive distal thrombosis of deep and often superficial veins. In phlegmasia, the arterial pulses may not be palpable, although anatomically the arteries are patent, and in severe cases, gangrene occurs, which may necessitate amputation.[33]

Clinical signs may be helpful, but many of these are nonspecific indicators of venous thrombosis. For example, Homans' sign, which is dorsiflexion of the foot to elicit calf discomfort, occurs with equal frequency in those with and without

Table 4–1. Predisposing Risk
Factors to Thrombosis

Inherited:
  Antithrombin III deficiency
  Protein C deficiency
  Protein S deficiency
  Dysfibrinogenemia and plasminogen disorders
Acquired:
  Immobilization
  Congestive heart failure
  Myocardial infarction
  Malignancy (lung, breast, pancreas, prostate)
  Nephrotic syndrome
  Myeloproliferative disease
  Dysproteinemias
  Paroxysmal nocturnal hemoglobinuria
  Behçet's syndrome
  Pregnancy
  Prior history of venous thrombosis
  Hip fractures or orthopedic surgery
  Venous catheters—Swan-Ganz and Hickman
  Drugs—Oral contraceptives
Anesthesia risk: Age over 40
                   Duration of anesthesia >40 min

DVT. Trousseau's sign of migratory superficial thrombophlebitis may be an indicator of visceral carcinoma. Armand Trousseau, a Parisian physician, self-diagnosed this condition prior to his death in 1867 from stomach cancer.[34]

It is important also to consider other conditions that may mimic DVT (Table 4–2). A complete examination is necessary to look for both evidence of systemic disease and other causes of leg swelling. For example, cardiac examination may reveal signs of right- or left-sided heart failure. Elevated jugular venous pressure and waveform patterns such as a large V-wave of tricuspid regurgitation or rapid X and Y descents may signify constrictive pericarditis. Abdominal examination may reveal a pulsatile liver or ascites. The popliteal space should be examined to exclude a Baker's cyst or a popliteal aneurysm. Lymphedema classically involves the toes and may be nonpitting; however, it frequently cannot be clinically differentiated from venous insufficiency. Tender erythematous inflammation with swelling of the lower leg and fever may be due to cellulitis.

Although the prediction of DVT may be improved by the pressure of certain clinical correlates including swelling above or below the knee, recent immobilization, cancer, and/or fever,[35] the clinical diagnosis based solely on history and examination frequently is inaccurate. Even an experienced examiner may be correct only 50% of the time. In reviewing a series of 1000 people with suspected DVT, almost 70% were subsequently shown not to have this as a cause of their symptoms.[3] Thus, if empiric treatment were employed, only one out of three would be correctly treated. Although clinical acumen remains important in the initial assessment, ultimately the diagnosis of acute DVT must be confirmed by objective testing since treatment should not be based on clinical impression alone.

Table 4–2.
Differential
Diagnosis of
Deep Vein Thrombosis

Local factors:
    Arthritis
    Baker's cyst
    Bony tumors
    Cellulitis
    Hematoma
    Muscle strain
    External venous compression (pelvic tumor)
    A/V fistula
Systemic factors:
    Congestive heart failure
    Pericardial constriction
    Restrictive cardiomyopathy
    Nephrotic syndrome
    Renal failure
Other:
    Idiopathic edema
    Lipedema
    Lymphedema: Primary/secondary
    Postphlebitic syndrome
    Superficial thrombophlebitis
    Varicose veins
Drugs:
    Nifedipine
    Florinef

DIAGNOSTIC TESTS

Contrast venography, which has been used over the last 30 years, remains the definitive method of confirming the diagnosis of acute deep vein thrombosis.[36] However, venography is invasive and has disadvantages related to the need for intravenous contrast.[37] These include anaphylaxis, renal insufficiency, and pain at the injection site along with potential iatrogenic thrombosis due to intimal damage from the hypertonic contrast solution. The diagnosis is established by finding an intraluminal filling defect. Often nonfilling of a vein segment is taken as indirect evidence of an occluding thrombus. In 5% to 15% of studies, there is nonvisualization of the deep system.[38] Venography is therefore subject to the inherent inaccuracy of being dependent on the quality of the individual study and experience of the radiologist. Venography may not be the perfect gold standard.

Noninvasive testing therefore has gained much popularity, and many studies have confirmed the safety and efficacy of making diagnostic and therapeutic decisions based on these tests. Noninvasive tests include impedance plethysmography, ^{125}I fibrinogen uptake scanning, and continuous wave and real-time Doppler ultrasound.

In using noninvasive tests, one has to consider sensitivity and specificity. Sensitivity refers to the ability of a test to detect people with the disease. Specificity is the proportion of negative test results in patients who do not have the disease.

IMPEDANCE PLETHYSMOGRAPHY

Impedance plethysmography (IPG), which is the most widely used of several plethysmographic techniques, measures changes in the venous volume of the leg by electrical bio-impedance.[37,39-41] A pneumatic cuff applied around the midthigh and inflated to 45 to 60 mm Hg occludes venous outflow but does not impede arterial inflow. Blood accumulates in the veins distal to the cuff, and the calf volume increases by several percent. When the cuff is released suddenly, venous volume rapidly decreases as blood flows out of the leg. A proximal DVT will be detected if it produces significant obstruction to the return (outflow) of blood from the leg. A nonoccluding thrombus may not be detected. Below the knee, the IPG is insensitive to thrombosis. In the calf, paired tibial and peroneal veins run in parallel, and consequently if a DVT is limited to only one of these veins, it will not be detected. This limitation applies as well to the hand-held Doppler examination. Other factors affecting IPG reliability include false-positive results owing to extravascular compression by pregnancy, pelvic tumors, hematoma, popliteal cysts, or knee extension, which may cause compression of the popliteal vein. However, the IPG remains a valuable, inexpensive, reproducible, and sensitive test for the detection of proximal DVT, in which it is 95% sensitive and 95% specific.[3,42] Despite failing to detect calf vein thrombi, this deficiency may not be clinically significant unless the thrombus propagates into a more proximal vein, at which point serial IPG testing should become positive.[43] The value of serial IPG testing was confirmed by Huisman and coworkers.[44] Of 426 people referred because of suspected DVT, 117 had a positive initial IPG, and with serial testing over the next 10 days, another 20 became positive. Phlebography confirmed thrombosis in 92% of these patients. Anticoagulation was withheld from the 289 patients with negative serial IPG, and during the 6-month follow-up, there was only one minor pulmonary embolism. Other studies have confirmed the usefulness of serial IPGs for outpatients with suspected DVT.[45,46] It should be noted, however, that these results apply only to a low-risk group of ambulatory patients. Information on the safety of withholding anticoagulation in hospitalized patients with negative IPGs is not available.

125I-FIBRINOGEN LEG SCANNING

This is the most sensitive of all noninvasive techniques for early detection of DVT and the only test that reliably detects small calf vein thrombi.[47] Unfortunately, there is up to a 48-hour delay for a positive or negative result because 125I-labeled fibrinogen must be incorporated into a developing thrombus to be seen as a hot spot on the scan. It is insensitive to pelvic vein thrombi and unreliable in the upper thigh because of increased counts from the bladder and other structures. False positives occur with muscle tear, hematoma, and surgical wounds, and therefore this test is best reserved for prospective screening of high-risk patients or for identifying calf vein thrombi when other noninvasive tests are indeterminate.[37,48]

DOPPLER ULTRASOUND

The hand-held continuous wave Doppler ultrasound can complement the physical examination.[49] Unfortunately, this examination is highly dependent upon the operator's experience and skill and is also insensitive to calf vein thrombosis.

In 1982 the first reports were published on the use of real-time two-dimensional ultrasound.[50,51] Since then, Doppler ultrasound has been combined with two-dimensional imaging (duplex scanning), and this has become a widely used evaluation for the diagnosis of suspected acute venous thrombosis. Recently the addition of color flow imaging enhances visualization and identification of vascular structures along with providing further hemodynamic information.[52,53] Duplex ultrasound has been called the wave of the future[54] as it is relatively inexpensive, non-invasive, and highly accurate. It has been predicted that it will supplant both venography[38] and hemodynamic noninvasive tests.[55] A sensitivity of 100% and specificity of 99% has been reported in a recent large prospective study comparing duplex to venography in the diagnosis of proximal (common femoral to popliteal) DVT.[56] Two recent review articles have combined results from studies over the past 8 years and report combined sensitivities of 0.93 and 0.96 along with a specificity of 0.98 and 0.99.[38,54]

The presence of an intraluminal thrombus is diagnostic; however, because a thrombus usually has the same echogenicity as blood, it frequently cannot be visualized. Other criteria for a positive test therefore include incomplete compressibility or noncompressibility of a vein under ultrasound visualization. A 5.0- to 10.0-mHz linear transducer is used. The usual examination technique begins with the patient supine in a reverse Trendelenburg position to promote venous filling. The common femoral vein at the level of the inguinal ligament is visualized initially and followed to the level of the superficial femoral vein at the adductor hiatus. With the patient prone, the popliteal and trifurcation veins are examined. Veins in the calf are more difficult to visualize, and a small thrombus of a tibial or peroneal vein may be missed. Proximal to the inguinal ligament, the pelvic veins are often obscured by bowel gases. A negative duplex scan does not exclude a calf or iliac thrombosis. Poor venous visualization at the adductor area, iliac vein, and calf area may lead to false-negative scans. Alternatively, noncompressibility in the adductor and inguinal areas may lead to false-positive diagnosis. Anatomic variants such as a duplicated superficial femoral vein also may be a cause of error.[57]

Deep vein thrombosis is often incidentally discovered during pelvic computerized tomography (CT) scanning. In the future, other imaging modalities such as magnetic resonance imaging may become a standard test for confirming the diagnosis of acute DVT.[58]

FURTHER EVALUATION

Patients with unexplained episodes of DVT who have no obvious predisposing risk factors and those with recurrent episodes of thrombophlebitis should be evaluated further to search for evidence of underlying systemic disease. In older patients, this may necessitate a workup for occult malignancy,[59] beginning with screening tests including a chest roentgenogram, blood tests, mammogram, and a hemoccult. In selected patients, one should consider further evaluation with gastrointestinal roentgenograms, CT scan of the abdomen and pelvis, and prostate ultrasound.

Antiphospholipid antibodies are acquired autoantibodies found in patients with and without autoimmune disorders such as systemic lupus erythematosus (SLE). The significance of these antibodies relates to predisposition to thrombosis. The presence of either antibody is associated with an increased risk of thrombosis.

Both may be found in other diseases including syphilis and acute infection and especially with drugs known to cause a lupuslike syndrome including chlorpromazine, procainamide,[60] and hydralazine. The association with thrombosis in non-SLE disorders has not been conclusively determined.[61]

The lupus anticoagulant is a circulating immunoglobulin that prolongs clotting time but is paradoxically associated with a 20% to 28% incidence of thrombosis. Approximately one-third of patients with SLE may have evidence for a lupus anticoagulant, but only half of patients with a lupus anticoagulant have SLE. The presence of a lupus anticoagulant should be suspected with a spontaneously prolonged activated partial thromboplastin time (up to three times normal) and can be confirmed by demonstrating a prolonged plasma clot time. The prothrombin time is less likely to be significantly prolonged.[62]

An anticardiolipin antibody has been identified in 44% of SLE patients but also in non-autoimmune diseases. The clinical significance of a specific isotype such as IgM or IgG and the antibody titer level has yet to be determined, as levels in individuals may fluctuate.[61]

Young patients with a family history of thrombotic disorders and those with recurrent episodes of unexplained thrombosis may undergo further evaluation looking for an inherited or acquired coagulopathy. This includes deficiencies of antithrombin III, protein C, protein S, and plasminogen.

Antithrombin III deficiency was first described in a Norwegian family in 1965.[63] It has been estimated to occur in 1:2000 to 1:20,000 people and in up to 4% to 6% of patients with idiopathic venous thrombosis. Clinical presentation is often seen in younger patients, predominately aged 15 to 30, who may have a family history of venous thromboembolism, thrombosis in an unusual site, recurrent venous thromboembolism, or thrombosis resistant to heparin therapy.[64] The risk of an asymptomatic carrier developing a thrombosis has been estimated at 65% over 15 years.[64]

A recent study determined the prevalence of coagulation deficiencies associated with acute DVT in 277 consecutive patients compared with 138 controls. The overall prevalence of coagulation deficiencies was 8.3% in patients with venous thrombosis compared with 2.2% in the controls.[65] Individually the prevalence of protein C deficiency was 3.2%, protein S 2.2%, and antithrombin III 1.0%. In this study the presence of a coagulation abnormality could not be accurately predicted based on a history of either recurrent, familial, or juvenile thrombosis. However, when all three of these historical factors were present, these patients had a 30% probability of a coagulation deficiency. Conversely, 92% of all patients with venous thrombosis had normal coagulation studies. Therefore, evaluation of coagulopathies should be selective, as routine screening of all patients may not be cost effective.[65]

TREATMENT OF ACUTE DEEP VENOUS THROMBOSIS

Anticoagulants remain the mainstay of treatment for thromboembolic disease. The two goals of anticoagulation in DVT are to (1) prevent death from pulmonary embolism and (2) limit venous damage and subsequent postphlebitic syndrome. Heparin anticoagulation had been well documented to be an effective treatment for thromboembolic disease, acting to stabilize the thrombus so that no further propagation occurs. Despite having no fibrinolytic activity, it allows for natural fibri-

Table 4–3. Guidelines for Heparin Therapy

1. Draw pretreatment blood tests: hemoglobin, platelets, APTT, PT.
2. Bolus 5000 to 10,000 units of IV heparin when disease suspected.
3. Begin continuous IV heparin infusion at approximately 1000 units per hour.
4. Monitor APTT every 6 hr until stable with APPT maintained at 1.5 to 2 times control.
5. Begin warfarin early, day 1 or 2, at estimated maintenance dose (7.5 to 10 mg).
6. After at least 4 to 5 days of overlapping therapy, stop heparin and check PT.
7. If PT is adequate, maintain warfarin alone at 1.3 to 1.5 times control. If there are no continuing risk factors, continue warfarin for 3 months. Continuing risk factors may indicate indefinite therapy. If thrombosis recurs, continue warfarin for 3 months to 1 year.

Source: Adapted from Chest 95(2)(Suppl):47S, 1989.

nolysis, which relieves the acute symptoms in most patients although recanalization of the affected vein may be incomplete.[66]

When confirmatory testing is not immediately obtainable but DVT or pulmonary embolism is strongly suspected, the patient should be heparinized if there is no contraindication to anticoagulation. Heparin may be subsequently discontinued if further evaluation proves negative. Guidelines for heparin therapy are outlined in Table 4–3.[67]

HEPARIN

Small amounts of heparin occur naturally in the body. In 1916 an anticoagulant substance was first identified from the liver and subsequently called heparin.[68] At present, heparin is prepared for pharmaceutical use from bovine lung tissue and porcine intestines. Heparin became established therapy for venous thrombosis in the early 1940s, and following reports by Allen at the Mayo Clinic and others elsewhere, the sequential use of heparin followed by dicumarol became standard therapy.[69,70]

Heparin acts as an anticoagulant inhibiting thrombosis by inducing a conformational change in antithrombin III. Heparin is then released to act again as a catalyst on another molecule of antithrombin III. In the absence of antithrombin III, heparin has no activity. Antithrombin III neutralizes thrombin by slowly binding with it, forming a thrombin-antithrombin complex. Further binding of heparin accelerates this enzyme-inhibitor complex by 1000-fold.[32] The heparin-antithrombin system is a major pathway to neutralize activated coagulation factors.

The major risk of heparin is bleeding, and the incidence of bleeding is greater with increasing dosages. Questions should be addressed therefore regarding the optimal dosage and duration of heparin therapy in order to balance the risk of bleeding versus the risk of recurrent venous thromboembolism.

A minimum amount of heparin is necessary. In a prospective randomized trial, patients with proximal DVT had a 47% incidence of recurrence when treated with only 5000 units of heparin subcutaneously twice daily and the trial had to be stopped.[71] In another trial there was a high risk of recurrent thromboembolism if the APTT was less than 1.5 times the control value.[72] Currently, the accepted recommendation for heparin administration is to prolong the APTT to 1.5 to 2.0 times the control or baseline value.[67]

Regarding the duration of therapy, it is well known that 7 to 14 days of continuous IV heparin followed by long-term warfarin anticoagulation results in a low rate of recurrent DVT. Before discontinuing heparin, an overlap of 4 or 5 days with warfarin is necessary to allow for depletion of all vitamin K–dependent clotting factors. Recently several studies have shown that the duration of hospital stay for IV heparin anticoagulation can be shortened to as little as 5 days by beginning warfarin on the first or second day of admission.[67,73,74]

Heparin requirements are greatest initially with acute thrombosis, necessitating more frequent titration based on monitoring of the activated partial thromboplastin time. Early complications with heparin include thrombocytopenia and elevation of aspartate aminotransferase.[75,76] Benign thrombocytopenia is a common occurrence, with the platelet count dropping to 70,000 to 100,000 units per liter. Rarely a severe antibody-mediated thrombocytopenia occurs which may predispose to further thrombosis: in these patients heparin should be stopped immediately and other thromboembolic prophylaxis used such as warfarin anticoagulation or placement of an inferior vena cava filter.

WARFARIN

In 1939 dicumarol was discovered to be the causative agent of hemorrhage in cattle eating spoiled sweet clover.[70] Warfarin (Coumadin) acts to inhibit the liver synthesis of vitamin K–dependent coagulation factors II, VII, IX, and X. The effect is delayed until these coagulation factors are cleared from the circulation. Although factor VII has the shortest half-life (7 hours), resulting in a prolongation of the prothrombin time, coagulation is not inhibited until other clotting factors are depleted. Warfarin also depletes natural inhibitors of coagulation including protein C and protein S. Initially, the rapid depletion of protein C may aggravate the thrombotic state. A loading dose of warfarin therefore is no longer recommended, as this may have a procoagulant effect during the first 2 days of therapy.[67,77]

The prothrombin time (PT) ratio (patient's PT/control's PT) is used to monitor the effectiveness of warfarin therapy. It is performed by adding a mixture of calcium and tissue thromboplastin to the patient's citrated plasma. Unfortunately prothrombin times from different laboratories may be variable owing to differences in the type and potency of the tissue thromboplastin used in the assay. For example, in the United States thromboplastin derived from rabbit brain is much less responsive by a factor of up to 2.6 times compared with the bovine thromboplastin used in the United Kingdom.[78] Since the 1970s, North American thromboplastins also have become less responsive, which could result in larger dosages of warfarin to prolong the prothrombin time test to the same degree. In 1982, the World Health Organization developed the International Normalized Ratio (INR) in order to standardize reporting of the prothrombin time. This incorporates the relative potency or responsiveness of a given thromboplastin reported as an International Sensitivity Index (ISI). The prothrombin time ratio can then be reported as the INR, which is the prothrombin time ratio to the ISI power. For example, a prothrombin time of 1.3 to 1.5 using a typical North American thromboplastin with an ISI of approximately 2.4 equates to an INR of 2.0 to 3.0.[78]

Warfarin is not without significant side effects inasmuch as hemorrhagic complications in long-term anticoagulation therapy occur in 10% to 40% of patients.[79,80] Major bleeding occurring in 7% and fatal hemorrhages in more than 5% of patients has been reported in a number of studies.[79] Another review study found the cumulative incidence of major bleeding at 1, 12, and 48 months to be 3%, 11%, and 22%. High-risk patients were those with a previous history of stroke, gastrointestinal bleeding, or serious coexisting disease, and the chance of major bleeding in this group increased to 63%.[81] As this risk of bleeding may increase with prolongation of prothrombin time, the lowest effective level of anticoagulation should be achieved.[81]

Over the past decade a series of trials by Hull and associates have helped to establish a more objective basis for current approaches to anticoagulation treatment.[3,71,82,83] Following heparin therapy, prolongation of prothrombin time to a mean of 19 seconds with warfarin is highly effective in proximal DVT in reducing the frequency of thromboembolism to approximately 2%. However, this was complicated by a 22% incidence of bleeding.[71] In another randomized prospective trial using less intensive warfarin therapy with a mean prothrombin time of 15 seconds, the incidence of bleeding was much lower without sacrificing therapeutic effectiveness.[82] In 1986 a joint subcommittee meeting on antithrombotic therapy of the American College of Chest Physicians (ACCP) and the National Heart, Lung, and Blood Institute concluded that the intensity of oral anticoagulation in many conditions should be reduced.[83] From the recommendations of the second ACCP conference in 1989, titrating the dosage of warfarin to prolong the prothrombin time to 1.3 to 1.5 times control is the currently recommended therapeutic range for the treatment of venous thromboembolic disease in the United States. This equates to approximately 15 to 18 seconds, with a control value of 11 to 12 seconds.[78,84]

In general, warfarin anticoagulation is continued for 3 months. Discontinuation of heparin at this time is associated with a 5% to 10% recurrence rate during the following year.[3,85] Those with an uncomplicated single episode of DVT have an even lower recurrence rate. Thus after a period of 3 months' anticoagulation, the risk of bleeding in general outweighs the risk of recurrent DVT. In patients who do have a recurrent episode of venous thrombosis, anticoagulation should be continued for at least 1 year. If there are continuing risk factors such as immobilization with bed rest, cancer, or a coagulation deficiency predisposing to thrombosis, anticoagulation should be continued indefinitely.

A rare complication of warfarin therapy is skin necrosis, as has been noted in some patients with protein C deficiency.[86] Hemorrhagic skin necrosis often involves areas where there is extensive adipose tissue, such as breasts, buttock, thigh, or abdominal wall, and may be due to small vessel thrombosis perhaps related to the rapid reduction of protein C by warfarin.[3] Gradual initiation of warfarin with a graduated dosage may prevent this abrupt drop in protein C levels.[87]

The clinician also should be aware of difficulties in maintaining the ideal prothrombin time ratio because of variations in diet, patient compliance, and the multiple drug interactions with warfarin.

ALTERNATIVE TREATMENT APPROACHES IN ASSOCIATED DISEASES

Subcutaneous heparain may be as effective as warfarin anticoagulation in the long-term secondary prevention of venous thrombosis when given every 12 hours with doses adjusted to prolong the midinterval (6 hours after injection) partial thromboplastin time to 1.5 times the control value.[3,85] Because it may take 2 to 3 days to achieve a therapeutic APTT, this should be started with a course of intravenous heparin. Although dosages vary, the mean dose in one study[85] was found to be 10,000 units twice a day, although often greater than 20,000 units daily is required. In acute DVT, therapy should not be initiated solely with subcutaneous heparin as the delay in achieving a therapeutic APTT has been associated with a 17% incidence of recurrent thromboembolism during anticoagulation. Half of these episodes were due to an extension of the DVT, and the other half had symptomatic pulmonary embolism.[88]

In pregnancy the use of warfarin is contraindicated in the first trimester because of the teratogenic effects on the fetus and also during the third trimester because of an increased risk of bleeding during delivery.[89] Subcutaneous heparin in therapeutic doses is effective during these periods.

Neurosurgical patients as well as those with a recent cerebrovascular or gastrointestinal hemorrhage have a contraindication to anticoagulation, and alternative measures for thromboembolic prophylaxis are necessary. Surgical plication of the inferior vena cava today is rarely performed owing to the availability of a variety of devices that can be percutaneously placed in the inferior vena cava. The Greenfield filter, for example, is 95% effective in preventing significant pulmonary emboli.[90] Although it has a high rate of patency, lower extremity edema may be a persistent problem. Thrombectomy may be of benefit in some patients with massive proximal deep venous obstruction or impending phlegmasia.[91-93]

In antithrombin III deficiency, heparin may be ineffective. Alternative options include initiating warfarin anticoagulation, or in acute circumstances, giving plasma or antithrombin III concentrate and heparin.[94] Other coagulopathies such as protein S and protein C deficiency can be treated with heparin followed by long-term administration of warfarin. Clotting association with a circulating lupus anticoagulant or an anticardiolipin antibody also may mandate long-term therapy with warfarin.[62]

CALF VEIN THROMBOSIS

Treatment of calf vein thrombosis remains controversial. If a thrombus is isolated to the calf, the risk of pulmonary embolism or further venous damage is often considered to be low. However, the importance of untreated calf vein thrombi is that approximately 20% will extend into the popliteal vein, where there may be up to a 50% incidence of pulmonary embolism.[3] In a prospective controlled study of patients with symptomatic calf vein DVT in which heparin therapy was discontinued only after 5 days, there was a recurrence rate of 29%. Of this group, proximal extension of thrombosis occurred in 5 of 28 (18%). There were no recurrences in a similar group treated with conventional anticoagulation for 3 months.[95] A 6-week course of warfarin also has been shown to be an adequate length of treatment for isolated calf vein thrombosis.[3]

By contrast, in the majority of patients a calf vein thrombosis will resolve without sequelae. Noninvasive testing can be used to stratify the relative risk in these patients.[46,96] For example, it may be safe to withhold anticoagulation in symptomatic patients if serial IPG testing remains negative over a period of 10 to 14 days. It should be noted that over this time span approximately 6% of patients become positive, indicating extension into a proximal vein. Current recommendations therefore are that patients with symptomatic calf vein thrombosis should either be treated with conventional heparin and warfarin anticoagulation for 6 to 12 weeks or be monitored with a serial noninvasive test for a period of 10 to 14 days, selectively treating only those in whom the test becomes positive.[67]

THROMBOLYTIC THERAPY

Controversy continues regarding the therapeutic role of thrombolytic agents in the treatment of acute DVT. For more than three decades, anticoagulation has been used as the primary method of therapy for acute DVT. Whereas heparin and warfarin anticoagulants prevent extension of thrombosis, they do not remove the existing thrombus and thrombosis cannot prevent venous valvular damage and subsequent lower extremity venous hypertension. Over a 10-year period it is estimated that up to 80% of patients with a proximal DVT will develop a postphlebitic syndrome at a cost estimated at up to $40,000 per patient.[97]

In contrast, thrombolytic agents will rapidly dissolve fresh clots, less than 1 week old, and may restore patency of the obstructed vein. The potential benefit is to decrease long-term morbidity from venous damage by more rapid lysis of the thrombus. Unlike indications for pulmonary embolism, a reduction in mortality is not an issue in considering lytic therapy for the treatment of DVT as heparin alone is effective in preventing recurrent thromboembolic disease. While there have been important advances in the use of thrombolytic agents in myocardial infarction, there have been few advances in therapy for DVT. Currently, thrombolytic agents are not used routinely but may be indicated in the case of a massive proximal DVT or impending phlegmasia. Thrombolysis also should be considered for young, otherwise healthy patients with extensive proximal thrombosis and threat of permanent residual disability.[98] A reduced incidence of postthrombotic sequelae and postphlebitic syndrome, however, has yet to be demonstrated consistently.[99,100] In deciding to use a thrombolytic agent, the potential benefits must be balanced against the increased risk of bleeding.

THROMBOLYTIC AGENTS

In 1933 Tillett and Garner[101] first reported on the fibrinolytic activity of hemolytic streptococci, having noted its ability to lyse clotted fibrin of normal human plasma. In 1959 streptokinase was used intravenously for venous thrombosis.[102] Subsequently, urokinase, tissue plasminogen activator (t-PA), and a number of other currently investigational thrombolytic agents have been developed including pro-urokinase (scu-PA), and acetylated plasminogen–streptokinase complex (APSAC). All these thrombolytic agents are plasminogen activators that convert an inactive plasma enzyme, plasminogen, to plasmin, which degrades fibrin.[67] Plasminogen activators also decrease levels of plasminogen and fibrin. Approximately 5% of circulating plasminogen becomes bound to fibrin during clot formation, and this may be activated selectively by "clot-specific" agents. t-PA and scu-PA are fibrin-selective agents due to either an affinity of the enzyme for fibrin-bound plasminogen (scu-PA) or direct binding to fibrin (t-PA). Streptokinase and urokinase do not bind preferentially to fibrin and thus equally activate circulating plasminogen. This leads to a systemic lytic state, which has been postulated to increase hemorrhagic complications. In clinical use, however, hemorrhagic complications are no less for fibrin-specific agents inasmuch as they are not as selective as anticipated.[103]

STREPTOKINASE

Streptokinase (SK) is the original and best known of the plasminogen activators. It combines with plasminogen to form an SK-plasminogen complex that converts any remaining unbound circulating plasminogen to active plasmin. The most common administration involves a bolus of 250,000 IU to overcome antigenicity followed by a continuous intravenous infusion of 100,000 U/h.[67] Premedication with 100 mg of hydrocortisone and acetaminophen may decrease allergic and febrile reactions.[104] The plasma half-life for SK is 30 minutes. For acute DVT it is often necessary to continue infusions for up to 48 to 72 hours. The risk of hemorrhage also increases with the length of infusion. Major side effects include febrile reactions in 15% to 50% of patients and allergic skin reactions in 6%. Anaphylaxis is rare. It is antigenic and cannot be repeated within 6 months.

Complete or partial lysis of acute thrombus may be expected with SK therapy in up to 70% to 80% of patients.[104,105] In comparison, the lack of any significant lysis with heparin (less than 10%) has been well documented in trials comparing SK and heparin therapy.[106,107] In 1984, Goldhaber and associates[108] did a pooled analysis of randomized trials of SK and heparin and found that thrombolysis was achieved 3.7 times more often among patients with SK than among those treated with heparin, but that major bleeding complications were 2.9 times more frequent with SK. The risk from hemorrhagic complications with SK has a wide range with a reported incidence of 8% to 25%.[108,109] In contrast, a recent review summarizing a series of 15 articles of SK therapy concluded that the incidence of major hemorrhagic complications was no greater in SK-treated patients than in those treated with heparin.[104] The most catastrophic event during thrombolytic therapy is an intracranial bleed. Compiling all studies reviewed, only 8 out of 874 patients suffered an intracranial hemorrhage, an incidence of only 0.9% (compared with an incidence of 0.5% often quoted during heparin therapy[97]). Less than 1% of patients died from lethal hemorrhage (7 of 874). They concluded that SK is beneficial when patients are properly selected and managed.

In this study, important factors in patient selection included the presence of a proximal thrombosis involving the thigh or pelvis, symptoms fewer than 7 days with fewer than 36 hours optimal, and no major contraindications such as a recent cerebral vascular accident (CVA), major surgery, or trauma including cardiopulmonary resuscitation, significant arterial hypertension, thrombus in the left side of the heart, or history of major bleeding or known bleeding disorder.[104] The most important factor determining effectiveness of thrombolysis is the duration of symptoms.

UROKINASE

Urokinase (UK) is currently derived from human urine and fetal kidney cells grown in culture. It directly activates circulating plasminogen and plasminogen bound to fibrin, producing a systemic lytic state. Many studies demonstrate that UK and SK are equally efficacious; however, fewer systemic allergic reactions, shorter infusion time, lesser systemic fibrinolytic activity, and fewer bleeding complications are some of the advantages cited for UK.[105] The cost of UK is sixfold higher than SK.[107] Urokinase is commonly administered as a loading dose of 4000 U/kg infused during a period of 10 minutes followed by 4400 U/kg per hour.[67,105,107]

A retrospective nonrandomized study of patients with acute, less than 7 days old, thigh or pelvic DVT found that SK and UK were equally efficacious, achieving complete clot lysis in approximately 80%.[105] In those patients with complete thrombolysis, this was achieved more rapidly with UK, requiring a mean infusion time of 32 hours (range, 2 to 48 hours). For SK therapy, a longer mean infusion time of 72 hours was required (48 to 106 hours). Compared with UK, greater fibrinogen depletion of fibrin occurred with SK, and in 60% of these patients, fibrinogen levels were less than 100 mg/dL. Low fibrinogen levels may be a major factor in bleeding during thrombolytic therapy.

Tissue Plasminogen Activator

Tissue plasminogen activator (t-PA) is formed in the vascular endothelium and is commercially produced by recombinant technology. It preferentially activates plasminogen associated with thrombus and is therefore more "clot-specific," although there is some activation of systemic plasminogen. A recent prospective multicenter randomized controlled trial of patients with proximal DVT treated with t-PA found that only 28% had complete or more than 50% lysis.[76] The addition of heparin made no difference to the lysis rate. No lysis occurred in 83% of patients treated with heparin alone and in 44% of the t-PA group. There were two neurologic events in 63 patients. In both patients, the total dose of t-PA was greater than 100 mg over 24 hours and functional fibrinogen levels were less than 1 g/dL. A fibrinogen level less than 150 mg/dL increases the risk of hemorrhage by 1.4 times.[110]

The low lysis rate in the aforementioned study may be due to inadequate lytic therapy incorporating a low dosage of 0.05 mg/kg/hr over a period of 24 hours. Verhaeghe and colleagues[109] evaluated two dosage regimens of t-PA in heparinized patients with either a 50- or 100-mg t-PA infusion over 8 hours followed by a 50-mg t-PA on the second day. A high rate of bleeding complicated this study, with major hemorrhages in 32% of patients.[109] In another study, thrombolysis was achieved in 58% of patients with an infusion of 0.5 mg/kg of t-PA over 4 hours with concurrent heparin.[111] With this infusion regimen there was evidence of a systemic lytic state with a 60% drop in fibrinogen levels. In contrast, a lower dose of t-PA infused over a longer period of time had minimal effect on fibrinogen but was less effective as only 21% of patients had significant clot lysis. There was also a trend toward reduction in postphlebitic syndrome in those patients with significant clot lysis.

Presently, anticoagulation remains the standard therapy used in over 90% of patients in the United States for venous thrombosis.[111] The potential benefit of thrombolytic therapy is to restore vein patency, to maintain normal valve function, and to protect patients from the postphlebitic syndrome. Further refinement and development of newer agents leading to greater efficacy with decreased risk of bleeding along with better patient selection and changes in administration protocols is needed in the future. Ultimately any advantages of lytic therapy over conventional anticoagulation will need to be defined by further prospective studies.

REFERENCES

1. Kakkar, VV, Flanc, C, Howe, CT, et al: Natural history of postoperative deep vein thrombosis. Lancet 2:230, 1969.
2. Jay, R, Hull, R, Carter, C, et al: Outcome of abnormal impedance plethysmography results in patients with proximal vein thrombosis. Frequency of return to normal. Thrombosis Res 36(3):259, 1984.
3. Hirsh, J and Hull, RD: Venous Thromboembolism: Natural History, Diagnosis, and Management. CRC Press, Boca Raton, Florida, 1987.
4. Rosenow, EC, Osmundson, PJ, and Brown, ML: Pulmonary embolism. Mayo Clin Proc 56:161, 1981.
5. Browse, NL, Clemenson, G, and Croft, DN: Fibrinogen detectable thrombosis in the legs and pulmonary embolism. Br Med J 1:603, 1974.
6. Browse, NL and Thomas, M, Lea: Source of nonlethal pulmonary emboli. Lancet 1:258, 1974.
7. Kakkar, V: Prevention of venous thrombosis and pulmonary embolism. Am J Cardiol 65:50C, 1990.
8. Huisman, MV, Buller, HR, ten-Cate, JW, et al: Unexpected high prevalence of silent pulmonary embolism in patients with deep venous thrombosis. Chest 95(3):498, 1989.
9. Dalen, JE and Alpert, JS: Natural history of pulmonary embolism. Prog Cardiovasc Dis 17:259, 1975.
10. Strandness, DE, Langlois, Y, Cramer, M, et al: Long-term sequelae of acute venous thrombosis. JAMA 250(10):1289, 1983.
11. Nicholaides, AN, Kakkar, VV, Field, ES, et al: The origin of deep vein thrombosis: A venographic study. Br J Radiol 44:653, 1971.
12. McLachlin, AD, McLachlin, JA, Jory, TA, and Rawling, EG: Venous stasis in the lower extremities. Ann Surg 152:678, 1960.
13. Karino, T and Motomiya, M: Flow through a venous valve and its implication for thrombus formation. Thrombosis Res 36:245, 1984.
14. Ogston, D: Venous Thrombosis: Causation and Prediction. John Wiley & Sons, New York, 1987.
15. Robbins, SL and Angell, M: Basic Pathology. Saunders, Toronto, 1976.
16. Stamatakis, JD, Kakkar, VV, Lawrence, D, et al: The origin of thrombi in the deep veins of the lower limb: A venography study. Br J Surg 65:449, 1978.
17. Stamatakis, JD, Kakkar, VV, Sagar, S, et al: Femoral vein thrombosis and total hip replacement. Br Med J 2:223, 1977.
18. Cockett, RB, Lea Thomas, M, and Negus, D: Iliac vein compression—Its relation to iliofemoral thrombosis and the post-thrombotic syndrome. Br Med J 2:14, 1967.
19. Goldhaber, SZ, Buring, JE, Lipnick, RJ, and Hennekens, CH: Pooled analysis of randomized trials of streptokinase and heparin in phlebographically determined acute deep venous thrombosis. Am J Med 76:393, 1984.
20. Watz, R and Savidge, GF: Rapid thrombolysis and preservation of valvular venous function in high deep vein thrombosis. Acta Medica Scandinavica 205:293, 1979.
21. Esmon, NL, Owen, WG, and Esmon, CT: Isolation of a membrane-bound cofactor for thrombin-catalyzed activation of protein C. J Biol Chem 257:859, 1982.
22. Gryglewski, RJ, Botting, RM, and Vane, JR: Mediators produced by the endothelial cell. Hypertension 12:530, 1988.
23. Moncada, S, Cryglewski, R, Bunting, S, and Vane, JR: An enzyme isolated from arteries transforms prostacyclin endoperoxidase to an unstable substance that inhibits platelet aggregation. Nature 263: 663, 1976.
24. Vane, JR, Anggard, EE, and Botting, RM: Regulatory functions of the vascular endothelium. N Engl J Med 323:27, 1990.
25. Furchgott, RF: Role of endothelium in responses of vascular smooth muscle. Circ Res 53:557, 1983.
26. Todd, AS: The histological localization of fibrinolysin activator. J Pathol Bacteriol 78:281, 1959.
27. Collen, D and Lijnen, HR: Tissue-type plasminogen activator-mechanism of action and thrombolytic properties. Haemostasis 16 (suppl 3):25, 1986.
28. Cohen, RA, Shepherd, JT, and Vanhoutte, PM: Inhibitory role of the endothelium in the response of isolated coronary arteries to platelets. Science 221:273, 1983.
29. Houston, DS, Shepherd, JT, and Vanhoutte, PM: Adenine nucleotides, serotonin and endothelium-dependent relaxations to platelets. Am J Physiol 248:H389, 1985.

30. Levin, EG, Marzec, U, Anderson, J, and Harker, LA. Thrombin stimulates tissue plasminogen activator release from cultured human endothelial cells. J Clin Invest 74:1988, 1984.

31. Gelehrter, TD and Sznycer-Laszuk, R: Thrombin induction of plasminogen activator-inhibitor in cultured human endothelial cells. J Clin Invest 77:6096, 1986.

32. Rosenberg, RD: Biochemistry of heparin antithrombin interactions, and the physiologic rule of this natural anticogulant mechanism. Am J Med 78(suppl 3B):3B25, 1989.

33. Brockman, SK and Vasko, SJ: Phlegmasia cerulea dolens. Surg Gynecol Obstet 1211:1347, 1965.

34. Rains, AJH and Ritchie, HD: Baily and Love's Short Practice of Surgery. HK Lewis and Company, London, 1975.

35. Landefeld, CS, McGuire, E, and Cohen, AM: Clinical findings associated with acute proximal deep vein thrombosis: A basis for quantifying clinical judgment. Am J Med 88:382, 1990.

36. Neiman, HL: Phlebography in the diagnosis of venous thrombosis. In Bergan, JJ and Yao, JST (eds): Venous Problems. Year Book Medical Publishers, Chicago, 1987.

37. Summer, DS: Diagnosis of deep venous thrombosis. In Rutherford, RB (ed): Vascular Surgery. WB Saunders, Philadelphia, 1989.

38. White, RH, McGahan, JP, Daschbach, MM, and Harling, RP: Diagnosis of deep-vein thrombosis using duplex ultrasound. Ann Intern Med 11:297, 1989.

39. Wheller, HB, O'Donnell, JA, and Mullick, SC: Impedance phlebography: Technique, interpretation and results. Arch Surg 104:164, 1972.

40. Barnes, RW, Collicott, PE, Mozersky, DJ, et al: Non-invasive quantitation of maximum venous outflow in acute thrombophlebitis. Surgery 72:971, 1972.

41. Hull, R, van Aken, WG, Hirsch, J, et al: Impedance plethysmography using the occlusive cuff technique in the diagnosis of venous thrombosis. Circulation 53:696, 1976.

42. Kempczinski, RE and Yao, JST (eds): Practical Noninvasive Diagnosis, ed 2. Year Book Medical Publishers, Chicago, 1987.

43. Hull, RD, Hirsh, J, Carter, CJ, et al: Diagnostic efficacy of impedance plethysmography for clinically suspected deep-vein thrombosis: A randomized trial. Ann Intern Med 102:21, 1985.

44. Huisman, MV, Buller, HR, Ten Cate, JW, and Vreeken, J: Serial impedance plethysmography for suspected deep venous thrombosis in outpatients. N Engl J Med 314(13):823, 1986.

45. Hull, RD, Raskob, GE, and Carter, CJ: Serial impedance plethysmography in pregnant patients with clinically suspected deep-vein thrombosis. Ann Intern Med 112:663, 1990.

46. Huisman, MV, Buller, HR, Ten Cate, JW, et al: Management of clinically suspected acute venous thrombosis in outpatients with serial impedance plethysmography in a community hospital setting. Arch Intern Med 149:511, 1989.

47. Kakkar, VV, Nicolaides, AN, Renney, JTG, et al: ^{125}I-labelled fibrinogen test adapted for routine screening of deep vein thrombosis. Lancet 1:540, 1970.

48. Hull, R, Hirsch, J, Sackett, DL, et al: Replacement of venography in suspected venous thrombosis by impedance plethysmography and ^{125}I-fibrinogen leg scanning. Ann Intern Med 94:12, 1981.

49. Turnbull, TL, Dymowski, JJ, and Zalut, TE: A prospective study of hand-held Doppler ultrasonography by emergency physicians in the evaluation of suspected deep-vein thrombosis. Ann Emerg Med 19(6):691, 1990.

50. Talbot, SR: Use of real-time imaging in identifying deep venous obstruction: A preliminary report. Bruit 6(6):41, 1982.

51. Coelho, JC, Sigel, B, Ryva, JC, et al: B-mode sonography of blood clots. JCU 10:323, 1982.

52. van Bemmelen, PS, Bendford, G, and Strandness, DE: Visualization of calf veins by color flow imaging. Ultrasound Med Biol 16(1):15, 1990.

53. Rose, SC, Zwiebel, WJ, Nelson, BD, et al: Symptomatic lower extremity deep venous thrombosis: Accuracy, limitations and role of color duplex flow imaging in diagnosis. Radiology 175(3):639, 1990.

54. Becker, DM, Philbrick, JT, and Abbitt, PL: Real-time ultrasonography for the diagnosis of lower extremity deep venous thrombosis. The wave of the future. Arch Intern Med 149:1731, 1989.

55. Comerota, AJ, Katz, ML, Greenwald, LL, et al: Venous duplex imaging: Should it replace hemodynamic tests for deep venous thrombosis? Vasc Surg 11(1):53, 1990.

56. Lensing, AW, Prandoni, P, Brandjes, D, et al: Detection of deep vein thrombosis by real-time B-mode ultrasonography. N Engl J Med 320:342, 1989.

57. Quinn, KL and Vandeman, FN: Thrombosis of a duplicated superficial femoral vein. Potential error in compression ultrasound diagnosis of lower extremity deep venous thrombosis. Ultrasound Med 9(4):235, 1990.

58. Francis, CW, Foster, TH, Totterman, S, et al: Monitoring of therapy for deep vein thrombosis using magnetic resonance imaging. Act Radiol 30(4):445, 1989.
59. Gore, JM, Appelbaum, JS, Greene, HL, et al: Occult cancer in patients with acute pulmonary embolism. Ann Intern Med 96:556, 1982.
60. List, AF and Doll, DC: Thrombosis associated with procainamide-induced lupus anticoagulant. Acta Haematol (Basel) 82(1):50, 1989.
61. Love, PE and Santoro, SA: Antiphospholipid antibodies: Anticardiolipin and the lupus anticoagulant in systemic lupus erythematosus (SLE) and in non-SLE disorders. Ann Intern Med 112(9):682, 1990.
62. Gastineau, DA, Kazmier, FJ, Nichols, WL, et al: Lupus anticoagulant: An analysis of the clinical and laboratory features of 219 cases. Am J Hematol 19:265, 1985.
63. Egeberg, O: Inherited antithrombin deficiency causing thrombophilia. Thromb Diath Haemorrh 13:516, 1965.
64. Hirsh, J, Piovella, F, and Pina, M: Congenital antithrombin III deficiency: Incidence and clinical features. Am J Med 87(3B):34S, 1989.
65. Heijboer, J, Brandjes, DPM, Buller, HR, et al: Deficiencies of coagulation-inhibition and fibrinolytic proteins in outpatients with deep-vein thrombosis. N Engl J Med 323:1512, 1990.
66. Killewich, LA, Bedford, GR, Beach, KW, et al: Spontaneous lysis of deep venous thrombi: Rate and outcome. J Vasc Surg 9(1):89, 1989.
67. Hyers, TM, Hull, RD, and Weg, JG: Antithrombotic therapy for venous thromboembolic disease. Chest 95(suppl):37S, 1989.
68. Schwartz, BS: Heparin: What is it? How does it work? Clin Cardiol 13(suppl V):12, 1990.
69. Best, CH: Preparation of heparin and its use in the first clinical cases. Circulation 19:79, 1959.
70. Deykin, D: Antithrombotic therapy in historical perspective. Am J Cardiol 65:2C, 1990.
71. Hull, R, Delmore, T, Genton, E, et al: Warfarin sodium versus low-dose heparin in the long-term treatment of venous thrombosis. N Engl J Med 301:855, 1979.
72. Hull, R, Hirsch, J, Jay, R, et al: Different intensities of anticoagulation in the long-term treatment of proximal vein thrombosis. N Engl J Med 307(27):1676, 1982.
73. Gallus, A, Jackaman, J, Tillett, J, et al: Safety and efficacy of warfarin started early after submassive venous thrombosis or pulmonary embolism. Lancet 2:1293, 1986.
74. Hull, RD, Raskob, GE, Rosenbloom, D, et al: Heparin for 5 days as compared with 10 days in the initial treatment of proximal venous thrombosis. N Engl J Med 322(18):1260, 1990.
75. Cines, DB, Maske, A, and Tennenbaum, S: Immune endothelial cell injury in heparin associated with thrombocytopenia. N Engl J Med 316:5, 1987.
76. Goldhaber, SZ, Meyerovitz, MF, Green, D, et al: Randomized controlled trial of tissue plasminogen activator in proximal deep venous thrombosis. Am J Med 88(3):235, 1990.
77. O'Reilly, RA, and Aggeler, PM: Studies on Coumadin anticoagulant drugs: Initiation of therapy without a loading dose. Circulation 38:169, 1968.
78. Hirsh, J, Poller, L, Deykin, D, et al: Optimal therapeutic range for oral anticoagulants. Chest 95(2):5S, 1989.
79. Levine, M, Raskob, G, and Hirsh, J: Hemorrhagic complications of long-term anticoagulant therapy. ACCP-NHLBI national conference on antithrombotic therapy. Chest 2(suppl):16S, 1986.
80. Landfeld, CS, Rosenblatt, MW, and Goldman, L: Bleeding in outpatients treated with warfarin: Relationship to the prothrombin time and important remediable lesions. Am J Med 87:153, 1989.
81. Landefield, S, and Goldman, L: Major bleeding in outpatients treated with warfarin: Incidence and prediction by factors known at the start of outpatient therapy. Am J Med 87:144, 1989.
82. Hull, R, Hirsh, J, Jay, R, et al: Different intensities of oral anticoagulant therapy in the treatment of proximal-vein thrombosis. N Engl J Med 307:1676, 1982.
83. Hyers, TM, Hull, RD, and Weg, JG: Antithrombotic therapy for venous thromboembolic disease. ACCP-NHLBI National Conference on antithrombotic therapy. Chest 89(suppl):26s, 1986.
84. Hyers, TM: Venous thromboembolic disease: Diagnosis and use of antithrombotic therapy. Clin Cardiol 13(4)(suppl VI):23, 1990.
85. Hull, R, Delmore, T, Carter, C, et al: Adjusted subcutaneous heparin vs. warfarin sodium in the long-term treatment of venous thrombosis. N Engl J Med 306:189, 1982.
86. Kazmier, FJ: Thromboembolism, coumarin necrosis, and protein C. Mayo Clin Proc 60:673, 1985.
87. Enzenauer, RJ, Berenbert, JL, and Campbell, J: Progressive warfarin anticoagulation in protein C deficiency: A therapeutic strategy. Am J Med 88:697, 1990.

88. Hull, RD, Raskob, GE, Hirsh, J, et al: Continuous intravenous heparin compared with intermittent subcutaneous heparin in the initial treatment of proximal-vein thrombosis. N Engl J Med 315:1109, 1986.
89. Hall, JG, Pauli, RM, and Wilson, KM: Maternal and fetal sequelae of anticoagulant during pregnancy. Am J Med 68:122, 1980.
90. Greenfield, L: Current indications for and results of Greenfield filter placement. J Vasc Surg 1:503, 1984.
91. Ganger, KH, Nachbut, BH, Ris, HB, and Zurbrugg, H: Surgical thrombectomy versus conservative treatment for deep venous thrombosis: functional comparison of long-term results. Eur J Vasc Surg 3(6):529, 1989.
92. Shionoya, S, Yamada, I, Sakurai, T, et al: Thrombectomy for acute deep venous thrombosis: Prevention of postthrombotic syndrome. J Cardiovasc Surg (Torino) 30(3):484, 1989.
93. Rutherford, RB: The role of thrombectomy in the management of iliofemoral venous thrombosis. In Rutherford, RB (ed): Vascular Surgery. WB Saunders, Philadelphia, 1989.
94. Schwartz, RS, Bauer, KA, Rosenberg, RD, et al: Clinical experience with antithrombin III concentrate in treatment of congenital and acquired deficiency of antithrombin. Am J Med 87:535, 1989.
95. Lagerstadt, CI, Fagher, BO, Olsson, CG, et al: Need for long-term anticoagulant treatment in symptomatic calf-vein thrombosis. Lancet 2:515, 1985.
96. Hull, R, Hirsh, J, Carter, C, et al: Diagnostic efficacy of impedance plethysmography for clinically suspected deep-vein thrombosis. Ann Intern Med 102:21, 1985.
97. Sherry, S, Bell, WR, Duckert, FH, et al: Thrombolytic therapy in thrombosis: A National Institute of Health consensus development conference. Ann Intern Med 93:141, 1980.
98. Goldhaber, SZ: Thrombolysis in venous thromboembolism. An International Perspective. Chest 97:176S, 1990.
99. Fiessinger, JN: Thrombolytic therapy for venous thrombosis. Ann Vasc Surg 1:522, 1987.
100. Kakkar, W and Lawrence, D: Hemodynamic and clinical assessment after therapy for acute deep vein thrombosis: A prospective study. Am J Surg 150(4A):54, 1985.
101. Tillett, WS and Garner, RL: The fibrinolytic activity of hemolytic streptococci. J Exp Med 58:485, 1933.
102. Johnson, AJ and McCarty, WR: The lysis of artificially induced intravascular clots in man by intravenous infusions of streptokinase. J Clin Invest 38:1627, 1959.
103. Loscalzo, J: An overview of thrombolytic agents. Chest 97(suppl 4): 117S, 1990.
104. Rogers, LQ and Lutcher, CL: Streptokinase therapy for deep vein thrombosis: a comprehensive review of the English literature. Am J Med 88(4):389, 1990.
105. Graor, RA, Young, JR, Risius, B, and Ruschhaupt, WF: Comparison of cost effectiveness of streptokinase and urokinase in the treatment of deep vein thrombosis. Ann Vasc Surg 5(1):524, 1987.
106. Sherry, S: Thrombolytic therapy for deep venous thrombosis. Semin Intervent Radiol 2:331, 1985.
107. Klatte, E, Becker, G, Holden, R, and Yune, H: Fibrinolytic therapy. Radiol 159:619, 1986.
108. Goldhaber, SZ, Buring, JE, Lipnick, RJ, and Hennekens, CH: Pooled analyses of randomized trials of streptokinase and heparin in phlebographically documented acute deep venous thrombosis. Am J Med 76:393, 1984.
109. Verhaeghe, R, Besse, P, Bounameaux, H, and Marbet, GA: Multicenter pilot study of the efficacy and safety of systemic rt-PA administration in the treatment of deep vein thrombosis of the lower extremities and/or pelvis. Thromb Res 55:5, 1989.
110. Hirsch, DR and Goldhaber, SZ: Bleeding time and other laboratory tests to monitor the safety and efficacy of thrombolytic therapy. Chest 97(suppl 4):124, 1990.
111. Turpie, AG, Levine, MN, Hirsh, J, et al: Tissue plasminogen activator (rt-PA) vs heparin in deep vein thrombosis. Results of a randomized trial. Chest 97 (suppl 4):172S, 1990.

CHAPTER 5

Chronic Venous Insufficiency

Wayne L. Miller, M.D., Ph.D.

Chronic venous insufficiency (CVI) of the lower extremity is most commonly the consequence of previous (years before) acute deep venous thrombosis. The pathologic state is characterized by aching leg pain with standing, edema, varicose veins, lipodermatosclerosis (stasis changes with tender induration of the subcutaneous tissue most commonly on the medial aspect of the lower leg), and ulceration. It can be estimated from some studies[1] that as many as 85% of patients with acute iliofemoral thrombophlebitis will develop venous ulceration by the 10th postevent year. The cost to society in terms of productive work hours lost and the persistent pain and discomfort experienced by the patient make this syndrome (the postphlebitic syndrome) a logical target for clinical and basic research. Although there has been considerable progress in the noninvasive laboratory assessment and diagnosis of CVI, there remain fundamental questions in prevention and management to be addressed.

ANATOMY AND PATHOGENESIS

A careful history and physical examination will usually confirm the presence of a venous problem but will not necessarily indicate the specific etiology or severity of the underlying pathology. The symptoms and findings of CVI are the consequence of venous hypertension, which results from venous outflow obstruction, reflux (venous valvular incompetence), or a combination of the two. Physiologic compensatory mechanisms attempt to minimize the effects of venous hypertension. Lymphatic drainage, which is significantly increased in postphlebitic extremities, and the inherent fibrolytic action, which removes pericapillary fibrin, become important. Therefore, the balance between the venous hypertension and the compensatory mechanisms may in part dictate the development of edema, dermal changes, and ulceration (Fig. 5–1). Venous ulcers also can develop in patients with isolated superficial venous disease in the absence of deep venous insufficiency, but these are a minority (15% to 20%) of patients presenting with venous ulcers.[2]

The most common sequence of events is the occurrence of acute obstructive venous thrombosis with subsequent recanalization, which results in venous valve

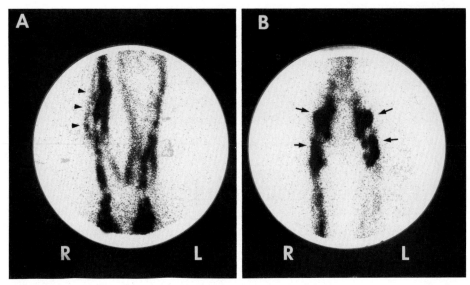

Figure 5–1. 18-year-old male with chronic venous insufficiency and accelerated lymphatic flow secondary to chronic venous hypertension. Lymphoscintigraphy (anterior views) of both legs after interdigital tracer injection (1 hour) followed by exercise demonstrates normal appearance time but prominent collateral lymph channels with rapid transport throughout the legs *(A, arrowheads)* and an exuberant visualization of nodes and lymph channels in the groin *(B, arrows)*. Patient presented with 3-year history of left ankle edema which had progressed to midcalf and recent development of right ankle swelling.

scarring and incompetence. As a consequence, venous hypertension develops in the deep venous system during ambulation.

The veins in the lower extremity are separated anatomically into the deep, the superficial, and the communicating or perforating veins. The deep veins carry the bulk of venous blood (85% to 90%) toward the heart, with small veins in the foot and ankle joining to form the paired posterior tibial, anterior tibial, and peroneal veins; these veins then empty into the popliteal vein at the knee level, which empties in turn into the superficial femoral vein, the common femoral vein, and the iliac vein, which continues as the inferior vena cava into the right atrium of the heart. The superficial veins in the subcutaneous tissue are the greater saphenous and lesser saphenous systems, which carry blood to the deep venous system (common femoral and popliteal veins, respectively). The communicating veins connect the superficial venous system with the deep venous system with blood being conducted inward from superficial to deep veins. This is assured by the presence of venous valves, which normally permit unidirectional flow only. Venous return to the heart while the patient is upright is possible because of the pumping action of the calf muscle in the presence of competent functioning venous valves. This mechanism is rendered ineffective in the postphlebitic syndrome because of damage to the valve from thrombophlebitis and the recanalization process. Iliofemoral thrombophlebitis is a common cause of severe CVI; other causes include structural weakness of the vein wall (as with varicose veins), which results in dilation of the vein and failure of the valve cusps to work properly, and congenital absence of venous valves.

Venous pressure is normally low during ambulation (25 mm Hg) because of the aforementioned pumping mechanism (Fig. 5–2). In the postphlebitic leg, however, the ambulatory pressure is high (sometimes 80 to 100 mm Hg) because of the incompetence of the deep venous valves (venous hypertension). Venous hypertension also can occur from persistent proximal venous occlusion,[3] but the principal determinant of ambulatory venous pressure and, therefore, the sequela of events (stasis changes, edema, ulceration) in the postphlebitic leg is incompetence of valves, most notably of the popliteal vein. The popliteal vein valve has particular importance because of its location in relation to the calf muscle pumping mechanism.[4] Incompetence of this valve is highly correlated with the development of venous ulceration.[5] Another result of the transmission of high venous ambulatory pressures to the superficial veins by incompetent communicating veins is the development of secondary varicose veins. The mechanism, however, that results in venous ulceration is more complex than simply venous hypertension. The cellular consequences of sustained ambulatory venous hypertension, namely impaired oxygen and nutrient transport, have been demonstrated to be due to pericapillary fibrin deposition.[6] Reduced endogenous fibrinolytic activity in the blood and vein wall has been observed in patients with stasis changes and ulceration. Histology has demonstrated dense pericapillary fibrin cuffing, which acts as a barrier to gas exchange producing cellular hypoxia and tissue necrosis.[6] A postulated sequence of events, therefore, is altered capillary permeability leading to fibrinogen leak into the pericapillary space with formation of fibrin by the extrinsic coagulation system and failure to clear the fibrin because of inadequate fibrinolysis. This interferes with

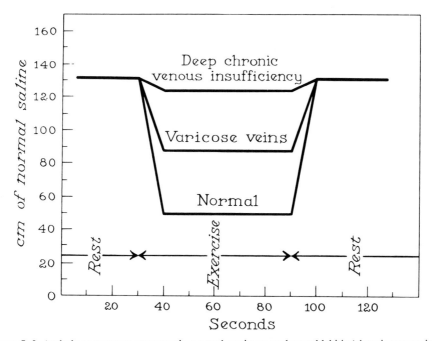

Figure 5–2. Ambulatory venous pressures in normal, varicose, and postphlebitic (chronic venous insufficiency) conditions. (From Fairbairn, JF, II, Juergens, JL, and Spittell, JA, Jr (eds): Peripheral Vascular Diseases, ed 5. WB Saunders, Philadelphia, 1980, with permission.)

gas and nutrient exchange, which leads to compromised cell function and eventually death of the cell. The etiology of the impaired fibrinolysis remains unknown, but a primary deficit may reflect a predisposition (in a subgroup of patients) to develop venous thrombosis.

In most instances the development of the postphlebitic syndrome follows the failure to detect or to adequately treat acute venous thrombosis. Recent studies have focused on the natural history of acute deep venous thrombosis (DVT) in symptomatic patients[7] in order to predict which patients are at highest risk of developing the sequelae of DVT. A previous history of DVT was the greatest risk factor (also age and obesity) for acute recurrent DVT in outpatients as well as inpatients. Many DVTs are silent (history of DVT in only 19% of patients in this study), and controversy continues over the origin and distribution of thrombi in the lower extremity. Thrombi were confined to the calf veins in 42.5% of limbs and isolated to proximal deep veins in 10% of limbs. Several studies suggest that thrombi begin most often in the calf veins and extend proximally by forming a thrombous column.[8] The calf veins, therefore, appear to be the anatomic site at greatest risk for thrombosis. Philbrick and Becker[9] reviewed the literature to assess the natural history of calf DVT and found that thrombus propagated to the thigh in only 20% of cases and that embolization does not occur from the calf (i.e., no fatal emboli with isolated calf DVT). Also, these authors offered no convincing evidence that calf DVT predisposes to chronic deep venous insufficiency. A management strategy of serial impedance plethysmography (IPG) was suggested with treatment (anticoagulation) only if proximal extension of thrombus occurred. Widmer and coworkers[10] reported a 21% incidence of postthrombotic syndrome at 5 years. There was a significant correlation between location of initial thrombus and incidence of postphlebitic syndrome; no postphlebitic syndrome was observed in the subgroup of patients with thrombus limited to below the knee, whereas there was a 34% incidence of postphlebitic syndrome with multilevel thrombi.

Venous reflux also has been used qualitatively to gauge the potential severity of postphlebitic sequelae, but quantitatively the degree of reflux necessary to produce symptoms is not clear. Christopoulos and associates[11] investigated the quantitation of venous reflux using air plethysmography to measure average venous filling rate (venous filling index, mL/s). A correlation between venous filling index and the incidence of chronic swelling, skin changes, and ulceration was demonstrated, although overlap among subgroups was present. A venous filling index above 2 mL/s (normal is 0.6 to 1.7 mL/s) indicated the presence of venous reflux, but the incidence of venous disease sequella was low for indices less than 5 mL/s. McEnroe and coworkers[2] reported on the correlation of severity of clinical findings with venous refill time (seconds) as measured by quantitative photoplethysmography (light reflection rheograph) in patients with known chronic venous insufficiency. Eighty percent of patients with severe (stage III) disease had venous refill times of less than 15 seconds. In the population studied (386 patients) the incidence of deep venous insufficiency alone was 65%, whereas that of superficial venous insufficiency alone was 21%; the combination was present in 14%. The cause of deep venous insufficiency was valvular incompetence in the majority (95%) and deep venous obstruction in the remainder. Forty percent of the patients had severe chronic venous insufficiency (stage III with ulcers), and of particular note is that 13% of these patients had involvement of the superficial venous system alone without deep venous insufficiency. The recognition that venous ulceration can occur without deep venous involvement is critical because these patients need to be identified as candidates not for deep reconstructive procedures but for simpler saphenous or perforating vein procedures. Patient assessment, therefore, by these techniques (and photoplethysmography) and others may help detect those patients at increased risk of developing severe postphlebitic syndrome and those who would benefit from early reconstructive surgical treatment.

CLINICAL FINDINGS

One of the earliest clinical manifestations of chronic deep venous insufficiency is orthostatic edema involving the ankles and dorsum of the feet. With chronic edema comes the more worrisome features of stasis dermatitis, liposclerosis, indurated cellulitis (Fig. 5–3), and ulceration. Hyperpigmentation due to hemosiderin deposition may occur above the ankles, as well as eczema resulting from the persistent scratching of pruritus (Fig. 5–4). Subcutaneous fibrosis with inflammation occurs in the lower leg and ankle regions, and with chronic induration the tissue retracts, producing pain and sometimes a disabling deformity. Ulceration is also an often disabling manifestation of chronic venous insufficiency. Ulcers develop at

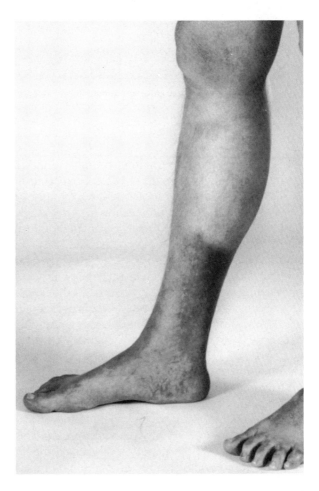

Figure 5–3. Chronic indurated cellulitis in a 50-year-old woman with history of recurrent DVT of the left leg and resulting chronic deep venous insufficiency.

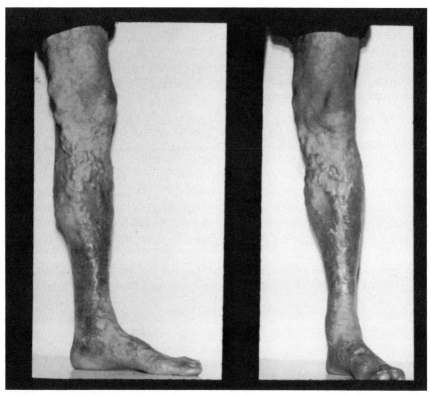

Figure 5–4. 67-year-old man with prominent lower extremity varicose veins, stasis pigmentation changes, and recurrent venous ulcers in the setting of a 20-year history of deep venous insufficiency.

sites of minor trauma, dermatitis, or induration. The most common location is the area of the medial malleolus, but ulcers can occur in any area of stasis pigmentation including the lateral and posterior surfaces, although this is more rare. Ulcers may be extensive in size and nonhealing if neglected (Fig. 5–5). Ulcers associated with CVI rarely occur on the upper leg or thigh and do not involve the toes or distal foot. Venous stasis ulcers may be painful, particularly when the leg is dependent, and the pain is improved with leg elevation (in contrast to ischemic arterial ulcers). Intercurrent conditions such as pregnancy, heart failure, or nephrosis may worsen the existing symptoms and predispose to the development of recurrent DVT.

A complication in patients with chronic iliofemoral venous obstruction is the development of severe thigh pain and a sensation of tightness (fullness) with exercise, which in many respects is similar to arterial claudication and was first described by Cockett and colleagues.[12] Venous claudication occurs only with chronic iliofemoral obstruction and does not occur with valvular incompetence or obstruction of peripheral deep veins, and edema is not present. Because of the obstruction, venous collaterals develop, which have a high and fixed outflow resistance.[13] Therefore, with exercise, venous and probably interstitial volumes increase to near maximum level but venous capacitance is inadequate, resulting in thigh pain, cyanosis, and the sensation of leg swelling. Prolonged rest with leg elevation (15 to 20 minutes) is often required to obtain relief in contrast to the pain of occlu-

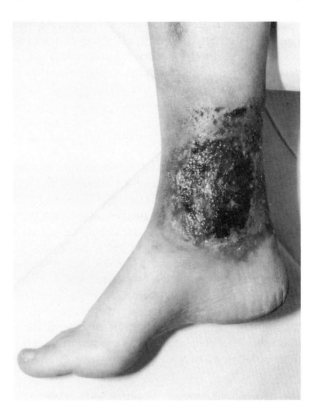

Figure 5–5. 41-year-old woman with nonhealing stasis ulceration as a complication of chronic deep venous insufficiency. Patient experienced trauma to the leg 8 years earlier and subsequently developed recurrent episodes of ulceration with failed skin grafting in setting of inadequate stocking support and long periods of standing without leg elevation.

sive arterial disease, which is most often relieved immediately with rest. Generally this condition is tolerated and venous bypass graft surgery to decompress the venous system is not necessary.

Other conditions must be distinguished from chronic venous insufficiency to prevent misdiagnosis and to prevent delaying appropriate treatment. Squamous cell carcinoma may develop at the edge of chronic venous ulcers. Although this is rare, the presence of long-standing unhealed ulcers should prompt the consideration of biopsy. Chronic lymphedema results in thick, firm skin and subcutaneous tissue, and the pitting edema, which is firm, involves the foot and toes. Leg elevation usually gives prompt benefit for the edema of chronic venous insufficiency, whereas chronic lymphedema requires several days of leg elevation for reduction in leg size to occur and, even then, restoration of normal size is not achieved. Also, pigmentation dermatitis and ulceration rarely occur with lymphedema. Recurrent lymphangitis and cellulitis resulting from local inflammation or injury to tissues can mimic the effects of deep venous insufficiency with leg swelling and the production of edema (lymphedema). Orthostatic edema of legs and ankles also may occur in the absence of local venous or systemic disease and is often bilateral and symmetric. The swelling of lipedema of the legs (excess fat accumulation in subcutaneous tissue) spares the feet and toes but also may have associated orthostatic edema. Severe, chronic uncompensated right heart failure also can result in bilateral and symmetric lower extremity edema and can induce stasis changes but usually can be distinguished from CVI by the presence of other readily recognized signs and symptoms.

Acquired or congenital arteriovenous fistulae (or malformations) can result in the clinical manifestations of CVI with lower extremity swelling, stasis pigmentation, and even ulcer formation. This occurs because venous hypertension develops secondary to the direct artery to vein communication. Findings of arterial ischemia including digital gangrene also may occur. In this setting, a history of a penetrating injury should be sought to support the presence of a traumatic-induced fistula. Unilaterally increased limb length, skin warmth, sweating, and hair growth in the presence of varicosities, particularly in a younger patient, suggests a congenital arteriovenous malformation.

Severe occlusive arterial disease and the associated ischemia commonly results in tissue infarction and ulcer formation of the toes and feet and on the lower leg with trauma to this area. In contrast to ulcers of CVI, ulcers due to arterial disease are more painful and have discrete edges with eschar and a pale base. In addition, other findings of arterial disease should be noted, particularly the absence of distal and proximal pulses, the presence of dependent rubor, elevation pallor, and increased venous filling time (greater than 45 to 50 seconds). Other, less common, etiologies of chronic ulceration of the legs need to be considered if venous insufficiency remains in doubt. Simple trauma, unattended burns as a complication of radiation therapy, and the indolent ulcers of pyoderma gangrenosum (associated with inflammatory bowel disease) are among the possible mimics of the manifestations of CVI. The absence of a history of deep venous thrombosis, varicosities, or edema help to exclude venous disease as an etiology.

ASSESSMENT

Considerable and appropriate attention has been given to the diagnosis of acute DVT but only recently has there been interest in an organized and comprehensive approach to the diagnosis of CVI. This in part has been stimulated by the development of surgical procedures to benefit superficial, perforator, and deep venous disease. Specific surgical procedures are available for valve incompetence, and bypass surgery can be done for venous obstruction. Diagnostically there has been difficulty in distinguishing perforator problems from deep venous abnormalities, deep venous obstruction from venous valve incompetence, and primary valve incompetence from postthrombotic valve destruction. These pathologic processes must be assessed in the patient for relative severity by quantitative measurements of the superficial, communicating (perforator), and deep venous systems.

A number of diagnostic techniques have been developed over the past few years that provide qualitative and quantitative information to the clinician in the assessment of chronic venous insufficiency. The purpose of this discussion is not to provide an exhaustive account of invasive and noninvasive investigations but rather to provide an outline of their usefulness in appropriate patients. Recent reviews are available.[14,15]

Methods for the evaluation of CVI are divided fundamentally into those techniques that provide anatomic information and those that provide hemodynamic information. Heretofore, the methods of assessing CVI have been primarily invasive (venography or measurements of direct venous pressure). Noninvasive methods are generally directed toward evaluating large vessel hemodynamics by detecting elevated venous blood pressure, abnormal limb-volume changes, valvular reflux (incompetence), or abnormal venous blood flow (direction and magnitude). Ultrasound (B-mode) has been the principal noninvasive method for anatomic assessment of CVI and permits definition of venous obstruction, valvular incompetence, and recanalization changes. Transcutaneous oxygen measurements provide information on the cellular consequences of CVI of impaired oxygen and nutrient exchange.

Ascending venography defines anatomy and gives an indication of the basic abnormality but cannot provide quantitative data. Therefore, venograms are performed to confirm the presence and extent of outflow obstruction with visualization of the anatomic level of obstruction and the extent of collateral vessel development. Descending venography can be performed to assess the degree of reflux and by inference the extent of valvular damage in the deep veins. The development, however, of duplex ultrasonic scanning (real-time ultrasound imaging combined with Doppler ultrasound) has provided a noninvasive means of quantitatively assessing the severity of obstruction and reflux in individual veins. As a result, venography needs to be performed in fewer patients.

Continuous wave (CW) Doppler ultrasound is effective in detecting reflux at the saphenofemoral and saphenopopliteal junctions. It is a quick, inexpensive, and noninvasive method of assessing veins of the leg but is of limited usefulness in the detection and localization of incompetence veins below the knee. Duplex scanning has largely overcome these deficiencies because not only can it detect the presence or absence of reflux at specific anatomic sites, but it can also provide quantitative measurement of the severity of the reflux. The ability of duplex scanning to detect reflux in individual veins has demonstrated that reflux confined to the superficial gastrocnemius vein can result in symptoms compatible with DVI and may account for as much as 5% false-positive popliteal vein reflux by continuous wave Doppler ultrasound.

Color flow imaging provides immediate visualization of blood flow and its direction. After the veins are identified initially by real-time B-mode imaging, the color is turned on and the pulsatile arterial flow is demonstrated in red (flow away from the transducer). Distal compression of the extremity augments venous flow in blue (flow toward the transducer). Sudden release of the compression will reveal reflux, if present, by a reversal in flow (away from the transducer), and therefore, a change to red color of normally blue venous blood flow. With this approach the detection of reflux at the saphenofemoral junction can be very efficient and even without the need for pulsed volume Doppler assessment.

Quantitative (calibrated) air plethysmography makes possible the detection of whole leg volume changes resulting from exercise in absolute units (milliliters). With the patient changing from supine to standing position, an increase in leg volume is observed as a result of venous filling (100 to 150 mL in normal limbs and 100 to 350 mL in limbs with chronic venous insufficiency[15]). A venous filling index is calculated as a measure of the average filling rate (mL/s). An index of 2 mL/s or less suggests no reflux, whereas values above 7 mL/s are associated with the findings of CVI. The placement of a tourniquet to occlude the superficial veins above the knee will reduce the index to less than 5 mL/s in the presence of primary varicose veins and competent popliteal veins but will not be changed if deep venous incompetence is present.

Quantitative photoplethysmography as by light-reflection rheography is a noninvasive method of providing information on venous emptying and venous filling. Diodes emit light through the skin which is reflected back from red blood cells to photoelectric sensors in proportion to the blood content of the subdermal venous system; this gives a measure of dermal venous volume. With exercise the blood content of the subdermis of the leg decreases and then recovers postexercise over 25 seconds or longer. A venous refill time of less than 25 seconds suggests venous insufficiency, and as with air or strain-gauge plethysmography, normalization with tourniquet placement indicates a diagnosis of superficial venous insufficiency. No improvement suggests isolated deep venous insufficiency. Improvement of venous filling time but not normalization suggests combined deep and superficial venous insufficiency.

A number of other techniques have been employed to evaluate venous outflow obstruction and valvular incompetence to include impedence and mercury Silastic strain-gauge plethysmography. Developed primarily for the detection of acute DVT, these techniques are relatively insensitive in CVI. The low sensitivity of IPG, for example, relates to the extensive collateral vessel formation that occurs with iliofemoral occlusions, resulting in minimal net outflow resistance detectable by IPG. Strain-gauge plethysmography also has a disadvantage of variability in sequential measurements and provides only segmental (calf veins) information, which may not reflect changes in the overall venous system of the limb.

MANAGEMENT

The mainstay in the management of chronic venous insufficiency is prevention with timely diagnosis and effective treatment of acute thrombotic events. This is undertaken to avoid the crippling effects of chronic venous hypertension, which results when valves are impaired in their function by excessive dilation (varicose veins) or destruction (iliofemoral-popliteal thrombophlebitis). In addition, vessel walls become less elastic in part because of the process of recanalization and less frequently because of frank obstruction. The standard therapy of acute venous thrombosis has been intravenous heparin followed by oral anticoagulation for 3 to 6 months. Heparin, however, has no lytic properties and may not uniformly protect against clot propagation and, therefore, does not influence the subsequent development of the postphlebitic syndrome. Ideal therapy would assure the removal of all thrombi, the maintenance of venous valvular function, and the prevention of rethrombosis. Two approaches have been employed with these goals in mind: venous thrombectomy and thrombolytic therapy.

Controversy exists regarding which mode of therapy, if any, more effectively limits or prevents the manifestation of the postphlebitic syndrome after acute DVT. Lack of adequate randomized prospective studies, difficulties in duration and completeness of followup, appropriate dosage of thrombolytics, and adequate venographic or ultrasound controls have limited the critical analysis necessary to establish the best treatment. Even with treatment, the desired optimal result is not clear. Kakkar and coworkers,[16] using ascending venography to evaluate valves in the upright patient, observed clinical improvement with resolution of venous thrombi but without necessarily preserving anatomic valve function. Thrombectomy for the iliofemoral vein segment has met with mixed results. Early findings were encouraging, but followup studies indicated a high incidence of postphlebitic syndrome.[17,18] Shionoya and colleagues[19] recently reported that thrombectomy within 7 days of the onset of symptoms of iliofemoral-popliteal venous thrombosis was more effective than lytic therapy with urokinase in preventing stasis ulceration. In the thrombolytic-treated group, the cumulative incidence of pigmentation at 15 years of followup was 41% and for ulceration was 27%. In contrast, the thrombectomy-treated group demonstrated an incidence of pigmentation at 15 years of 15% with no occurrence of stasis ulceration. This, however, was a nonrandomized study with bias expressed for the treatment selected based upon the extent of venous insufficiency.

Thrombolytic therapy remains a promising treatment made for proximal venous thrombosis when used with conventional anticoagulation. Such therapy has been shown to maintain valve function,[20] but it remains to be shown conclusively that patients will remain symptom-free. Uncertainties as to optimal dosage regimen, bleeding complications, expense (urokinase), and the complications of antigenic response (streptokinase) have perhaps undermined the utilization of this therapy. Tissue plasminogen activator (rt-PA) has been compared with heparin in randomized trials in the treatment of proximal DVT. In one study,[21] greater than 50% thrombus lysis was achieved in 58% of patients treated with rt-PA compared with none in heparin-only treated patients. Followup at a maximum of 3 years demonstrated that of the patients with greater than 50% clot lysis, 25% had symptoms consistent with postphlebitic syndrome whereas 56% were symptomatic in those patients in whom lysis was less than 50% (to include no lysis in the heparin-treated patients). Other well-designed studies have shown clot lysis of 50% or greater in only approximately one-third of rt-PA treated patients.[22] This relatively low lysis rate may be due to suboptimal dosing, duration of administration, or time to treatment after thrombosis formation. As a result, conflicting evidence exists with regard to the efficacy of thrombolytic therapy in the prevention of postphlebitic sequelae. Additional studies are needed to clarify issues of effective dose, route and duration of administration, and documentation of development of postphlebitic syndrome.

The need for management of patients with CVI is indicative of the inadequacies in the management of the acute predisposing thrombotic events. For the majority of these patients the postphlebitic syndrome is an incurable problem that is treated symptomatically with the goal of preventing the worst manifestations of venous ulceration. Knee-high elastic support stockings are an integral part of a good management program. Elastic support promotes venous flow by compressing the leg and increasing interstitial pressure and also compressing dilated superficial and intramuscular veins. This aids in the efficiency of the calf muscle pump mechanism and prevents edema, and often stasis changes in the skin. Support stockings are best applied when the leg is not edematous, which is usually in the morning before arising after a period of leg elevation. The heavy type of stocking fitted to provide graduated compression (30 to 40 mm Hg) from ankle to knee gives the best support at the ankle where it is most needed to counteract the venous hypertension of increased hydrostatic pressure. Effective support also may require foam-rubber pads fashioned to cover and extend slightly beyond the area of stasis changes. The hollow of the ankle is a particularly vulnerable area because of the anatomic configuration; therefore, it is difficult to provide adequate support with just stockings alone, which often do not compress this area. Custom-shaped padding held in place with elastic bandages is often necessary for this area in patients with severe venous insufficiency (Fig. 5–6). Hemodynamic assessment using photoplethysmography has demonstrated graded high-compression (40 mm Hg) support hosiery to be effective in significantly reducing ambulatory venous pressure in patients with post-

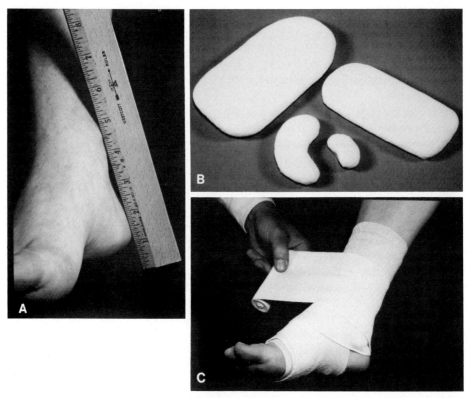

Figure 5–6. The malleolar hollow (*A*) is vulnerable and requires particular attention to providing adequate elastic support. Foam-rubber pads (*B*) can be shaped to provide support over healing or skin-grafted ulcer. Application of elastic bandage and foam-rubber pad (*C*) can be accomplished by the patient once properly instructed.

phlebitic limbs.[23] In addition, periodic elevation of the legs during the day with the ankles above heart level effectively relieves edema. Also, exercise of leg musculature (walking, bicycling, or swimming) develops calf muscle tone which enhances venous outflow.

Skin care is also important. Scratching of the involved area should be prevented and often local application of an emollient such as lanolin ointment will be effective with dry eczema. Antipruritic lotions or cortisone may be necessary in some instances. Care should be taken to avoid those substances that are irritating and that might superimpose a dermatitis and thus potentially lead to chronic non-healing lesions.

The majority of patients with symptoms of venous insufficiency will have perforator vein incompetence with varying degrees of deep venous damage. A significant subgroup of patients, however, will have only superficial varicosities with superficial venous incompetence, which, in general, is amenable to surgical correction. Surgery is recommended for incompetent superficial veins that are causing symptoms (aching, swelling, pruritus), complications (such as pigmentation, dermatitis, or ulceration), or are large and cosmetically troublesome. Vein stripping surgery has provided significant improvements in the long-term management of varicose veins. Recurrent varicosities after surgery are described, but are most often caused by incomplete removal or faulty high ligation during the surgery permitting collateral development from above down to the lower leg.

Surgical management of chronic deep venous insufficiency involves split-thickness skin grafting of large (greater than 3 cm in diameter) stasis ulcers and is done to shorten the duration of healing and disability. Prevention of recurrent ulceration after healing has occurred requires scrupulous long-term attention to adequate elastic support and its application. Subfascial ligation of medial and lateral ankle perforating veins has been advocated to interrupt the transmission of high deep venous pressures to the skin and subcutaneous tissue in ulcer-prone areas. Controversy exists as to the effectiveness of this procedure, but reported recurrent ulceration rates after perforation ligation suggest a role in the management of refractory venous stasis ulcers. Cikrit and associates[24] reported an ulcer recurrence rate of 22% in a 15-year experience with a modified Linton procedure. It also should be noted that ulcer recurrence rates as high as 43% have also been recorded.[25]

Venous bypass surgery has been done in the relative minority of symptomatic patients with venous claudication and iliac vein occlusions and patent distal vessels. Femorofemoral crossover bypass grafting has demonstrated acceptable results in this select group of patients.[26,27] Other approaches such as superficial femoral to greater saphenous venous bypass have been employed but await appropriate followup.[28]

In contrast, surgical approaches aimed at the more common problem of venous reflex have involved venous valve procedures such as reconstruction of incompetent valves by valvuloplasty, transposition of a venous segment possessing a functioning valve, or autograft of a valve segment of axillary or brachial vein. Vein valve transplants into the popliteal vein position for severe popliteal vein incompetence have resulted in a sufficient lowering of ambulatory venous pressure to promote healing of ulcers or damaged skin.[29] Femoral venous valve repair (valvuloplasty) also has shown good results in two-thirds of patients at 2 to 5 years of follow-up.[30]

After the assessment of all treatment modalities for chronic venous insufficiency has been completed, it is apparent at this juncture that no type of medical or surgical management is curative but rather palliative and then only with conscientious long-term care and follow-up.

REFERENCES

1. O'Donnell, TF, Browse, NL, Burnand, KG, et al: The socioeconomic effects of an iliofemoral venous thrombosis. J Surg Res 22:483, 1977.
2. McEnroe, CS, O'Donnell, TF, and Mackey, WC: Correlation of clinical findings with venous hemodynamics in 386 patients with chronic venous insufficiency. Am J Surg 156:148, 1988.
3. Ludbrook, J: Post thrombotic venous obstruction in the lower limb. Arch Surg 106:11, 1973.
4. O'Donnell, TF, Mackey, WC, Shepard, AD, et al: Clinical hemodynamic and anatomic follow-up of direct venous reconstruction. Arch Surg 122:474, 1987.
5. Schull, KC, Nicolaides, AN, Fernandes, É, et al: Significance of popliteal reflux in relation to ambulatory venous pressure and ulceration. Arch Surg 114:1304, 1979.
6. Burnand, KG, Whimster, I, Naidoo, A, et al: Pericapillary fibrin in the ulcer-bearing skin of the leg: The cause of lipodermatosclerosis and venous ulcerations. Br Med J 285:1071, 1982.
7. Rollins, DL, Semrow, CM, Friedell, ML, et al: Origin of deep vein thrombi in an ambulatory population. Am J Surg 156:122, 1988.

8. Nicolaides, AN and O'Connel, JD: Origin and distribution of thrombi in patients presenting with clinical deep venous thrombosis. In Nicolaides, AN (ed): Thromboembolism. University Park Press, Baltimore, 1975.

9. Philbrick, JT and Becker, DM: Calf deep venous thrombosis. Arch Intern Med 148:2131, 1988.

10. Widmer, LK, Zemp, E, Widmer, MT, et al: Late results in deep vein thrombosis of the lower extremity. VASA 14:264, 1985.

11. Christopoulos, D, Nicolaides, AN, and Szendro, G: Venous reflux: Quantification and correlation with the clinical severity of chronic venous disease. Br J Surg 75:352, 1988.

12. Cockett, FB, Thomas, ML, and Negus, D: Iliac vein compression—Its relation to ileofemoral thrombosis and the postthrombotic syndrome. Br Med J 2:14, 1967.

13. Killewich, LA, Martin, R, Cramer, M, et al: Pathophysiology of venous claudication. J Vasc Surg 1:507, 1984.

14. O'Donnell, TF, McEnroe, CS, and Heggerick, P: Chronic venous insufficiency. Surg Clin North Am 70:159, 1990.

15. Nicolaides, AN, Christopoulos, D, and Vasdekis, S: Progress in the investigation of chronic venous insufficiency. Ann Vasc Surg 3:278, 1989.

16. Kakkar, VV, Howe, CT, Laws, JW, et al: Late results of treatment of deep venous thrombosis. Br Med J 1:810, 1969.

17. Johansson, E, Nordlander, S, and Zetterquist, S: Venous thrombectomy in the lower extremity: Clinical phlebographic and plethysmographic evaluation of early and late results. Acta Chir Scand 139:511, 1973.

18. Lansing, AM, and Davis, WM: Five year follow-up study of iliofemoral venous thrombectomy. Ann Surg 168:620, 1968.

19. Shionoya, S, Yamada, I, Sakurai, T, et al: Thrombectomy for acute deep vein thrombosis: Prevention of postthrombotic syndrome. J Cardiovasc Surg 30:484, 1989.

20. Elliott, MS, Immelman, EJ, Jeffery, P, et al: A comparative randomized trial of heparin versus streptokinase in the treatment of acute proximal venous thrombosis: An interim report of a prospective trial. Br J Surg 66:838, 1979.

21. Turpie, AGG, Levine, MN, Hirsh, J, et al: Tissue plasminogen activator (rt-PA) vs heparin in deep vein thrombosis: Results of a randomized trial. Chest 97:172S, 1990.

22. Goldhaber, SZ, Meyerovitz, MF, Green, D, et al: Randomized controlled trial of tissue plasminogen activator in proximal deep venous thrombosis. Am J Med 88:235, 1990.

23. Noyes, LD, Rice, JC, and Kerstein, MD: Hemodynamic assessment of high-compression hosiery in chronic venous disease. Surgery 102:813, 1987.

24. Cikrit, DF, Nichols, WK, and Silver, D: Surgical management of refractory venous stasis ulceration. J Vasc Surg 7:473, 1988.

25. Johnson, WC, O'Hara, ET, Corey, C, et al: Venous stasis ulceration: Effectiveness of subfascial ligation. Arch Surg 120:797, 1985.

26. Halliday, P, Harris, J, and May, J: Femoro-femoral crossover grafts (Palma Operation): A long-term follow-up study. In Bergan, JJ and Yao, JST (eds): Surgery of the Veins. Grune & Stratton, New York, 1985.

27. Dale, WA: Venous bypass surgery. Surg Clin North Am 62:391, 1982.

28. Annous, MO, and Queral, LA: Venous claudication successfully treated by distal superficial femoral-to-greater saphenous venous bypass. J Vasc Surg 2:870, 1985.

29. Nash, T: Long term results of vein valve transplants placed in the popliteal vein for intractable postphlebitic venous ulcers and pre-ulcer skin changes. J Cardiovasc Surg 29:712, 1988.

30. Eriksson, I, Almgren, B, and Nordgren, L: Late results after venous valve repair. Int Angiol 4:413, 1985.

CHAPTER 6

Surgical Treatment of Venous Disease

Peter Gloviczki, M.D.
Steven W. Merrell, M.D.

In the past, surgical therapy for venous disease mainly consisted of varicose vein removal and the ligation of perforating veins between the deep and superficial venous systems. More recently, some of the traditional concepts of venous disease have been dispelled, and new aspects of the pathogenesis of venous disorders have been defined.[1-7] Recent studies have shown that a significant proportion of patients with chronic venous insufficiency have no history or phlebographic evidence of previous deep venous thrombosis.[2,5] These patients have primary valvular incompetence, and not "postphlebitic syndrome." Many cases that were previously thought to represent isolated superficial venous incompetence have been shown to be associated with concurrent deep venous insufficiency.[1] Furthermore, the frequency of isolated perforator incompetence has been shown to be as low as 3% in one recent review,[4] which is much less frequent than that described in older literature.[8,9]

With the changing concepts of venous disease, there have been renewed efforts to design and improve operations that address the underlying pathophysiology. Diagnostic techniques have been developed to more precisely determine whether a given case of deep venous insufficiency is caused by obstruction or valvular incompetence. More accurate diagnosis permits better patient selection for surgical therapy. Refined surgical techniques to treat obstruction and valvular incompetence have improved results to the point that these procedures can now be considered for patients who fail nonoperative therapy.[4,5,10-13]

This chapter will review the various surgical approaches to treat acute venous thrombosis and chronic venous insufficiency. To fully understand the procedures discussed, a brief review of the pertinent surgical anatomy is included. The majority of the chapter will focus on venous disorders of the lower extremities, but a short discussion of surgical options for the treatment of axillary-subclavian venous thrombosis also will be presented.

SURGICAL ANATOMY OF THE VEINS OF THE LOWER EXTREMITY

SUPERFICIAL VENOUS SYSTEM

There are two major superficial veins: the greater and the lesser saphenous veins. Both originate from the dorsal venous arch at the level of the foot. The greater saphenous vein ascends along the anteromedial aspect of the calf and joins the femoral vein at the groin, traversing the superficial fascia in the fossa ovale (Fig. 6–1). The lesser saphenous vein collects its tributaries from the posterolateral and posterior aspects of the leg and is in close contact with the sural nerve. Although the number of anatomic variations is significant, the lesser saphenous vein usually joins the popliteal vein about 3 to 5 cm proximal to the popliteal fossa.[14]

DEEP VENOUS SYSTEM

The deep veins are paired vessels at the level of the calf and accompany the peroneal, the posterior tibial, and the anterior tibial arteries. In the majority of cases, the gastrocnemius and soleal veins enter the popliteal vein just distal to or at the junction of the lesser saphenous vein. The superficial femoral vein is frequently paired, but duplication of the popliteal vein is less frequent. The superficial and deep femoral veins form the common femoral vein, which drains through the iliac veins into the inferior vena cava. Most patients have a single valve in either the external iliac or common femoral vein, but up to 37% of patients have no valve on one or both sides.[6,15] Because the common iliac vein and vena cava are valveless, this anatomy may predispose a significant proportion of the population to unusually high pressures on the valve at the saphenofemoral junction, which increases the likelihood of developing superficial venous insufficiency. There are usually four valves in the superficial femoral vein and at least one valve in the popliteal vein of every normal person. The calf veins each contain several valves.

PERFORATING VENOUS SYSTEM

These veins connect the superficial venous system with the deep venous system. At the level of the ankle and the lower half of the calf, Cockett's perforators connect the posterior arch vein with the posterior tibial veins (Fig. 6–1).[8] Perforating veins at the knee or thigh communicate directly between the greater saphenous vein and the popliteal or femoral veins. In patients who are about to undergo perforator ligation, preoperative localization by venography or duplex scanning is helpful, because the anatomy of some of the perforators is inconsistent.

SURGICAL TREATMENT OF ACUTE VENOUS THROMBOSIS

ACUTE SUPERFICIAL VENOUS THROMBOSIS

Nonsuppurative thrombophlebitis of the superficial veins may develop due to local trauma, prolonged inactivity, fungal infection, or the use of oral contraceptives. Underlying varicose veins may predispose to thrombophlebitis, independent of other causes.[16] Migratory superficial thrombophlebitis may be associated with chronic ischemia of the extremities in Buerger's disease, or it may develop in patients with occult or known malignancy.

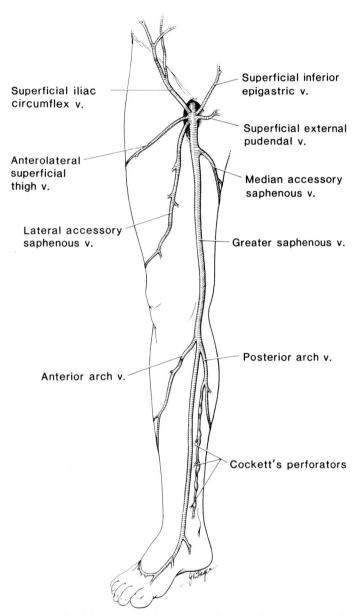

Superficial iliac circumflex v.

Superficial inferior epigastric v.

Superficial external pudendal v.

Anterolateral superficial thigh v.

Median accessory saphenous v.

Lateral accessory saphenous v.

Greater saphenous v.

Posterior arch v.

Anterior arch v.

Cockett's perforators

Figure 6–1. Normal anatomy of the greater saphenous vein and its tributaries.

The thrombosed vein is warm, red, and tender. A firm cord is frequently palpable. Conservative management with hot compresses, nonsteroidal anti-inflammatory medications, and elevation of the extremity is effective in most cases. Anticoagulation is usually not required. Rarely, excision of the acutely thrombosed greater saphenous vein is indicated to prevent progression of the thrombosis to the saphenofemoral junction and into the deep venous system.[16]

Suppurative thrombophlebitis may occur as a complication of intravenous line placement or self-inflicted injections from intravenous drug abuse. The clinical presentation is similar to nonsuppurative thrombophlebitis in terms of local findings, although high fever, leukocytosis, and bacteremia also may be present. The diagnosis is confirmed by spontaneous or expressed drainage of purulent material from the venipuncture site.

Suppurative phlebitis is treated with intravenous antibiotics and complete resection of the involved vein segment through multiple small incisions, which are packed open for postoperative drainage. Suppurative thrombophlebitis of large central veins is rare and usually is associated with prolonged use of central venous catheters. Standard treatment consists of intravenous antibiotics, removal of the central lines, and anticoagulation.[17] Persistent sepsis or recurrent septic pulmonary emboli from central veins are indications for balloon catheter thrombectomy.[18]

ACUTE DEEP VENOUS THROMBOSIS

Standard therapy for acute deep venous thrombosis consists of anticoagulation, bed rest, and elevation of the extremity. Surgical thrombectomy for acute iliofemoral deep venous thrombosis has been controversial and is not widely accepted. The potential benefits of the procedure include prevention of pulmonary embolization, reduction of early morbidity related to pain, swelling or tissue loss, and reduction of the incidence of late postthrombotic sequelae.[19]

The iliofemoral thrombus is removed with balloon catheters through a transverse incision in the common femoral vein. Distal thrombi are expressed through the same incision with the aid of an Esmarch bandage placed on the extremity. Positive pressure ventilation during thrombectomy decreases the chances of pulmonary embolization, and use of the cell saver decreases the need for blood transfusion. There have been six published series since 1980 which confirm early patency of the operated veins in up to 93% of patients.[20] Unfortunately, long-term follow-up is lacking and none of the currently available studies have proven superiority of venous thrombectomy over standard nonoperative therapy. There is also no controlled study comparing venous thrombectomy with thrombolytic therapy in a large number of patients with adequate long-term follow-up.

The best results of thrombectomy are obtained in young patients with a first episode of proximal (iliofemoral) thrombosis. Optimally, thrombectomy should be performed within 72 hours of the onset of symptoms. At present, we recommend venous thrombectomy for patients with threatened limb loss or venous gangrene caused by massive deep venous thrombosis, which is associated with high compartment pressures and arterial insufficiency (phlegmasia cerulea dolens).[21]

SURGICAL TREATMENT OF CHRONIC VENOUS INSUFFICIENCY

Chronic insufficiency of the venous circulation of the extremities is usually the result of congenital or acquired valvular incompetence or, less frequently, obstruction of the veins. The clinical picture ranges from severe pain and recurrent ulcerations to no symptoms at all. The site of involvement appears to be critical, because varicosity of the superficial venous system is usually benign and the incidence of significant complications is low. In contrast, insufficiency of the deep veins or of the perforators is more frequently associated with pain, swelling, ulceration, and long-term disability of the patients.

VARICOSE VEINS

The diagnosis of varicosity in the lower extremity is established by physical examination, with superficial veins that are dilated and tortuous (Fig. 6–2). Varicosity may be present in the so-called stem veins, the greater and lesser saphenous veins, or in their tributaries. "Spider veins" are small intradermal varicose veins.

The etiology of varicose veins should be clear before deciding for surgical treatment. In *primary varicosity,* no definite cause is identified, although age, female sex, pregnancy, obesity, and a positive family history are predisposing factors for the development of varicosity. As mentioned earlier, the lack of a competent valve above the saphenofemoral junction may increase the incidence of saphenous vein varicosity.[6,15] However, at least one study failed to show convincing evidence of this association.[22] Saphenous vein bypass grafts used for arterial reconstruction rarely develop varicose degeneration, so the pathogenesis of varicosity probably involves an intrinsic abnormality of the vein wall, in addition to the higher pressures generated by valvular incompetence.[3]

The causes of *secondary varicosity* include incompetence or obstruction of the deep veins owing to previous deep venous thrombosis, tumor, trauma, or high venous pressures due to congenital or acquired arteriovenous fistulas.

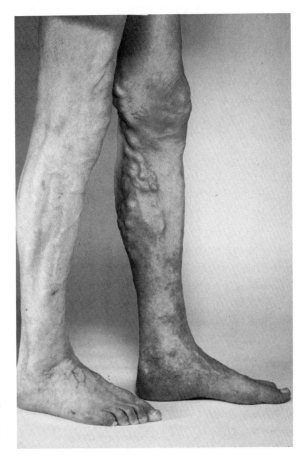

Figure 6–2. Primary varicosity of the left lower extremity with incompetence of the greater saphenous veins and its tributaries.

Indications for Surgical Treatment

The most frequent indications for operation on varicose veins are aching, swelling, and the feeling of heaviness in the legs, especially after prolonged standing. Surgical treatment also may be indicated for cosmetic reasons in a good-risk patient. Table 6–1 shows the signs and symptoms in a series of patients at the Mayo Clinic who underwent operation for varicose veins.[23]

Skin erosion, with varicose vein rupture and hemorrhage, is the most dramatic acute complication of varicose veins. Bleeding may be significant, and in rare cases even may be fatal.[16] However, hemorrhage from varicose veins may be easily controlled by compression of the ruptured vein and elevation of the extremity. Semielective removal of the varicose veins should then be performed to prevent recurrent bleeding.

Surgical treatment is contraindicated in elderly patients who are considered at high risk due to concurrent medical conditions, as well as in patients with arterial insufficiency of the lower extremities, lymphedema, skin infection, or coagulopathy and in pregnant patients. Resection of varicose veins is also contraindicated in patients with an arteriovenous fistula. If the arteriovenous communication is acquired, it should be repaired surgically, preserving the continuity of the arterial and the venous circulation whenever possible. Percutaneous transcatheter embolization of some acquired fistulas also may be an option. If the varicosity is secondary to a high-flow congenital arteriovenous malformation, embolization via subselective catheterization is the preferred mode of therapy,[24] and surgical excision is recommended only for superficial, well-localized malformations.

Table 6–1. Indications for Surgery in 350 Patients with Varicose Veins[23]

Sign or Symptom	Patients	
	#	%
Aching	250	71.4
Swelling	210	60.0
Heaviness	165	47.1
Cramps	136	38.9
Itching	106	30.3
Cosmetic	86	24.6
Stasis dermatitis	56	16.0
Pigmentation	55	15.7
Burning	55	15.7
Ulcer	29	8.3
Cellulitis	21	6.0
Erosion of skin	4	1.1
Fatigue	2	0.6
Restless legs	1	0.3
No symptoms	8	2.3

(From Lofgren EP: Present-day indications for surgical treatment of varicose veins. Mayo Clin Proc 1966; 41:515, with permission.)

Symptomatic congenital varicose veins in patients with Klippel-Trenaunay syndrome can be treated by excision of the involved vein segment, but careful preoperative evaluation is absolutely necessary.[25] In the absence of deep veins, removal of even short segments of the superficial venous system may lead to disaster in these patients.

Preoperative Evaluation

If the history, physical examination, and audible Doppler examination confirm the diagnosis of primary varicosity, treatment can proceed without additional studies. Patients with congenital arteriovenous fistula or congenital venous malformations need detailed imaging with venography and magnetic resonance imaging before any invasive treatment is undertaken.[24,25] Figure 6–3 describes the evaluation and management of patients with varicose veins.

Sclerotherapy

In the last several years, sclerotherapy of varicose veins has gained increasing popularity in the United States. It is now the treatment of choice for spider veins and small distal varicose veins.[16,26] Sclerotherapy also may be used to ablate recurrent varicose veins after stripping.

Depending on the size of the vessel, 1% or 3% sodium tetradecyl sulfate is injected into the lumen of the vein with a small syringe and a 25-gauge needle. The patient is placed in a slight reverse Trendelenburg position to distend the veins and facilitate injection. Compression is immediately applied to keep the sclerosing solution in the lumen of the vessel. After cotton balls or dental rolls are secured with paper tape over the site of the injection, an elastic wrap is applied to the extremity. Approximately 0.25 to 0.5 mL is injected into each vein, and usually 5 to 10 injections are performed per session. Elastic compression is suggested for at least 6 weeks after treatment.

Complications are rare, and usually minor. The most frequent morbidities include skin discoloration, thrombophlebitis, and hematoma formation. Allergic or anaphylactic reactions to the sclerosing agent are very rare but have been observed. Skin or fat necrosis may occur if a large amount of concentrated solution is injected outside the vein. Intra-arterial injection and ischemic gangrene have been described, but these are very rare complications. Some authors have reported a higher rate of recurrence with sclerotherapy than with surgical excision, especially when treating larger varicosities.[16]

Surgical Treatment

In recent years, the surgical approach to varicose veins has changed in two major ways: First, there has been an increasing awareness that a competent saphenous vein should not be removed in patients with isolated branch varicosity. Second, development of the "avulsion" technique allows varicose vein removal through small stab wounds, with excellent cosmetic results.

If there is valvular incompetence of the saphenous vein, stripping of the incompetent portion of the greater and lesser saphenous veins together with avulsion of the superficial varicose veins of the thigh and calf is the treatment of choice (Fig. 6–4). Ligation of the greater saphenous vein should be flush with the femoral vein to avoid formation of a cul de sac, which could become a source of deep venous thrombosis or pulmonary embolization. Ligation and division of all saphe-

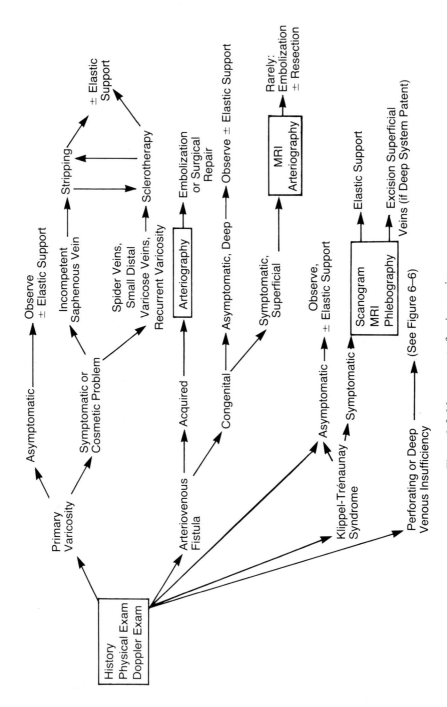

Figure 6–3. Management of varicose veins.

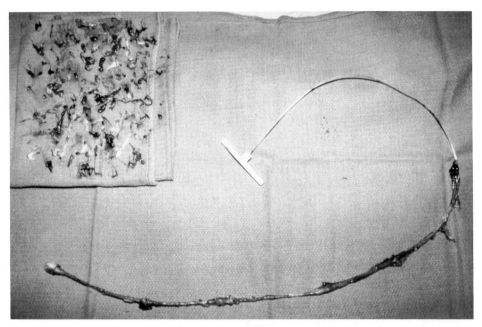

Figure 6–4. Photograph of an operative specimen showing greater saphenous vein stripped with a disposable stripper. The pieces of varicose veins were avulsed through small stab wounds.

nous vein tributaries at the saphenofemoral junction is important to prevent recurrence.[15] All of the previously marked varicose veins are avulsed through small stab wounds, and the incisions are closed with paper tape strips. The incompetent portion of the greater saphenous vein is stripped at the end of the procedure with a disposable intraluminal plastic stripper, and an elastic wrap is applied to the extremity to prevent hematoma formation.

If all varicose veins are compulsively removed and the incompetent segment of saphenous vein is stripped, 85% of the patients will have good to excellent results at the time of late follow-up.[27]

CHRONIC DEEP VENOUS INSUFFICIENCY

Indications for Surgical Treatment

Patients with chronic deep venous insufficiency may present with pain, swelling, varicosity, and a variety of stasis skin changes including induration, pigmentation, dermatitis, and ulcerations (Fig. 6–5). Most symptoms respond well to conservative management, which includes elastic compression, elevation of the extremity, and topical treatment of the ulcerations. Failure of medical management is an indication for surgical treatment.

Preoperative Evaluation

Noninvasive evaluation of the venous circulation with Doppler examination and impedance plethysmography usually confirms the clinical diagnosis of chronic venous insufficiency and helps to differentiate between occlusion and valvular incompetence. However, patients considered for deep venous reconstruction

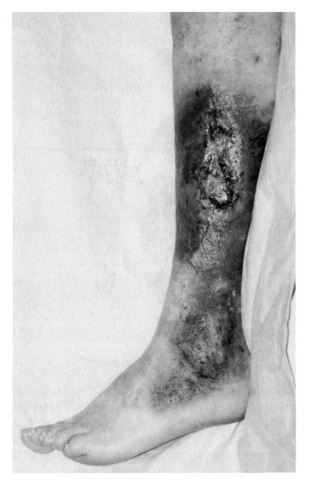

Figure 6–5. Severe manifestations of chronic venous insufficiency with induration, pigmentation, and large nonhealing venous ulcer.

should undergo additional evaluation with direct venous pressure measurements and ascending and descending phlebography using the technique of Kistner.[28] Figure 6–6 shows our current algorithm for evaluation and management of patients with chronic deep venous insufficiency.

Surgical Treatment

SKIN GRAFTING. Although most venous stasis ulcers heal after elevation of the extremity and elastic compression, skin grafting is indicated for large ulcers to accelerate healing and shorten the hospitalization time. The ulcer bed must be dry and free of infection before the procedure is performed. Split-thickness skin grafts are usually preferred for wound coverage.

LIGATION OF PERFORATORS. Removal of the incompetent superficial veins and ligation of incompetent perforators are best performed when the ulcer, if present, has completely healed. Incompetent perforating veins should be ligated only if the deep veins are patent. The classic approach of Linton,[9] with a long incision extending from the knee down to the ankle, is rarely used in current practice. If the quality of the skin overlying the perforators prevents a direct approach, subfascial ligation

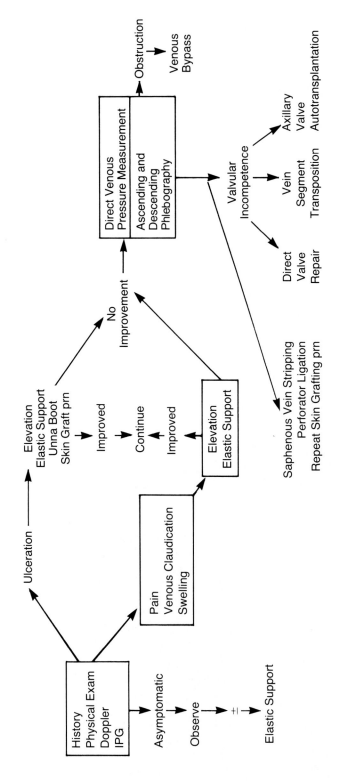

Figure 6–6. Management of chronic deep venous insufficiency.

of the perforators may be performed through a short, posterior midline incision. The greater or lesser saphenous veins are removed only if obvious incompetence is demonstrated preoperatively and patency of the deep system has been confirmed. Venous ulcers recur in 30% of patients after surgical therapy, and ulcerations persist for a prolonged period in 15% of patients.[29] These data underscore the importance of continued patient compliance with extremity elevation and elastic compression in the postoperative period.

Direct Venous Reconstruction

The results of direct venous reconstruction for obstruction or valvular incompetence have improved considerably in recent years,[30] largely owing to improved patient selection, accurate preoperative diagnosis, and atraumatic surgical technique. The use of perioperative pneumatic compression boots and continuous postoperative anticoagulation have decreased the incidence of thrombotic complications.[4,13,30,31] The reported frequency of deep venous thrombosis following venous reconstruction is between 0% and 8%, and no mortality or significant episodes of pulmonary embolization have been reported in several recent series.[4,5,10–13,32–34]

OPERATION FOR VENOUS OBSTRUCTION. Factors influencing patency of grafts after venous reconstruction are low flow, low pressure, increased thrombotic potential of the host, and the thrombogenic surface of the graft material.[35] Of the available prosthetic grafts, expanded polytetrafluoroethylene has given the most satisfying results (Fig. 6–7).[13,30,34] Autologous vein, however, appears to be the best venous graft. When large-caliber veins have to be replaced, a spiral vein graft prepared from the greater saphenous vein is an excellent alternative.[13,36,37] Preparation of the spiral graft is simple, and the graft may be tailored for reconstruction of vein of any diameter (Fig. 6–8). It can be useful for replacement of an injured femoral

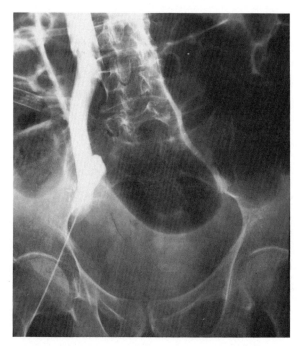

Figure 6–7. Postoperative venogram of a right iliocaval ePTFE graft, performed for severe symptoms of venous congestion in a male patient with chronic common iliac vein thrombosis. The graft has been patent for 3 years, and the patient has had almost complete relief of the symptoms.

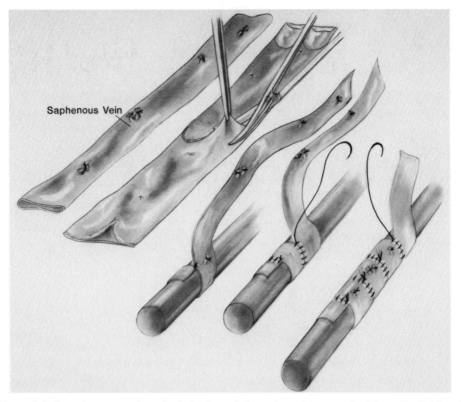

Figure 6–8. Steps in construction of spiral vein graft from the saphenous vein. (From Gloviczki and Pairolero,[36] with permission.)

vein (Fig. 6–9) or for construction of the occluded superior vena cava and innominate veins (Fig. 6–10).

The patency of prosthetic grafts in the venous system appears to be better when a temporary distal arteriovenous fistula is added to increase flow through the graft.[30,35] After 3 to 6 months the fistula is occluded by direct ligation or placement of an occlusive balloon by a percutaneous catheterization technique. However, results of venous bypass for obstruction are still inferior to those obtained with arterial grafting.[13]

The *cross-femoral saphenous vein bypass* was originally described by Palma and Esperón,[38] and it became popular in this country because of the pioneer work of Dale.[32,39] The procedure is indicated for unilateral iliac venous occlusion in patients who typically present with swelling and venous claudication. The saphenous vein from the healthy side is dissected, tunneled to the contralateral side, and anastomosed to the common femoral vein (Fig. 6–11). Some authors recommend the use of an additional arteriovenous fistula at the groin to enhance flow through the vein graft.[2] In a small group of operated patients, O'Donnell[12] achieved excellent results. Dale[32] reported the largest experience with cross-femoral bypass, with improvement in 77% of his patients. Such good results, however, were not duplicated by others.[2]

Other variations of the Palma procedure include the *saphenopliteal bypass* and the *saphenotibial bypass*.[2,39,40] The saphenopopliteal bypass may be useful for

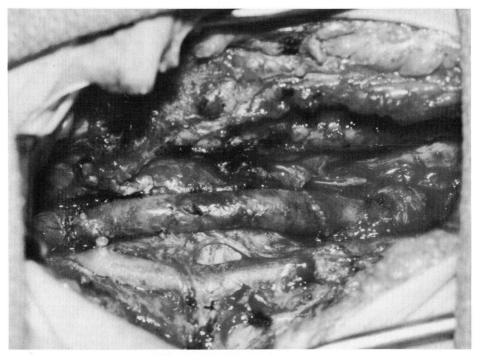

Figure 6–9. Reconstruction of the femoral vein with a 6-cm-long spiral vein graft.

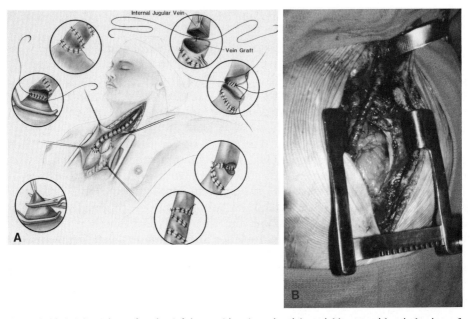

Figure 6–10. (*A*) Steps in performing left internal jugular vein–right atrial bypass with spiral vein graft, for left innominate vein obstruction. (*B*) Intraoperative photograph of spiral vein graft. (From Gloviczki and Pairolero,[36] with permission.)

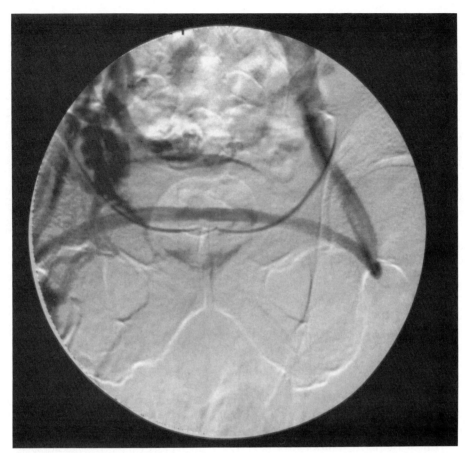

Figure 6–11. Postoperative venogram of a patent cross-femoral saphenous vein graft, performed for symptomatic right iliac vein occlusion.

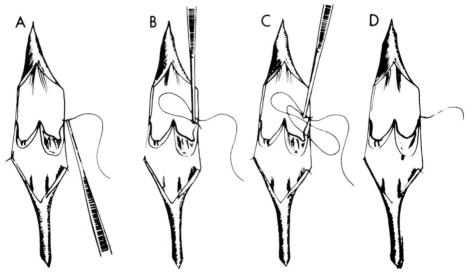

Figure 6–12. Direct valve repair in the femoral vein by the technique of Kistner. (From Kistner, RL: Transvenous repair of the incompetent femoral vein valve. In Bergan, JJ and Yao, JST (eds): Venous Problems. Year Book Medical Publishers, Chicago, 1978, p. 493, with permission.)

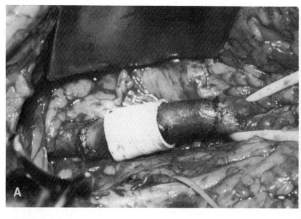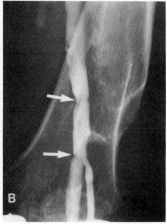

Figure 6–13. Same patient as in Figure 6–5. (*A*) Axillary vein with a competent valve transplanted into the popliteal vein. Note expanded polytetrafluoroethylene cuff around the vein graft to prevent dilatation and secondary incompetence. (*B*) Ascending phlebography confirms patency of the vein graft. Arrows indicate sites of anatomoses. (From Gloviczki and Pairolero,[36] with permission.)

the patients with superficial femoral vein occlusion and involves an end-to-end or end-to-side venovenous anastomosis between the midportion of the saphenous vein and the popliteal vein. Dale[39] and Husni[40] have independently reported patency rates of up to 60%. The saphenotibial bypass was introduced by Raju to treat femoropopliteal venous obstruction and bypass the resistance of residual functioning perforator valves.[2] Although the concept is appealing, significant clinical experience with this operation is not available.

All of the aforementioned saphenous vein bypasses have the advantages of requiring only one venovenous anastomosis and of using a nonthrombogenic, autogenous bypass conduit. However, the number of symptomatic patients who have the appropriate anatomy to undergo these procedures is relatively small.

OPERATIONS FOR VALVULAR INCOMPETENCE. The pioneering work of Kistner[5] has led to an increased interest in this subject during the last decade. Direct venous valve repair, venous transposition, and vein valve transplantations are the types of valvular reconstruction that have been used clinically.

Venous valve repair can be performed only in patients who have incompetent valves and no history of deep venous thrombosis (Fig. 6–12). Kistner[5] and Raju[4] have both reported encouraging results, but they have had difficulty with the correlation of clinical improvement and objective changes in hemodynamic measurements. Nonetheless, Raju reported excellent clinical results in over 60% of the patients 2 years after the operation.[4]

Vein segment transfer was introduced by Kistner[5] in 1982. In this procedure, the incompetent superficial femoral vein is anastomosed end-to-end to the saphenous vein or the deep femoral vein, depending on which has a competent proximal valve. Unfortunately, Kistner's good experience could not be repeated by Johnson and coworkers[41], who reported deterioration in 10 of 12 operated patients.

Valve Transplantation. Autotransplantation of a segment of arm vein with a competent valve into the femoral or popliteal vein has been used with increasing frequency in recent years. The valve-containing segment of axillary or brachial vein

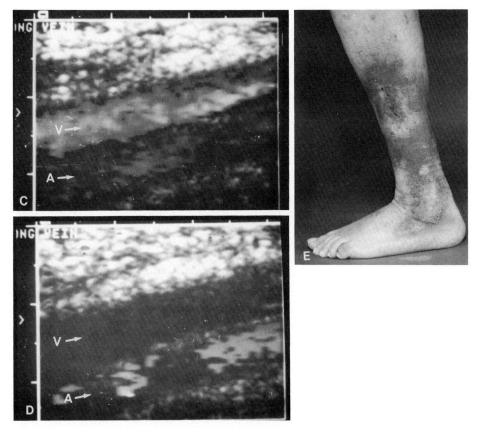

Figure 6–13 (continued). (*C*) Color-flow Doppler examination of popliteal area during expiration shows normal arterial (A) and venous (V) flow patterns. (*D*) Same segment during Valsalva maneuver shows normal arterial flow (A) and competence of transplanted venous segment (V—black, no signal). (*E*) At 3 months after valve transplantation ulcer was completely healed.

is implanted into the proximal popliteal vein using loupe magnification and a no-touch atraumatic technique (Fig. 6–13). In postthrombotic syndrome, attention should be paid to anastomosing the graft to the true lumen, carefully avoiding the false lumen of the recanalized vein. Table 6–2 summarizes the current results of vein valve transplantations.

Table 6–2. Results of Valve Transplantation for Chronic Venous Insufficiency

| Authors | Patients, Number | Follow-up, Month | Outcome, Number (%) | |
			Improved	No Change
Taheri et al[33]	48	Up to 60	38 (79%)	10 (21%)
Raju and Fredericks[4]	18	>24	9 (50%)	9 (50%)
O'Donnell[12]	10	>24	10 (100%)	0 (0%)
Sottiurai[45]	8	34	8 (100%)	0 (0%)
Total	84		65 (77%)	19 (23%)

To date, reports of clinical improvement following operations for valvular incompetence have not been accompanied by improvement in venous hemodynamics. As a result, Bergan and coworkers[30] stated that longer follow-up and objective evidence of late valvular competence will be needed before these procedures can be recommended for routine surgical practice. However, the published results are sufficient to justify venous reconstructive surgery for selected patients who fail nonoperative treatment.

AXILLARY-SUBCLAVIAN VENOUS THROMBOSIS

The incidence of venous thrombosis in the upper extremities is low, accounting for 2% of all cases of venous thrombosis.[42] However, with the widespread use of diagnostic and therapeutic catheterizations, the incidence of this disease seems to be increasing.[43,44] Occlusion of the axillary or subclavian vein may be spontaneous, but it is usually related to injury or effort in otherwise healthy young people. In a recent Mayo Clinic study[43] of 95 patients with axillary-subclavian venous occlusion, thoracic outlet compression was evident in 34 patients. Conversely, clinically significant venous thrombosis was found in only 3.5% of the 969 patients treated for thoracic outlet syndrome.[43]

The clinical syndrome of axillary-subclavian venous thrombosis was described more than a century ago by Paget and von Schroetter. The chief complaints include pain and swelling of the arm. The superficial veins are distended, and there is a prominent venous collateral pattern over the anterior chest. In the acute phase, pain and tenderness over the axillary vein is frequently present. Duplex scanning or venography is necessary to confirm the diagnosis.

Pulmonary embolization is an uncommon complication of acute axillary-subclavian thrombosis, occurring in less than 5% of these patients.[42] The embolus is usually small and nonfatal. It appears that the frequency of significant postphlebitic symptoms is higher in patients who do not receive adequate anticoagulation for at least 3 months after the acute thrombosis.[43]

There is no consensus regarding the role of surgical treatment for chronic symptoms that do not respond to elastic compression. If the patient has intermittent signs of venous compression and the axillary vein is narrowed or recanalized, thoracic outlet decompression may be helpful. If the disease is bilateral and extends into the innominate veins or into the superior vena cava, direct venous bypass with prosthetic grafts or, as a better alternative, with spiral vein graft may be necessary (Fig. 6–13). Our favorable experience with the use of spiral vein grafts for superior vena cava replacement has recently been reported.[13] Certainly, the best treatment for chronic venous insufficiency of the upper extremity is prevention.[43] Prevention is best accomplished by early recognition of acute axillary-subclavian venous thrombosis, adequate anticoagulation, and the selected use of early thrombolytic therapy, or thrombectomy in severe cases.

REFERENCES

1. Raju, S: Venous insufficiency of the lower limb and stasis ulceration: Changing concepts and management. Ann Surg 197:688, 1983.
2. Raju, S: New approaches to the diagnosis and treatment of venous obstruction. J Vasc Surg 4:42, 1986.

3. Rose, SS and Ahmed, A: Some thoughts on the aetiology of varicose veins. J Cardiovasc Surg 27:534, 1986.
4. Raju, S and Fredericks, R: Valve reconstruction procedures for nonobstructive venous insufficiency: Rationale, techniques, and results in 107 procedures with two- to eight-year follow-up. J Vasc Surg 7:301, 1988.
5. Kistner, RL: Deep venous reconstruction (1968–1984). Int Angiol 4:429, 1985.
6. Browse, NL, Burnand, KG, and Thomas, ML (eds): Diseases of the Veins: Pathology, Diagnosis, and Treatment. Hodder & Stoughton, London, 1988.
7. Raju, S: Venous reconstruction for chronic venous insufficiency of the leg. In Ernst, CB, and Stanley, JC (eds): Current Therapy in Vascular Surgery, ed 2. BC Decker, Philadelphia, 1991.
8. Cockett, FB and Jones, DEE: The ankle blow-out syndrome: A new approach to the varicose ulcer problem. Lancet 1:17, 1953.
9. Linton, RR: The post-thrombotic ulceration of the lower extremity: its etiology and surgical treatment. Ann Surg 138:415, 1953.
10. Sottiurai, VS: Technique in direct venous valvuloplasty. J Vasc Surg 8:646, 1988.
11. Taheri, SA, Heffner, R, Budd, T, and Pollack, LH: Five years' experience with vein valve transplant. World J Surg 10:935, 1986.
12. O'Donnell, TF Jr, Mackey, WC, Shepard, AD, et al: Clinical, hemodynamic, and anatomic follow-up of direct venous reconstruction. Arch Surg 122:474, 1987.
13. Gloviczki, P, Pairolero, PC, Cherry KJ Jr, and Hallett JW Jr: Reconstruction of the vena cava and its primary tributaries: A preliminary report. J Vasc Surg 11:373, 1990.
14. May, R: Anatomy. Major Prob Clin Surg 23:1, 1979.
15. Villavicencio, JL: Excision of varicose veins. In Ernst, CB and Stanley, JC (eds): Current Therapy in Vascular Surgery, ed 2. Philadelphia, BC Decker, 1991.
16. Lofgren, EP: Chronic venous insufficiency. In Spittell, JA Jr (ed): Clinical Vascular Disease. Cardiovascular Clinics. FA Davis, Philadelphia, 1983.
17. Verghese, A, Widrich, WC, and Arbeit, RD: Central vein septic thrombophlebitis—The role of medical therapy. Medicine 64:394, 1985.
18. Hoffman, MJ and Greenfield, LJ: Central venous septic thrombosis managed by superior vena cava Greenfield filter and venous thrombectomy: A case report. J Vasc Surg 4:606, 1986.
19. Rutherford, RB: The role of thrombectomy in the management of iliofemoral venous thrombosis. In Rutherford, RB (ed.): Vascular Surgery, ed 3. WB Saunders, Philadelphia, 1989.
20. Bergan, JJ: Surgical management of acute superficial and deep femoral venous thrombosis. In Ernst, CB and Stanley, JC (eds.): Current Therapy in Vascular Surgery, ed 2. BC Decker, Philadelphia, 1991.
21. Gloviczki, P, Hollier, LH, Cherry, KJ Jr, et al: Phlegmasia cerulea dolens: The continuing morbidity. Int Angiol 1:127, 1982.
22. Basmajian, JV: The distribution of valves in the femoral, external iliac, and common iliac veins and their relationship to varicose veins. Surg Gynecol Obstet 95:537, 1952.
23. Lofgren, EP: Present-day indications for surgical treatment of varicose veins. Mayo Clin Proc 41:515, 1966.
24. Gloviczki, P and Hollier, LH: Arteriovenous fistulas. In Haimovici, H (ed): Vascular Surgery: Principles and Techniques, ed 3. Appleton-Century-Crofts, New York, 1989.
25. Gloviczki, P, Stanson, AW, Stickler, GB, et al: Klippel-Trenaunay syndrome: The risks and benefits of vascular interventions. Surgery 110:469, 1991.
26. Bergan, JJ: Varicose veins: Chronic venous insufficiency. In Moore, WS (ed.): Vascular Surgery: A Comprehensive Review. WB Saunders, Philadelphia, 1991.
27. Larson, RH, Lofgren, EP, Myers, TT, et al: Long-term results after vein surgery: Study of 1,000 cases after 10 years. Mayo Clin Proc 49:114, 1974.
28. Kistner, RL, Ferris, EB, Randhawa, G, et al: A method of performing descending venography. J Vasc Surg 4:464, 1986.
29. Lofgren, KA, Lauvstad, WA, and Bonnemaison, MFE: Surgical treatment of large stasis ulcer: Review of 129 cases. Mayo Clin Proc 40:560, 1965.
30. Bergan, JJ, Yao, JST, Flinn, WR, and McCarthy, WJ: Surgical treatment of venous obstruction and insufficiency. J Vasc Surg 3:174, 1986.
31. Hobson, RW II, Lee, BC, Lynch, TC, et al: Use of intermittent pneumatic compression of the calf in femoral venous reconstruction. Surg Gynecol Obstet 159:284, 1984.
32. Dale, WA: Reconstructive venous surgery. Arch Surg 114:1312, 1979.
33. Taheri, SA, Pendergast, DR, Lazar, E, et al: Vein valve transplantation. Am J Surg 150:201, 1985.

34. Dale, WA, Harris, J, and Terry, RB: Polytetrafluoroethylene reconstruction of the inferior vena cava. Surgery 95:625, 1984.
35. Gloviczki, P, Hollier, LH, Dewanjee, MK, et al: Experimental replacement of the inferior vena cava: factors affecting patency. Surgery 95:657, 1984.
36. Gloviczki, P, and Pairolero, PC: Venous reconstruction for obstruction and valvular incompetence. In Goldstone, J (ed): Perspectives in Vascular Surgery. Quality Medical Publishing, St. Louis, 1988.
37. Doty, DB: Bypass of superior vena cava: Six years' experience with spiral vein graft for obstruction of superior vena cava due to benign and malignant disease. J Thorac Cardiovasc Surg 83:326, 1982.
38. Palma, EC and Esperón, R: Vein transplants and grafts in the surgical treatment of the postphlebitic syndrome. J Cardiovasc Surg 1:94, 1960.
39. Dale, WA: Management of Vascular Surgical Problems. McGraw-Hill, New York, 1985.
40. Husni, EA: Reconstruction of veins: The need for objectivity. J Cardiovasc Surg 24:525, 1983.
41. Johnson, ND, Queral, LA, Flinn, WR, et al: Late objective assessment of venous valve surgery. Arch Surg 116:1461, 1981.
42. Barker, NW, Hygaard, KK, Walters, W, et al: A statistical study of postoperative venous thrombosis and pulmonary embolism. IV. Location of thrombosis: relation of thrombosis and embolism. Proc Staff Meet Mayo Clin 16:33, 1941.
43. Gloviczki, P, Kazmier, FJ, and Hollier, LH: Axillary-subclavian venous occlusion: The morbidity of a nonlethal disease. J Vasc Surg 4:333, 1986.
44. Lokich, JJ and Becker, B: Subclavian vein thrombosis in patients treated with infusion chemotherapy for advanced malignancy. Cancer 52:1586, 1983.
45. Sotturai, VS: Surgical management of post-phlebitic syndrome. J Vasc Surg (in press).

PART 3

Pulmonary Vascular Disorders

CHAPTER 7

Acute Pulmonary Embolism

Jay H. Ryu, M.D.
Edward C. Rosenow, III, M.D.

The diagnosis of acute pulmonary embolism remains one of the most challenging diagnostic dilemmas the clinician faces. There are no typical or characteristic historical, physical, or routine laboratory findings in pulmonary embolism (PE). Thus, the clinical diagnosis of this disorder is inaccurate. There is more than a 50% chance that the high-risk patient with acute onset of pleuritic chest pain and dyspnea has *not* had an acute embolic episode to the lungs.[1,2] It is a potentially fatal disorder that is often misdiagnosed. A high degree of alertness and suspicion along with an appropriate use of objective testing methods are required to avoid this problem.

The true incidence of PE is unknown. Dalen and Alpert[3] estimated that more than one-half million people per year in this country suffer acute PE, with approximately 10% (13,000) dying within 1 hour of the event. Many are recovering from elective surgery, orthopedic procedures, or uncomplicated myocardial infarction, or are in the postpartum period, only to die from the consequences of PE.

Of the several hundred thousand persons who survive a PE for more than 1 hour, two-thirds are estimated to go undiagnosed and one-third of this undiagnosed, untreated group will die. Thus, there may be between 50,000 and 100,000 preventable deaths from pulmonary embolism every year in this country. Despite these staggering estimates, the overall evidence points to an increasing incidence of the disorder for several reasons: an increasing number of extensive surgical procedures, particularly in older people; an increase in the older population; prolongation of the life of the patient with inoperable malignancy; and greater use of oral contraceptives.

Over 95% of PEs are thrombi that originate in the deep veins of the thigh and pelvis. Deep venous thrombi of the upper extremities, right-sided cardiac chambers, and renal veins can occasionally be the source of thromboemboli as well. Other possible sources of embolic material can be air, fat, amniotic fluid, and tumor. These usually occur under readily identifiable circumstances with the exception of tumor emboli, which may present insidiously or acutely even in patients with no prior history of cancer.

DEEP VENOUS THROMBOSIS

Pulmonary embolism is not a disease but a complication of deep venous thrombosis. Deep venous thrombosis (DVT) involving the lower extremities occurs commonly but is frequently misdiagnosed on the basis of history and physical examination alone, both of which are insensitive and nonspecific in the diagnosis of DVT.[4,5] Approximately half of the patients with clinical signs compatible with venous thrombosis have normal venograms, that is, false-positive physical findings.[6,7] In addition, most venous thrombi are clinically unsuspected.

It is estimated that approximately 50% of deep venous thrombi in the iliofemoral venous system will embolize if untreated.[2] Calf vein thromboses are thought to embolize rarely, but this remains controversial.[8,9] However, it should be realized that 5% to 20% of patients with calf vein thrombosis will have subsequent clot propagation to the deep veins of the thigh and pelvis, which then do constitute a source for PEs.[10]

It is essential for proper management to corroborate the clinical impression of DVT with objective tests. A number of different diagnostic tests are available to aid in the diagnosis of DVT. Each has its advantages and disadvantages, and no one test will be best for all circumstances. A thorough discussion of these testing methods is included elsewhere in this volume. The favored noninvasive diagnostic tests are impedance plethysmography (IPG) and duplex ultrasonography. Venography remains the reference standard in the diagnosis of DVT.

CLINICAL FEATURES OF PULMONARY EMBOLISM

Pulmonary embolism most commonly presents in an acute manner. However, one should also beware of its chronic and insidious presentation. In addition, there may be a significant number of patients who present either with none of the usual symptoms or with atypical features, who may go undiagnosed or eventually diagnosed on procedures performed for unrelated reasons or only at autopsy.

Of the three acute varieties of presentation, the acute onset of dyspnea with or without chest pain and an abnormal chest roentgenogram is the most common (see Table 7–1).[11] The same acute onset of symptoms with a normal chest roentgenogram occurs in about 15% to 20% of cases. The third presentation is that of acute cor pulmonale occurring in massive embolism, that is, more than 40% of the vascular system occluded. It is not uncommon for a patient to exhibit sequentially two or all three of these presentations with the occurrence of subsequent emboli over a period of hours or days.

The fourth variety of presentation of pulmonary emboli is the occurrence of repeated small emboli over a period of weeks and months until enough vascular occlusion has occurred for pulmonary hypertension to develop. It is very unusual

Table 7–1. Possible Presentations of Pulmonary Emboli

1. Acute onset of symptoms with normal chest radiograph
2. Acute onset of symptoms with abnormal chest radiograph
3. Acute cor pulmonale with dyspnea, anginoid chest pain, and normal or abnormal chest radiograph
4. Insidious onset of dyspnea over months with normal or abnormal chest radiograph
5. No symptoms or atypical symptoms

for this to occur as a result of acute pulmonary embolism that has been appropriately treated.

Atypical presenting features may include fever, syncope, confusion, coma, wheezing, arrhythmias, and others. We have also encountered patients who have presented with chest roentgenographic abnormalities in the absence of symptoms.

A thromboembolus is a thrombus that has migrated downstream to a new location and consists of a mesh of fibrin, red blood cells, and platelets, which coat the surface of the thrombus. The sequelae of a pulmonary embolus relate to both the degree of mechanical obstruction and to the degranulation of platelets on the surface of the thrombi with the release of a number of vasoactive and bronchoactive substances. The reactions to these mediators probably account for many of the nonspecific signs and symptoms of pulmonary emboli.

There are three factors that tend to predict the cardiovascular response to a pulmonary embolus: (1) the extent of the mechanical obstruction, (2) the degree of smooth muscle constriction of the pulmonary arteries and arterioles, and (3) the presence or absence of underlying cardiopulmonary disease. In normal individuals, it is not possible for the mean pulmonary artery pressure to exceed 40 mm Hg because the normal right ventricle cannot generate greater pressures even if massive embolism has recently occurred. Thus, if the pulmonary artery pressure is above 40 mm Hg at the time of embolization, pre-existing cardiopulmonary disease likely is present.

Cardiovascular collapse rarely occurs with less than 40% obstruction (submassive), unless there is underlying cardiopulmonary disease or another coexisting process is present. Systemic hypotension occurs in fewer than 20% of patients with acute pulmonary embolism.

Bronchoconstriction occurs in most patients with PE, but it is limited to the small peripheral airways which are perfused only by the pulmonary artery that is occluded by the embolus. This peripheral airway constriction contributes to an appreciable loss of lung volume (pneumoconstriction), producing one of the more common findings on the chest roentgenogram in pulmonary embolism—an elevated hemidiaphragm. Untreated, this peripheral airway bronchoconstriction persists for 24 to 48 hours, but it can be blocked or quickly reversed with heparin.

Pulmonary infarction, the necrosis of lung tissue from a lack of blood supply, occurs in fewer than 5% of patients with pulmonary emboli. A pulmonary infiltrate or pleural effusion with an embolus is not synonymous with pulmonary infarction. Infarction is more likely to occur with smaller, subsegmentally located emboli than with larger, more proximal ones. A pulmonary infiltrate consisting of either hemorrhage or edema, or both, occurs in about one-half of the patients with pulmonary emboli in the absence of infarction. An infarction may take weeks or months to clear, whereas noninfarction infiltration clears usually in less than 1 week.

Dyspnea and chest pain, acute in onset and frequently pleuritic, are the most common symptoms of acute pulmonary embolism.[12,13] Less common symptoms include apprehension, cough, sweats, and syncope. Hemoptysis is present in 20% to 30% of patients and is not necessarily related to the occurrence of infarction.

A relative increase in the respiratory rate (tachypnea) occurs in almost all patients with pulmonary embolism, probably on the basis of mediator stimulation of lung receptors. Tachycardia or rales over an area of infarction or infiltration are less common. Fever is present in approximately half of the patients and may rise as high as 40°C; chills are uncommon. An increase in the intensity of the pulmonic component of the second sound occurs not uncommonly, depending on the pulmonary artery pressure, but is a very subjective finding and of little relative value. A right ventricular S_3 gallop is heard in most patients with acute cor pulmonale.

The electrocardiogram is abnormal in up to 85% of patients with acute pulmonary embolism, but the changes tend to be nonspecific and generally transient.[14] The classic S_1, Q_3, T_3 pattern is observed in approximately 10% of patients. The two most common abnormalities are QRS changes and ST-segment and T-wave changes, each occurring in about half of the patients. Except for sinus tachycardia, arrhythmias are relatively uncommon and when present are usually atrial in origin. Pulmonary embolism always should be suspected as a potential cause in anyone with electromechanical dissociation.

The chest roentgenogram is read as normal in 20% to 30% of patients with pulmonary embolism, but once the diagnosis is confirmed, it is not difficult in retrospect to identify changes that are thought by some to be typical of pulmonary embolism, particularly when they occur acutely.[1,15,16] However, the usual abnormalities are generally so nonspecific that they rarely lead to the suggestion of the correct diagnosis.

In order to appreciate some of the subtle changes that may be present on a chest radiograph, the current radiography must be compared with a recent pre-embolism radiograph, if available. One of the more common abnormalities observed on a chest radiograph is an elevated hemidiaphragm, which occurs in up to one half. But this, like many other findings mentioned up to this point, is not diagnostic. However, it may strengthen the suspicion enough to pursue further studies. Platelike atelectasis may occur above this elevated hemidiaphragm or in the absence of this elevation.

A parenchymal infiltrate is found in nearly half of those with PE, but in fewer than 5% of these does this represent true infarction. An infarction that takes the form of a pyramidally shaped infiltrate with the peak directed toward the hilus (Hampton's hump) is very uncommon. Otherwise, the appearance of an infarct is nonspecific and may mimic a neoplasm.

Pleural effusions are found in nearly one-third of the patients with PE, but more may be detected if decubitus views are obtained on all patients with proven pulmonary embolism.[17] The pleural effusion is bilateral in fewer than 10% and rarely massive. The effusion is bloody in the majority of cases when it is associated with infarction and less commonly so when there is no infarction. There are no diagnostic studies of value on this fluid; rarely, a false-positive cytology occurs in an effusion associated with infarction. The fluid is usually an exudate. Pulmonary embolism should be suspected when a patient has a pleural effusion that spontaneously clears, especially a bloody effusion.

Enlargement of the pulmonary artery may occur as a result of an embolus. The enlargement is not necessarily due to pulmonary hypertension; it may be due to the actual thrombus. An increased radiolucency due to decreased vascular filling, referred to as oligemia or Westermark's sign, is a common finding, but it is often a retrospective observation, particularly when comparison is made with a pre-embolism radiograph.

The assessment of the partial pressure of arterial oxygen (Pao_2) is unfortunately of little value in the diagnosis of pulmonary embolism; hypoxemia is nonspecific. And a normal Pao_2 (80 mm Hg or greater at sea level) is found in up to 15% of patients with pulmonary embolism. The alveolar-arterial Po_2 [$P(A - a)o_2$]

gradient may be more useful as a screening test than the Pao_2 alone. Cvitanic and Marino [18] found a widened $P(A - a)o_2$ gradient in 95%, a low $Paco_2$ (<36 mm Hg) in 74%, a low Pao_2 in 76%, and widened $P (A - a)o_2$ gradient *or* a low $Paco_2$ in 98% of patients with an acute PE. Thus, only 2% of patients with acute PE had a normal $P(A - a)o_2$ gradient and normal $Paco_2$ breathing room air.

At this point, it should be apparent that symptoms and signs are not adequately sensitive nor specific in the diagnosis of PE in suspected patients. Screening laboratory test results are also unlikely to be helpful. In some of these patients, careful clinical evaluation may allow a diagnosis other than PE. In many other patients, further objective testing is necessary to document the presence or absence of DVT or PE.

LUNG SCAN

Ventilation-perfusion lung scan is frequently used as the sole determinant of whether or not PE has occurred. However, it must be remembered that an abnormal lung scan is nonspecific in the diagnosis of acute PE, but a normal six- or eight-view perfusion scan virtually rules out the possibility of PE, providing it has been done within 48 to 72 hours of the event. The lung scan should be interpreted by an experienced reader who has available all the pertinent facts related to the patient, including the chest radiograph.

Although a normal perfusion scan virtually excludes the diagnosis of acute PE, it does not eliminate the possibility of DVT.[2] As always, if the results of a test do not fit the clinical situation, further studies should be considered. If a lung scan is not normal, then it is interpreted as either high, indeterminate, or low probability for PE. There is considerable controversy regarding the accuracy of these separate categories. For example, the incidence of angiographic-proven PE ranges form 12% to 40% with a "low probability" scan.[2,19-22] This variability in predictive value appears to result from difference in patient population studied and types of lung scan abnormalities included in this category.

The principle of perfusion lung scanning is based on trapping radioactively tagged particulate matter in the pulmonary capillary bed. Macroaggregates of albumin or albumin microspheres labeled with technetium 99m are injected into a peripheral vein and imaged with a γ-camera. A radioactive inert gas such as xenon 133 is used in a ventilation scan. The procedure is performed by having the patient take an initial first breath followed by rebreathing to equilibrium through a closed system; then the washout of the radioactive material from the lungs is monitored for 3 to 5 minutes. A normal ventilation scan will show a uniform distribution of radioactive gas in the first breath and equilibrium views with a uniform washout from the lung fields. The most common cause of an abnormal ventilation scan is chronic obstructive pulmonary disease.

There are several ways of performing ventilation-perfusion scans. In some institutions the perfusion scan is done first, and, if it is normal, no further studies are done. If it is abnormal, a ventilation scan is immediately performed. However, others prefer to begin with the ventilation scan inasmuch as there is background radioactivity if the [^{99m}Tc] albumin perfusion scan is done first.

As with so many features already discussed in regard to the diagnosis of pulmonary embolism, the major limiting factor in ventilation-perfusion lung scans is the nonsepcificity of the findings. To compound the problem even further, in nearly one third of the cases in the urokinase-streptokinase pulmonary embolism trial (USPET),[23] three experts could not agree on the interpretation of the extent of perfusion defects. This appeared to be less of a problem in the recent major study, Prospective Investigation of Pulmonary Embolism Diagnosis (PIOPED).[21]

Many different clinical conditions, such as pulmonary infiltrates of any kind, obstructive lung disease, and centrally located lung tumors, may cause perfusion abnormalities. Approximately 5% of the normal population have an abnormal ventilation-perfusion (non–high-probability) scan.

If the perfusion scan is abnormal, the sizes and numbers of defects are assessed and compared with the ventilation scan and chest radiograph. A "high-probability" scan result will prove to be pulmonary embolism by pulmonary angiogram in 85% to 90% of cases.[19,21] In general, this category includes one or more segmental (or greater) perfusion defects with no corresponding ventilation or chest roentgenogram abnormalities ("mismatch") or multiple moderate segmental (25% to 75% of a segment) or larger perfusion defects with no corresponding ventilation or roentgenographic abnormalities or substantially larger than either matching ventilation or roentgenographic abnormalities.

The finding of a high-probability lung scan is usually sufficient to make a diagnosis of acute pulmonary embolism, providing the clinical situation fits, that is, a high prior clinical probability. Angiography will confirm pulmonary emboli in 96% of these patients.[19,21] However, the recent PIOPED[21] study showed that only 41% of patients with angiographically proven PE had high-probability scans. Thus, the sensitivity of a high-probability lung scan in PE is relatively low, inasmuch as the majority of patients with PE will have non–high-probability scans. A high-probability scan in a patient with a previous history of PE is less useful inasmuch as only three-fourths of these patients will have pulmonary emboli on angiography.[21]

In patients suspected of having PE with lung scan results that do not belong in either the normal or high-probability category, further testing is required. A possible exception may be a patient with a low-probability scan who has a low prior clinical probability for PE. The chance of pulmonary angiogram showing PE in this group was 4% on the PIOPED study.[21]

Lung scans should be performed as soon as possible in the course of the workup of a suspected pulmonary embolus, preferably within 48 hours, because the intrinsic fibrinolytic system will reduce the size of the thrombus. As the thrombus shrinks, the perfusion defects will get smaller with time. Even when pulmonary angiography is contemplated, a properly performed perfusion scan can be used to guide the angiographer to the specific areas of abnormality.

PULMONARY ANGIOGRAPHY

Pulmonary angiogrpahy is the reference standard, but it is by no means a perfect test. As with lung scans, it should be done within 24 to 48 hours of the suspected embolism; otherwise, resolution of the thrombi may make interpretation of the angiogram erroneous. A pulmonary angiogram that is positive for emboli shows either intraluminal filling defects or cutoffs of pulmonary arteries or both. Asymmetry of blood flow and oligemia are suspicious but not diagnostic findings, inasmuch as these changes can occur with other conditions. The results of the angiogram are indeterminate in 3% to 15% of patients.[19,21] A preceding perfusion scan might allow the angiographer to narrow the area of investigation. A negative pulmonary arteriogram appears to eliminate the possibility of pulmonary embolism.

However, one may question the sensitivity of pulmonary angiogram inasmuch as up to 18% to 30% of suspected PE patients with a negative pulmonary angiogram have proximal DVT detected by IPG or venogram.[2,19]

The mortality with the procedure is approximately 0.2% and the morbidity is around 4%;[21,24] allergy to the contrast media is a contraindication to the procedure, but the use of the new nonionic contrast media should be considered. Relative contraindications include left bundle branch block (because the procedure may cause right bundle branch block and thus complete heart block), ventricular irritability, renal insufficiency, and severe pulmonary hypertension.

Cine computerized tomography, digital subtraction angiography, and magnetic resonance may detect central, large thromboemboli but are not yet sophisticated enough to give the resolution necessary for detecting peripheral pulmonary emboli. Angioscopy may have a role in certain clinical situations but it is not widely available.[25]

We recommend considering a pulmonary angiogram in the following situations: (1) when the ventilation-perfusion lung scan is of low or indeterminate probability and the clinical picture is moderate to highly suspicious for PE; (2) when there is suspected PE in the presence of significant parenchymal lung disease, making a ventilation-perfusion lung scan difficult to interpret; (3) when there is probable PE by ventilation-perfusion lung scan (high-probability scan) but a low prior clinical suspicion or a high risk for the use of anticoagulants; (4) when there is a past history of unconfirmed "recurrent pulmonary emboli," especially if the events occur while on anticoagulants; and (5) when massive PE and/or hemodynamic instability occurs and the use of fibrinolytic therapy, pulmonary embolectomy, or inferior vena caval interruption is contemplated. In summary, if there is uncertainty about whether or not PE has occurred in the last 72 hours, it is best to proceed with pulmonary angiography. In some of the aforementioned situations, confirmed diagnosis of DVT by objective testing of the lower extremity veins may make pulmonary angiogram unnecessary.

DIAGNOSIS

In patients suspected of PE, there are several diagnostic pathways available. In patients who are hemodynamically unstable and suspected of having massive embolism, a pulmonary angiogram should be performed. This would provide the quickest route to a definitive diagnosis. It would also facilitate the use of fibrinolytic agents, IVC interruption, or pulmonary embolectomy if the situation warrants. If the pulmonary angiogram is negative, evaluation of veins of the lower extremities should be considered.

In most other patients who are suspect for PE after the initial clinical evaluation, noninvasive evaluation of the deep veins of the lower extremities (IPG or duplex ultrasonography) or lung scan can be undertaken. Although a positive IPG or ultrasonography does not prove the presence of pulmonary emboli, it does provide an endpoint to treat, that is, DVT. If the results of IPG or ultrasonography are equivocal, the diagnosis of DVT could be pursued further with a venogram.

If the perfusion lung scan is normal, the diagnosis of PE is virtually excluded. However, in some cases, evaluation of the lower extremities may be required to further settle any doubt about the presence or absence of venous thromboembolism. If the ventilation-perfusion lung scan is abnormal and shows a high-probability result in a patient highly suspected (high prior clinical probability) of PE, the diagnosis of PE is likely secure and anticoagulant treatment can proceed. It may be prudent to undertake pulmonary angiography to confirm the presence of PE in a patient at high hemorrhagic risk from anticoagulant treatment. Conversely, with a low-probability scan in a patient with low prior clinical probability, the presence of PE is very unlikely and no further investigations may be necessary.

In the remaining patients in whom neither the lung scan nor the noninvasive evaluation of the lower extremities has adequately resolved the clinical dilemma, for example, a patient with an indeterminate lung scan and no evidence of DVT, a pulmonary angiogram should be performed to document the presence or absence of PE. The chance of PE in these patients is neither high nor low enough to adequately rule in or out the possibility of PE without an angiogram. This also applies to patients in whom the degree of clinical suspicion for PE and the lung scan results are disparate, for example, a patient with a low prior clinical probability but a high-probability scan, or vice versa, who does not have evidence of DVT on objective testing. Although the clinical diagnosis of venous thromboembolism is inaccurate, the clinical impression as to the likelihood of PE in a suspected patient can be coupled with lung scan findings in determining the predictive value as to the absence or presence of PE and the need for further testing.

TREATMENT

The objectives in treating acute pulmonary embolism are to prevent death from the acute event or recurrence and to reduce morbidity including pulmonary hypertension and postphlebitic syndrome. Patients who are diagnosed or highly suspected of acute PE should be immediately treated with intravenous heparin (in the absence of high hemorrhagic risk factors). In patients with highly suspected PE, treatment can be initiated while continuing the diagnostic investigation, which usually takes 2 to 6 hours; if venous thromboembolism is excluded, heparin therapy is discontinued. The treatment for PE requires higher doses of heparin during the first 24 hours than during the later phase. We recommend 5000 to 15000 U to be given by immediate IV bolus followed by a constant infusion of 1500 to 3000 U/h for the first 24 hours and then a maintenance infusion of 1000 to 1500 U/h. Activated partial thromboplastin time (APTT) should be checked two to four times during the first 24 hours, and it should be scheduled once or twice a day thereafter. The optimal therapeutic range of APTT on heparin therapy is 1.5 to 2.0 times the control value.[26] Heparin has been shown to reduce the mortality rate in pulmonary embolism. Complications of acute heparin therapy include hemorrhage and heparin-induced thrombocytopenia. The risk of recurrent thromboembolic events is significantly increased if an APTT of 1.5 times or greater than the control value is not achieved during the first 24 hours.[27] Heparin also can be given by intermittent IV injection or subcutaneous injection. If anticoagulation is absolutely contraindicated, a vena caval filter should be inserted in a patient with proven venous thromboembolism.

The optimal duration of initial IV heparin therapy in acute pulmonary embolism is not clearly known. The traditional approach advocates 7 to 10 days of heparin therapy with oral anticoagulants started after 4 or 5 days. This would provide an overlap on both drugs for 4 or 5 days. Recent studies of patients with submassive pulmonary embolism suggest that initiation of warfarin therapy on the same day or the day after starting heparin therapy is equally effective, with decreased hospitalization time and costs.[28]

Long-term anticoagulant therapy should be maintained for approximately 3 to 6 months after the first episode of venous thromboembolism, at least a year after a second episode, and indefinitely if three or more episodes occur.[26,29] Patients with irreversible risk factors such as antithrombin III or protein C or S deficiency also should continue anticoagulant therapy indefinitely. Warfarin is most commonly used for long-term anticoagulation. The optimal therapeutic range for prothrombin time on warfarin therapy for venous thromboembolism is 1.3 to 1.5 times the control or pretreatment value (North American Thromboplastin).[26,29] The adjusted-dose subcutaneous heparin given twice daily is the treatment of choice in pregnant patients in whom warfarin therapy is contraindicated.

Thrombolytic therapy with agents such a streptokinase, urokinase, and tissue plasminogen activator may be useful in patients with acute massive embolism who are hemodynamically unstable or have extensive ileofemoral venous thrombosis.[26,29] Although these agents appear to cause more rapid lysis of clots, reduction in mortality due to pulmonary embolism has not been shown. Given the higher risk of bleeding complications with thrombolytic therapy compared with heparin therapy, the use of thrombolytic agents should be individualized.

Interruption of the inferior vena cava should be considered in the following instances: (1) when there is a failure of heparin therapy; (2) if there is a contraindication to anticoagulant therapy; (3) in cases of recurrent thromboembolic events despite adequate anticoagulant therapy; (4) in patients with chronic thromboembolic hypertension; (5) with acute massive embolism; and (6) following pulmonary embolectomy. The Greenfield, Mobin-Uddin, and bird's nest filters are the devices most commonly used, and they are inserted percutaneously. Surgical ligation or plication can be employed in special situations.

Pulmonary embolectomy for acute pulmonary embolism is now rarely performed in this country. The mortality rate associated with this procedure varies from 30% to 70%.[30,31] However, pulmonary thromboendarterectomy has been effective in treating certain patients with chronic thromboembolic hypertension.[32]

Last, one needs to remember that the best treatment for acute PE is the prevention of DVT. Prophylactic regimens used to prevent DVT and PE include leg elevation, early ambulation, graduated compression stockings, intermittent pneumatic compression, low-dose heparin (with or without dihydroergotamine), adjusted-dose heparin, aspirin, dextran, oral anticoagulants, and combined modalities.[26,33,34] The optimal prophylactic regimen for an individual patient is chosen by estimating the degree of risk (low, moderate, or high) for developing venous thromboembolism based on the patient's disease and other clinical risk factors, versus the risk of serious bleeding complications in the given clinical setting.

REFERENCES

1. Urokinase Pulmonary Embolism Trial. A National Cooperative Study. Circulation 47 (Suppl 2):1, 1973.
2. Hull, RD, Hirsh, J, Carter, CJ, et al: Pulmonary angiography, ventilation lung scanning, and venography for clinically suspected pulmonary embolism with abnormal perfusion lung scan. Ann Intern Med 98:891, 1983.
3. Dalen, JE and Alpert, JS: Natural history of pulmonary embolism. Prog Cardiovasc Dis 17:259, 1975.
4. Hirsh, J: Diagnosis of venous thrombosis and pulmonary embolism. Am J Cardiol 65:45C, 1990.
5. Wheeler, HB and Anderson, FA, Jr: Diagnostic approaches for deep vein thrombosis. Chest 89(Suppl):407S, 1986.

6. Johnson, WC: Evaluation of newer techniques for the diagnosis of venous thrombosis. J Surg Res 16:473, 1974.
7. Sigel, B, Felix, R, Jr, Popky, GL, et al: Diagnosis of lower limb venous thrombosis by Doppler ultrasound technique. Arch Surg 104:174, 1972.
8. Moser, KM and LeMoine, JR: Is embolic risk conditioned by location of deep venous thrombosis? Ann Intern Med 94(part 1):439, 1981.
9. Mohr, DN, Ryu, JH, Litin, SC, et al: Recent advances in the management of venous thromboembolism. Mayo Clin Proc 63:281, 1988.
10. Kakkar, VV, Flanc, C, Howe, CT, et al: Natural history of postoperative deep vein thrombosis. Lancet 2:230, 1969.
11. Rosenow, EC, III, Osmundson, PJ, and Brown, ML: Pulmonary embolism. Mayo Clin Proc 56:161, 1981.
12. Moser, KM: Pulmonary embolism. Am Rev Respir Dis 115:829, 1977.
13. Bell, WR, Simon, TL, and DeMets, DL: The clinical features of submassive and massive pulmonary emboli. Am J Med 62:355, 1977.
14. Stein, PD, Dalen, JE, McIntyre, KM, et al: The electrocardiogram in acute pulmonary embolism. Prog Cardiovasc Dis 17:247, 1975.
15. Simon, M: Plain film and angiographic aspects of pulmonary embolism. In Moser, KM and Stein, M (eds): Pulmonary Embolism. Year Book Medical Publishers, Chicago, 1973.
16. Talbot, S, Worthington, BS, and Roebuck, EJ: Radiographic signs of pulmonary embolism and pulmonary infarction. Throax 28:198, 1973.
17. Bynum, LJ and Wilson, JE, III: Radiographic features of pleural effusions in pulmonary embolism. Am Rev Respir Dis 117:829, 1978.
18. Cvitanic, O and Marino, PL: Improved use of arterial blood gas analysis in suspected pulmonary embolism. Chest 95:48, 1989.
19. Hull, RD, Hirsh, J, Carter, CJ, et al: Diagnostic value of ventilation-perfusion lung scanning in patients with suspected pulmonary embolism. Chest 86:819, 1985.
20. Biello, DR: Radiological (scintigraphic) evaluation of patients with suspected pulmonary embolism. JAMA 257:3257, 1987.
21. The PIOPED Investigators: Value of the ventilation/perfusion scan in acute pulmonary embolism: Results of the Prospective Investigation of Pulmonary Embolism Diagnosis (PIOPED). JAMA 263:2753, 1990.
22. Webber, MM, Gomes, AS, Roe D, et al: Comparison of Biello, McNeil, and PIOPED criteria for the diagnosis of pulmonary emboli on lung scans. AJR 154:975, 1990.
23. Urokinase-Streptokinase Embolism Trial: Phase 2 results. JAMA 229:1606, 1974.
24. Mills, SR, Jackson, DC, Older, RA, et al: The incidence, etiologies, and avoidance of complications of pulmonary angiography in a large series. Radiology 136:295, 1980.
25. Shure, D, Gregoratos, G, and Moser, KM: Fiberoptic angioscopy: Role in the diagnosis of chronic pulmonary arterial obstruction. Ann Intern Med 103(part 1):844, 1985.
26. Hyers, TM, Hull, RD, and Weg, JG: Antithrombotic therapy for venous thromboembolic disease. Chest 95(Suppl):37S, 1989.
27. Hull, RD, Raskob, GE, Hirsh, J, et al: Continuous intravenous heparin compared with intermittent subcutaneous heparin in the initial treatment of proximal-vein thrombosis. N Engl J Med 315:1109, 1986.
28. Gallus, A, Jackaman, J, Tillett, J, et al: Safety and efficacy of warfarin started early after submassive venous thrombosis or pulmonary embolism. Lancet 1:1293, 1986.
29. Hirsh, J and Hull, RD: Treatment of venous thromboembolism. Chest 89:426S, 1986.
30. Greenfield, LJ: Vena caval interruption and pulmonary embolectomy. Clin Chest Med 5:495, 1984.
31. Gray, HH, Miller, GAH, and Paneth, M. Pulmonary embolectomy: Its place in the management of pulmonary embolism. Lancet 1:1441, 1988.
32. Moser, KM, Daily, PO, Peterson, K, et al: Thromboendarterectomy for chronic, major-vessel thromboembolic pulmonary hypertension: Immediate and long-term results in 42 patients. Ann Intern Med 107:560, 1987.
33. Consensus conference. Prevention of venous thrombosis and pulmonary embolism. JAMA 256:744, 1986.
34. Hull, RD, Raskob, GE, and Hirsh J: Prophylaxis of venous thromboembolism: An overview. Chest 89(Suppl):374S, 1986.

CHAPTER 8

Pulmonary Vascular Disease: Primary Pulmonary Hypertension

Robert G. Tancredi, M.D.

Primary pulmonary hypertension is a clinical syndrome associated with progressive and sustained elevation of pulmonary arterial pressure in association with distinct pathologic changes in the small pulmonary vessels. The cause of primary pulmonary hypertension is not known. Our knowledge of this disorder has not progressed much beyond the descriptive phase. Unfortunately, research in this area is hampered by the fact that this is rarely recognized disease in humans, especially in its early stages, and no suitable animal models have been identified for study.

Pulmonary vascular disease with pulmonary hypertension was first described in an autopsy case report by Romberg[1] in 1891. However, it was 60 years later, following the introduction of cardiac catheterization into clinical practice, that Dresdale[2] and associates were able to report the first group of patients with unexplained pulmonary hypertension. Wood[3] added to the clinical description of the disorder and speculated as to the possible role of vasoconstriction as a causative factor. Some features in the pathologic description are consistent with this hypothesis. Also, a report from Europe[4] documenting pulmonary hypertension in patients using the drug aminorex, an appetite suppressant with sympathomimetic properties, further supported a role for vasoconstriction. However, in some patients, pathologic studies suggested a possible role for microthromboembolism, and anticoagulant therapy seemed to have a beneficial effect.[5]

Despite intense interest in the pathogenesis of this disorder, none of the larger medical centers had encountered sufficient numbers of patients with primary pulmonary hypertension to conduct meaningful studies. For this reason, the National Heart, Lung, and Blood Institute (NHLBI) in 1981 started a registry for patients with primary pulmonary hypertension[6] in order to help characterize the clinical features of the disorder along with its natural history and long-term survival. Over 51 months, 32 medical centers entered 187 patients into the registry. This was the largest group of patients ever reported and the first group studied prospectively rather than retrospectively. From this and other studies, the clinical picture for primary pulmonary hypertension has been well characterized. Although symptoms

113

are vague and insidious at onset, dyspnea and decreased exercise capacity are generally the limiting symptoms at the time of diagnosis. Right ventricular failure is common in the later stages of the disease, and death usually occurs within 5 years of the time of diagnosis.

PATHOGENESIS

The basic cause of primary pulmonary hypertension is not known. It would appear that the syndrome of primary pulmonary hypertension represents the end-stage clinical expression of a number of different histopathologic entities. In most instances, the disease process is confined to the small muscular pulmonary arteries, with sparing of the lung parenchyma. Pathologic studies from patients dying of primary pulmonary hypertension have demonstrated three distinct histologic pictures, namely, plexogenic pulmonary arteriopathy, thrombotic pulmonary arteriopathy, and pulmonary veno-occlusive disease.[7] Although these histologic subtypes are characteristic of primary pulmonary hypertension, they are not pathognomonic of the disorder. For example, some patients with congenital heart disease associated with left-to-right shunts at the level of the ventricles or great vessels (e.g., ventricular septal defect, patent ductus arteriosus, aortopulmonary window) may develop plexiform lesions in association with sustained pulmonary hypertension.[8] Similar lesions have been seen in some patients with cirrhosis,[9] collagen vascular disease,[10] or aminorex ingestion. These different pathologic features found in association with primary pulmonary hypertension have raised speculation as to whether they are different responses to the same causative event or whether they represent totally different disease processes.

Pathologic features of plexogenic pulmonary arteriopathy are well described. Early lesions in small muscular arteries begin with medial hypertrophy and intimal thickening, which progress to fibroelastosis, usually concentric and laminar, with marked intimal proliferation. This ultimately becomes obstructive and nearly obliterative at the small vessel level. These early developmental pathologic changes support the hypothesis that elevated pulmonary artery pressure results from intense pulmonary vasoconstriction. In advanced disease, one finds complex plexiform lesions associated with multichannel aneurysmal dilatations in small vessels.

Rich[11] has emphasized that the vasoconstrictor response to various stimuli in the pulmonary arterial bed is quite heterogenous and may be modified by an inherent susceptibility to such agents. This may explain why only a small fraction of the population develops pulmonary edema at high altitudes or why some patients with mitral valve stenosis develop markedly elevated pulmonary artery pressures, whereas others with similar valve areas do not. The report of aminorex-induced pulmonary hypertension supported the vasoconstriction hypothesis, but the incidence of pulmonary hypertension was only 1:1000, suggesting an underlying predisposition or susceptibility in affected patients. Studies of the lungs in patients who died of this syndrome demonstrated plexogenic arteriopathy.

Although plexogenic arteriopathy is the most frequent pathologic picture encountered in patients with primary pulmonary hypertension, some patients do not develop plexiform lesions. Instead, one finds evidence suggesting recanalized thrombi in small arteries, manifested as eccentric intimal fibrosis. Although coagulation abnormalities have not been described in primary pulmonary hypertension, it seems likely that in situ thrombosis does occur in small pulmonary vessels. This could be the result of endothelial cell injury with alterations in the platelet-endothelial cell interaction, in which case thrombosis would be a secondary event rather than a primary cause. Of particular interest is a recent pathologic study of patients with familial pulmonary hypertension,[12] in which the full spectrum of plexogenic and thrombotic lesions was found within and among the same families, suggesting that they might be but different expressions of the same disease process. Finally, pulmonary veno-occlusive disease is a rare cause of pulmonary hypertension. In this disorder, one finds venous intimal proliferation and fibrosis with obliteration of some small venous vascular channels and thrombosis with or without recanalization in others. Fewer than a hundred cases have been reported in the literature. Generally, the diagnosis is made at postmortem examination.

Over time, some patients with collagen vascular diseases may develop pulmonary vasculitis with severe pulmonary hypertension. Usually this is associated with interstitial lung disease with obliterative vascular changes and associated hypoxia. Although these findings are not consistent with the diagnosis of primary pulmonary hypertension, there are some patients with collagen vascular disorders who develop elevated pulmonary artery pressures in the absence of pulmonary parenchymal involvement.[13] Also, 29% of the patients in the NHLBI registry study had positive antinuclear antibody tests. Perhaps, in some patients, primary pulmonary hypertension may result from a collagen vascular disease confined to the lungs.[11]

CLINICAL PICTURE

Primary pulmonary hypertension is generally a disease occurring in the third to fourth decade of life, with a mean age in the NHLBI study of 36.4 years. However, it has a broad age span, with 9% of the patients over the age of 60 years at first presentation. The overall female preponderance (1.7:1) was markedly exaggereated in the black population (4.3:1). Familial clustering has been noted in about 5% of the cases. The clinical course of the disease is highly variable. Although the mean survival is reported as 2 to 3 years from the time of diagnosis, some patients are alive 10 years later.

The most common presenting symptom is dyspnea. In retrospect, about 60% of the patients had this symptom in the early stages of the disease, and all patients complained of dyspnea at the time the diagnosis was established. Fatigue was also present in about three out of four patients, and chest pain in about half of them. Generally, by the time the diagnosis is made, patients already have clinical and hemodynamic findings of severe pulmonary hypertension. Because the presenting symptoms are vague and very subjective, one can understand why the patient or the physician might overlook the symptoms or attribute them to deconditioning without pursuing the matter further. Other symptoms at the time of presentation include syncope or near-syncope in about a third of the patients, and frank right ventricular failure in patients with advanced disease.

Dyspnea has been associated with the nearly universal finding of hypoxia in these patients. In the absence of intrinsic heart or pulmonary parenchymal disease, this is most likely related to the decreased cardiac output and marked ventilation-perfusion abnormalities noted in the later stages of the disease. It is generally thought that chest pain represents myocardial ischemia confined to the right ventricle because of the increase in right ventricular pressure and wall stress. The mechanism of syncope with exertion is similar to that encountered in aortic stenosis, namely, the inability to increase cardiac output in response to exercise-induced peripheral vasadilatation. Occasionally, patients may experience syncope at rest. This raises the possibility of an underlying cardiac dysrhythmia. However, cardiac dysrhythmias, either atrial or ventricular, are not generally part of the clinical picture of primary pulmonary hypertension.

Findings on physical examination usually reflect changes in the circulation of the right side of the heart which are secondary to severe pulmonary hypertension. Mean jugular venous pressure may be elevated, and a marked canonlike *a* wave in the jugular venous pulse contour reflects forceful right atrial contraction associated with elevated right ventricular end-diastolic pressure in the presence of intact atrial and ventricular septae. A right ventricular lift in the left parasternal area is often palpable, and occasionally the dilated pulmonary artery may be felt on the surface of the chest wall. The pulmonic component of the second heart sound is markedly accentuated, very narrowly split, and frequently palpable. A right ventricular third heart sound reflects an elevated right ventricular diastolic pressure, and a fourth heart sound is also commonly heard. Tricuspid regurgitation is noted in nearly 50% of these patients, and the systolic regurgitant murmur associated with this is frequently the most remarkable finding on physical examination. Pulmonary insufficiency secondary to sustained elevation in pulmonary artery pressure is less frequently heard. Despite the almost universal finding of arterial hypoxemia, cyanosis is infrequent, being seen in fewer than 20% of the patients. Clubbing is not a feature of primary pulmonary hypertension, and its presence should provoke a search for other pulmonary or cardiac disorders. In advanced stages of the disease, peripheral edema may reflect right ventricular failure.

DIFFERENTIAL DIAGNOSIS

Pulmonary artery pressure will rise passively in response to elevations in pulmonary venous pressure, thereby maintaining the arteriovenous pressure gradient for flow across the lungs. However, sustained pulmonary venous hypertension may cause reactive pulmonary vasoconstriction, which, in time, leads to medial hypertrophy and eccentric intimal proliferation in small muscular pulmonary arterioles. When this occurs, pulmonary artery pressure will rise to levels higher than one might expect from the level of mean left atrial pressure alone. Pulmonary capillaries are spared the effects of this marked rise in pulmonary arterial pressure. Instead, right ventricular dysfunction will develop, eventually leading to right ventricular failure, functional tricuspid regurgitation, and systemic venous congestion with edema, a clinical picture similar to that found in the latest stages of primary pulmonary hypertension.

The causes of pulmonary venous hypertension are listed in Table 8–1. Disorders affecting the pulmonary veins themselves, particularly primary veno-occlusive disease or congenital stenosis, are difficult to diagnosis ante-mortem and are probably considered clinically as patients with primary pulmonary hypertension. Acquired pulmonary venous stenosis might be expected in patients with granulomatous, fibrotic, or neoplastic involvement of the mediastinum who present with pulmonary hypertension. Aside from these rare exceptions, all of the disorders included in Table 8–1 can be diagnosed by history, physical examination, demonstration of an elevated pulmonary capillary wedge pressure by catheterization of the right side of the heart, and echo-Doppler study of the heart and great vessels.

Table 8–1. Causes of Pulmonary Hypertension Secondary to
Elevated Pulmonary Pressure

1. Pulmonary venous obstruction
   a. Primary veno-occlusive disease
   b. Congenital stenosis
   c. Acquired stenosis (granulomatous, fibrotic, or neoplastic disorders of the mediastinum)
2. Left atrial obstruction
   a. Tumor
   b. Blood clot
   c. Cor triatriatum
3. Left ventricular dysfunction
   a. Coronary artery disease
      (1) Acute myocardial infarction
      (2) Ruptured papillary muscle
      (3) Perforation of interventricular septum
      (4) Ventricular aneurysm
      (5) Ischemic dysfunction; fibrosis
   b. Primary nonobstructive cardiomyopathy
      (1) Congestive
      (2) Hypertrophic
      (3) Restrictive
   c. Hypertrophic obstructive cardiomyopathy
4. Aorta
      (1) Supravalvular aortic stenosis
      (2) Coarctation
      (3) Systemic hypertension
5. Valvular disease
   a. Mitral valve stenosis or regurgitation
   b. Aortic valve stenosis or regurgitation

In these diseases, pulmonary hypertension will respond to treatment of the primary underlying disorder, and secondary pathologic changes in small pulmonary arterioles may regress.

Structural or functional disorders of the lung and its circulation can also cause pulmonary hypertension through two mechanisms: (1) pulmonary arteriolar constriction due to hypoxia and acidosis and (2) obstruction and obliteration of small pulmonary vessels.

Chronic hypoxia is probably one of the most potent stimulants for pulmonary vasoconstriction and frequently is the major cause of pulmonary hypertension and cor pulmonale in patients with chronic lung disease (Table 8–2). For example, periodic exacerbations of chronic bronchitis are associated with marked heterogeneities in regional ventilation due to airway obstruction from copious tenacious secretions. Alveolar hypoventilation stimulates pulmonary vasoconstriction in association with hypercapnia and acidosis, leading to pulmonary hypertension. Adequate ventilation and oxygenation with improvement in airway mechanics can ameliorate the pulmonary hypertension associated with this disorder.

In a number of pulmonary disorders such as emphysema and diffuse interstitial pulmonary parenchymal disease, hypoxic vasoconstriction is superimposed on an underlying loss of functioning lung parenchyma and vessels. In these instances, the progression of pulmonary hypertension is related to the gradual obliteration of the vascular bed with constriction in the overall cross-sectional area available to

Table 8-2. Causes of Pulmonary Hypertension Secondary to
Functional or Structural Disorders of the Lung

1. Chronic hypoxia
   a. Upper airway obstruction
   b. Lower airway obstruction
      (1) Chronic bronchitis; bronchiectasis
      (2) Emphysema
      (3) Asthma
   c. Diffuse interstitial pulmonary disease
      (1) Interstitial fibrosis (idiopathic, toxic, pneumoconiosis)
      (2) Granulomatous
      (3) Collagen vascular disease
   d. Altered respiratory movements
      (1) Pickwickian syndrome; sleep apnea syndrome
      (2) Neuromuscular disorders affecting chest wall
      (3) Skeletal deformities of thoracic cage
      (4) Lung resection
   e. Residence at high altitude
2. Thromboembolic disorders
3. Increased pulmonary blood flow (left-to-right shunts)
4. Miscellaneous
      (1) Parasitic disorders (schistosomiasis)
      (2) Chronic liver disease
      (3) Drugs (aminorex) and toxins (rapeseed oil)
      (4) Crotalaria (in experimental animals)

flowing blood. The elevated pulmonary artery pressure encountered in association
with pulmonary emboli also results from the combined effects of hypoxic vasoconstriction and obliteration of vascular channels.

LABORATORY STUDIES IN PRIMARY PULMONARY HYPERTENSION

The electrocardiogram usually shows normal sinus rhythm with very little evidence for underlying atrial or ventricular irritability. This is in contrast to pulmonary hypertension and cor pulmonale associated with chronic lung disease, in
which arrhythmias are very prominent features in the clinical picture. As pulmonary artery pressure becomes elevated, the electrocardiogram shows a shift toward
right axis deviation with evidence for right ventricular hypertrophy and right ventricular strain. Prominent P waves reflect right atrial hypertrophy.

Posteroanterior and lateral roentgenograms of the chest, though not diagnostic
for the disorder, will show findings consistent with significant pulmonary hypertension. The cardiac shadow may be normal and the lung fields themselves will be
normal. The main pulmonary artery and proximal hilar vessels are dilated and
prominent, but the vessels decrease sharply in caliber toward the periphery.

The two-dimensional echo-Doppler study plays an important role in the evaluation of patients with pulmonary hypertension. Careful examination of the left
side of the heart will rule out any significant problems that might contribute to
pulmonary venous hypertension. The left atrial size is normal and the left ventricular internal dimensions in end-diastole are usually normal but may be reduced

owing to decreased volume loading from the low cardiac output. Ventricular septal motion is abnormal, consistent with right ventricular pressure overload. The pulmonary artery is enlarged, and early midsystolic closure of the pulmonary valve is a clue to the presence of pulmonary hypertension. Right ventricular internal dimensions are increased with associated right ventricular hypertrophy. Doppler evidence for pulmonary and tricuspid valve regurgitation may not always be associated with audible murmurs on the chest wall.

Doppler studies have been directed at analysis of the systolic flow velocity profile across the right ventricular outflow tract, evaluation of tricuspid regurgitant flow, and measurement of pulmonary regurgitant velocity in end diastole. These techniques have permitted noninvasive estimation of pulmonary artery and right ventricular systolic pressure. When done simultaneously with direct measurement, the correlation is reasonably good. As these techniques become refined with more experience, they may provide some of the critical tools necessary to detect pulmonary hypertension in its early stages when therapeutic efforts might be more effective. A recent study correlating echo-Doppler measurements with direct cardiac catheterization identified several Doppler-derived parameters that show some relationship to overall survival in patients with primary pulmonary hypertension.[14]

Pulmonary function studies generally show a mild restrictive pattern with decreased lung volumes but no evidence for significant airways obstruction or other parenchymal lung disease. However, despite the absence of significant pulmonary dysfunction, mild to moderate hypoxia is present in most patients with primary pulmonary hypertension. This has been attributed to ventilation-perfusion mismatches throughout both lungs. Also, the decreased cardiac output leads to a marked decrease in mixed venous oxygen content. Studies have shown a close correlation between mixed venous oxygen content and systemic arterial oxygen saturation in these patients. However, a marked drop in arterial oxygen saturation might provoke a search for right-to-left shunting through a patent foramen ovale.

Perfusion lung scans may demonstrate diffuse patchy abnormalities in lung perfusion throughout both lungs or may actually show normal perfusion. These perfusion patterns may provide clues to underlying lung pathology.[15] That is, normal perfusion patterns are generally found in patients with plexogenic pulmonary arteriopathy, whereas the patchy diffuse abnormalities suggest thrombotic arteriopathy or, rarely, veno-occlusive disease. Perhaps the most important reason for obtaining a perfusion scan is to rule out the presence of chronic recurrent pulmonary emboli. This distinction is critical and has important implications regarding therapy. If any question is raised in this regard, one should proceed directly to pulmonary angiography.

In the past, clinicians were hesitant to perform angiography or even perfusion scans in patients with primary pulmonary hypertension because of isolated case reports of adverse reactions in response to these tests. However, the experience reported in the NHLBI registry showed that 163 lung perfusion scans were performed without incident, and 50 pulmonary angiograms were obtained with only one episode of transient hypotension. Therefore, in experienced hands, these procedures can be performed safely.

When a patient with primary pulmonary hypertension is encountered for the first time, a complete workup must include cardiac catheterization. There are three major goals of the catheterization study: (1) measure directly the level of pulmonary artery pressure and estimate pulmonary vascular resistance, (2) rule out any left-to-right shunts or other significant cardiac disorders affecting the left side of the heart, and (3) test the response to various therapeutic agents.

When patients with primary pulmonary hypertension first present for complete evaluation, the mean pulmonary artery pressure is usually elevated to as high as three times the normal value, at about 60 mm Hg. Pulmonary vascular resistance will continue to rise over time as the disorder progresses. Because pulmonary artery pressure seems to stabilize at near systemic levels, the increasing pulmonary vascular resistance is reflected in a gradual drop in the cardiac index. This is also associated with a moderate increase in right atrial pressure. Numerous studies have shown that overall survival in this disorder is related to the level of right ventricular dysfunction as reflected through right atrial pressure and overall cardiac index.[16]

Antinuclear antibody titers were positive in about 29% of patients with primary pulmonary hypertension who were registered in the NHLBI study. However, the frequency of Raynaud's phenomenon (encountered primarily in women) was only slightly higher than that noted in the general population.

It is interesting to note that 6% of the patients in the NHLBI registry had normal chest roentgenograms, echocardiograms, and electrocardiograms despite the presence of significant pulmonary hypertension on cardiac catheterization study. This reflects the insensitivity of current methods for detecting this disorder and should encourage efforts to develop newer and better techniques for detecting pulmonary hypertension in its early stages.

TREATMENT OF PRIMARY PULMONARY HYPERTENSION

GENERAL MEASURES

The clinical course of primary pulmonary hypertension, though generally progressive, is quite variable, particularly with regard to the patient's sense of well-being on a day-to-day basis. Although it is difficult to relate this variability to changes in the level of pulmonary artery pressure, we do know that patients with primary pulmonary hypertension may exhibit rapid and severe elevations in pulmonary artery pressure in response to moderate exertion. Therefore, patients should be advised not to engage in strenuous physical activities or sports, especially those associated with isometric exercise or sudden changes in level of activity. On the other hand, modest aerobic activity such as walking or light bicycle riding can be encouraged within the limits of the patient's tolerance.

Primary pulmonary hypertension is often found in young women of childbearing age. Physiologic cardiovascular changes associated with pregnancy, along with the increased risk of deep venous thrombosis and embolism, may hasten the progression of the disease. Therefore, the physician must advise the patient against becoming pregnant, and surgical sterilization might be the best alternative to provide for this.

DRUG THERAPY

Anticoagulants

The role of anticoagulant therapy in the treatment of primary pulmonary hypertension follows from pathologic studies showing thrombosis in smaller muscular arterioles in almost half of the patients with primary pulmonary hypertension. A retrospective study from the Mayo Clinic[5] demonstrated improved survival in patients treated with anticoagulants. In addition, we know that patients with failure of the right side of the heart and systemic venous congestion with peripheral edema are at increased risk for developing deep venous thrombosis and subsequent embolization. Unfortunately, our current state of knowledge regarding primary pulmonary hypertension does not allow us to identify discrete subsets of patients who might be particularly suitable for anticoagulant therapy. For all of these reasons and in the absence of specific contraindications, all patients with primary pulmonary hypertension should be placed on a long-term oral anticoagulant therapy.

Pulmonary Vasodilators

In primary pulmonary hypertension, the major hemodynamic abnormality is the increase in pulmonary vascular resistance. Because this parameter cannot be measured directly, it is expressed (in arbitrary units) as the mean pulmonary artery pressure divided by pulmonary blood flow. Therefore, any pharmacologic intervention that increases pulmonary blood flow and/or decreases mean pulmonary artery pressure will lower pulmonary vascular resistance, presumably through vasodilatation of small pulmonary arterioles. However, in the lung, quantitation of pharmacologic vasodilatation may be complicated by the fact that the number of vascular channels being perfused by blood seems to increase as perfusion pressure is raised.[17] The converse also occurs.

Many different classes of drugs have been studied (Table 8–3) in attempts to achieve measurable hemodynamic and symptomatic improvement in patients with

Table 8–3. Vasodilators Studied in Patients with Primary Pulmonary Hypertension

1. α-Adrenergic blockers
    a. Tolazoline
    b. Phentolamine
    c. Phenoxybenzamine
    d. Prazosin
2. β-Receptor agonists
    a. Isoproterenol
    b. Terbutaline
3. Direct vasodilators
    a. Diazoxide
    b. Nitroprusside
    c. Hydralazine
    d. Isosorbide dinitrate
4. Angiotensin-converting enzyme inhibitor
    Captopril
5. Prostaglandin
    a. Prostaglandin E_1
    b. Prostacyclin
6. Calcium-channel blockers
    a. Diltiazem
    b. Nifedipine
    c. Verapamil
7. Anticholinergic
    Acetylcholine
8. Serotonin blockade
    Ketanserin
9. Oxygen

primary pulmonary hypertension.[18] For each of these agents, one can find reports in the literature demonstrating an improvement in hemodynamics, particularly in the acute testing situation. Unfortunately, the number of patients demonstrating decreases in pulmonary vascular resistance along with improvement in symptoms remains quite small. Such studies are complicated by the fact that, for most agents, vasodilatation is not restricted to the pulmonary vessels, and systemic hypotension and syncope may become significant problems. Also, a beneficial long-term effect, particularly regarding life expectancy, has not been demonstrated conclusively for any of the drugs studied. Our ignorance of the basic underlying pathophysiology of this disorder is highlighted by the fact that we have yet to identify those parameters that might assist a physician in selecting those patients who could expect to achieve some benefit from any particular intervention. Perhaps the disorder is already irreversible and "untreatable" when patients present themselves for medical evaluation. Earlier diagnosis may provide us with a totally new perspective regarding the effectiveness of various therapeutic alternatives. In the meantime, the fact that some patients do seem to improve when treated with dilating agents encourages our continuing efforts to identify the suitable therapeutic regimen for each patient on an individual basis.

Initial testing of pulmonary vasodilating agents must be performed in a hospital setting where pulmonary arterial pressure and systemic blood pressure can be monitored continuously and cardiac output determinations made at appropriate intervals. The principles and hazards of drug testing along with problems associated with data interpretation have been well described in a recent review.[11]

Of all the drugs studied in patients with this disorder, the calcium-channel blocking agents appear to show the best promise for providing sustained and symptomatic relief in some patients. However, the dosage required is considerably higher than those generally employed. In a recent study, Rich and Brundage[19] administered high oral doses of nifedipine or diltiazem as long-term treatment and noted sustained reductions in pulmonary arterial pressure and pulmonary vascular resistance over a 1-year follow-up in six patients. Regression of right ventricular hypertrophy was also documented by electrocardiographic and echocardiographic studies. Of interest was the fact that none of the patients experienced side effects requiring cessation of therapy.

Continuous intravenous prostacyclin[20] also has been reported to induce modest hemodynamic improvement that persists for at least 2 months. However, as with all of the vasodilators, long-term benefit in a significant fraction of patients has yet to be demonstrated.

Digitalis

Digitalis may be of value in the treatment of right ventricular failure associated with primary pulmonary hypertension. However, the response is likely to be modest, at best, and one must avoid the temptation to increase the dose to the point at which toxicity becomes a problem.

Diuretics

Diuretics may be helpful in managing the peripheral edema associated with right ventricular failure. However, complete resolution of edema may be difficult to maintain in advanced right ventricular failure of the right side of the heart. One might have to accept the persistence of mild edema in order to avoid the hypotension and electrolyte changes associated with aggressive diuretic therapy.

Oxygen

Although hypoxia-mediated pulmonary vasoconstriction plays an important role in the development of some forms of secondary pulmonary hypertension, it does not appear to be an important causative factor in primary pulmonary hypertension. Nevertheless, the fact that many patients with primary pulmonary hypertension have some arterial hypoxia has prompted the use of supplemental oxygen. To date, there are no published reports demonstrating a sustained objective benefit from the use of continuous supplemental oxygen in these patients, though some patients do experience subjective improvement.

ATRIAL SEPTOSTOMY

Atrial septostomy has been proposed as a palliative procedure for patients with primary pulmonary hypertension.[21] This approach evolved from the observation that patients with Eisenmenger's syndrome (left-to-right shunt with severe pulmonary hypertension) present with clinical and pathologic features similar to patients with primary pulmonary hypertension, but with longer overall survival.[22] Patients with primary pulmonary hypertension and patent foramen ovale may also live longer. This has been attributed to bi-directional shunting across the septal defect, thereby alleviating some of the load on the right ventricle. Reports of patients who have undergone atrial septostomy point out that the modest benefit is achieved at the expense of inducing systemic cyanosis and intermittent syncope.

HEART-LUNG TRANSPLANTATION

At present, heart-lung transplantation is the only procedure that can offer dramatic improvement in life style, sense of well-being, and survival for patients with primary pulmonary hypertension.[23] Although still investigational, this procedure is being performed at many medical centers throughout the world. Donor availability remains a problem, and patients often die before organs become available. Early mortality is related to hemorrhage and infection, but long-term survivors face problems associated with chronic rejection, infections related to immunosuppressive therapy, and coronary atherosclerosis in the grafted heart.

SUMMARY

Clinical and pathologic features of primary pulmonary hypertension have been well characterized, but little is known regarding the underlying cause and pathogenesis. The disorder is usually discovered in its late stage, when pulmonary vascular resistance is already severely compromised and the pathologic changes already well developed. It is not surprising, then, that most attempts at defining effective pharmacologic interventions have been disappointing. Some new approaches are clearly needed.

The past decade has witnessed the rapid growth of molecular techniques in areas applied to the study of the blood vessel wall, blood coagulation, and the platelet–endothelial cell interaction. Platelet-derived growth factors and other macrophage-derived factors may play important roles in the pathogenesis of the early proliferative lesions found in the small pulmonary arterioles. Other vascular-derived mediators may be important determinants in modulating the vasoconstrictor or vasodilator response in small vessels.[24] A recent brief but pertinent review[25] has highlighted some of the new directions being taken. It appears that the right questions are finally being asked, and we now may have the tools to answer them.

REFERENCES

1. Romberg, E: Uver sklerose der lungenarterien. Dtsch Arch Klin Med 48:197, 1891.
2. Dresdale, DT, Schultz, M, and Michtom, RJ: Primary pulmonary hypertension I. Clinical and hemodynamic study. Am J Med 11:686, 1951.
3. Wood, P: Pulmonary hypertension with special reference to the vaso-constrictive factor. Br Heart J 20:557, 1958.
4. Gurtner, HP: Aminorex and pulmonary hypertesion. Cor Vasa 27:160, 1985.
5. Fuster, V, Steele, PM, Edwards, WD, et al: Primary pulmonary hypertension: Natural history and the importance of thrombosis. Circulation 70:580, 1984.
6. Rich, S, Dantzker, DR, Ayres, S, et al: Primary pulmonary hypertension: A national prospective study. Ann Intern Med 107:216, 1987.
7. Hitano, S and Strasser, T (eds): Primary pulmonary hypertension. World Health Organization, Geneva, 1975.
8. Hoffman, JIE, Rudolph, AM, and Heyman, MA: Pulmonary vascular disease with congenital heart lesions: Pathologic features and causes. Circulation 64:873, 1981.
9. McDonnell, PJ, Toye, PA, and Hutchins, GM: Primary pulmonary hypertension and cirrhosis: Are they related? Am Rev Respir Dis 127:437, 1983.
10. Sullivan, WD, Hurst DJ, Harmon CE, et al: A prospective evaluation emphasizing pulmonary involvement in patients with mixed connective disease. Medicine 63:92, 1984.
11. Rich, S: Primary pulmonary hypertension. Progr Cardiovasc Dis 31:205, 1988.
12. Loyd, JE, Atkinson, JB, Pietra GG, et al: Heterogeneity of pathologic lesions in familial primary pulmonary hypertension. Am Rev Respir Dis 138:952, 1988.
13. Salerni, R, Rodnan, GP, Leon, DF, et al: Pulmonary hypertension in the CREST syndrome variant of progressive systemic sclerosis (scleroderma). Arch Intern Med 86:394, 1977.
14. Eysmann, SB, Palevsky, HI, Reichek, N, et al: Two-dimensional and Doppler-echocardiographic and cardiac catheterization correlates of survival in primary pulmonary hypertension. Circulation 80:353, 1989.
15. Rich, S, Pietra, GG, Kieras, K, et al: Primary pulmonary hypertension: Radiographic and scintigraphic patterns of histologic subtypes. Am Intern Med 105:499, 1986.
16. Rich, S, and Levy, PS: Characteristics of surviving and nonsurviving patients with primary pulmonary hypertension. Am J Med 76:573, 1984.
17. Maseri, A, Caldin, P, Howard, P, et al: Determinants of pulmonary vascular volume: Recruitment versus distensibility. Cir Res 31:218, 1972.
18. Weir, EK, Rubin LJ, Ayres, SM, et al: The acute administration of vasodilators in primary pulmonary hypertension. Experience from the National Institute of Health registry on primary pulmonary hypertension. Am Rev Respir Dis 140:1623, 1989.
19. Rich, S, and Brundage, BH: High dose calcium blocking therapy for primary pulmonary hypertension: Evidence for long-term reduction in pulmonary arterial pressure and regression of right ventricular hypertrophy. Circulation 76:135, 1987.
20. Rubin, LJ, Mendozo, J, Hood, M, et al: Treatment of primary pulmonary hypertension with continuous intravenous prostacyclin (epoprostenol): Results of a randomized trial. Am Intern Med 112:485, 1990.
21. Rich, S, and Lam, W: Atrial septostomy as palliative therapy for refractory primary pulmonary hypertension. Am J Cardiol 51:1560, 1983.
22. Rozkovic, A, Montanes, P, and Oakley, CM: Factors that influence the outcome of primary pulmonary hypertension. Br Heart J 55:449, 1986.
23. Jamieson, SW, Stinson, EB, Oyer, PE, et al: Heart-lung transplantation for irreversible pulmonary hypertension. Ann Thorac Surg 38:554, 1984.
24. Lerman, A, Hildebrand, FL, Jr, Margulies, KB, et al: Endothelin: A new cardiovascular regulatory peptide. Mayo Clin Proc 65:1441, 1990.
25. Newman, JH, and Ross, JC: Primary pulmonary hypertension: A look at the future. J Am Coll Cardiol 14:551, 1989.

PART 4

Arterial Disorders

CHAPTER 9

Arteriovenous Communications

P.J. Osmundson, M.D.

There are two basic types of arteriovenous communications: acquired arteriovenous fistulas and congenital arteriovenous malformations. The fundamental pathophysiologic abnormality in each is an abnormal communication between arteries and veins or arterioles and venules without an intervening capillary bed. Despite this simple concept regarding the pathophysiology, the clinical spectrum of arteriovenous communications is extremely broad and depends on the tissues involved, the anatomic location, the contiguous structures, and the magnitude of blood shunted from the arterial to the venous circulation.

ACQUIRED ARTERIOVENOUS FISTULAS

The majority of clinically significant acquired arteriovenous (AV) fistulas involving the extremities are single and the result of trauma. Acquired AV fistulas in the abdomen, pelvis, chest, and neck may also be traumatic in origin, but other causes must be considered. Erosions between an artery and a vein complicating aneurysms is a rare but important example because of the necessity of prompt diagnosis and treatment. Abdominal aortic aneurysms can rupture into the inferior vena cava[1] or renal vein.[2] Abdominal aortic aneurysms or iliac artery aneurysms may rupture into iliac veins.[3] Other rarer causes of acquired AV fistulas are erosions secondary to infections, tumors, or intravascular appliances such as an inferior vena cava filter.[4] Excluded from discussion in this chapter are iatrogenic, therapeutic, surgically created AV shunts such as those for hemodialysis, or to enhance limb growth, or to aid in sustaining graft patency.

The major hemodynamic effects of an acquired AV fistula are inversely related to the hemodynamic resistance associated with the AV communication. Thus the diameter of the communication is of great importance. There are both central and peripheral circulatory consequences of a fistula. If the AV communication is large, the resistance is low and the volume of blood shunted is very great. This may lead to huge compensatory increases in the cardiac output, and high output cardiac failure may ensue. The most dramatic and extreme clinical example of this phenomenon occurs with an aortocaval fistula secondary to erosion of an abdominal aortic

127

aneurysm and rupture into the inferior vena cava. Rupture of an aneurysm into an iliac vein is noteworthy because of the clinical triad of sudden high output cardiac failure, unilateral lower extremity ischemia or venous engorgement, and a thrill and bruit over an abdominal mass.[3]

Peripheral circulatory consequences of AV fistulas relate to relative ischemia distal to the shunt. A dual mechanism is involved with elevation of venous pressure and shunting of oxygenated blood into the venous circulation. The ischemia distal to a fistula in an extremity may result in ulceration or even gangrene in extreme cases.

The diagnosis of an acquired AV fistula is usually made with ease. The history of the initiating trauma is ordinarily quite apparent, and the abnormalities on physical examination are obvious. A palpable thrill and an audible bruit are present over the fistula. The skin temperature may be increased at the site of the fistula and reduced more distally. There may be locally prominent superficial veins. Continuous wave Doppler ultrasound interrogation is very clearly abnormal, with audible distortion of the Doppler signal, resulting in a loss of the normal biphasic arterial signal in conjunction with a prominent venous signal that is continuous; and the increase is clearly with systole, the so-called pulsatile venous signal.

The bradycardic sign, as described by Nicoladoni and Branham, is of less importance in current diagnosis than it is in elucidating mechanisms involved in the hemodynamic alterations. Pressure applied to the artery proximal to the AV fistula results in slowing of the heart rate more than 4 beats per minute. The blood pressure is temporarily increased. Atropine abolishes the Nicoladoni-Branham reflex. Alterations in baroreceptors in the carotid sinus and aortic arch occur, and the reflex is mediated by the vagus nerve.

Other abnormalities that occur with AV fistula include an increase in the oxygen saturation and venous blood near the fistula or proximal to it, an increase in venous pressure distal to the fistula, and an increase in the cardiac output that correlates with the size of the shunt. Though of interest in the pathophysiology of AV fistulas, it is rarely necessary to rely on these abnormalities for diagnosis.

ARTERIOGRAPHY

Arteriography is indicated for confirmation of the diagnosis of an acquired AV fistula and for accurate localization in preparation for surgical treatment. Although the communication between the involved artery and vein may not be visualized by arteriography, the site of the fistula can be determined by the site of the initial venous opacification of contrast media. When the fistula is large, there is rapid flow in the artery and vein proximal to the fistula, both of which vessels are enlarged, and there is slow flow in the distal arterial portion with possibly retrograde flow in the vein distal to the fistula.

TREATMENT

Surgery is indicated for virtually all acquired AV fistulas. The only exceptions would be tiny fistulas with minuscule shunts or in situations in which patients may have a more serious life-threatening illness. The goal of surgical treatment is to close the fistula and restore normal arterial and venous circulation. Quadruple ligation and excision of acquired AV fistulas should be reserved for lesions involving only minor vessels. Complications that may occur if acquired AV fistulas are left untreated are high output cardiac failure and bacterial endarteritis. In the extremity distal to the fistula, complications include ischemia, distal venous hypertension, and increased limb growth in younger patients. The results of surgical treatment are excellent.[1]

CONGENITAL AV MALFORMATIONS

Congenital AV malformations abnormally shunt blood from the arterial to the venous circulation without passing through an intervening capillary network. These pathologic conditions must be differentiated conceptually from normal communications between arterioles and venules that bypass the capillary bed, which are physiologically important for temperature regulation and adaptation to function. These normal AV communications are responsive to local autonomic and humoral controls in contrast to the pathologic AV communications, which are not.

Arteriovenous malformations are but one type of congenital vascular malformation. One widely recognized system of classifying congenital vascular malformations is based on the most dominant or serious component of the abnormality.[5] In this classification, the lesions of greatest potential for complications are those with macrofistulous communications, followed in turn by microfistulous AV malformations, and further by venous angiomas, and capillary and cavernous hemangiomas.

Congenital vascular malformations result from abnormal maturation of one or several of the embryologic stages in the development of blood vessels. The composition of the structures in the malformation varies greatly from those with predominant venous components and no hemodynamic consequences from AV shunting to those in which there is a major arterial component and marked shunting, the macrofistulous communications.

In the past, congenital vascular malformations were often classified by eponyms according to the original descriptions. W. B. Bean observed, "One rapidly gets lost in a sea of eponyms which designate bizarre vascular syndromes."[6] The syndromes that have warranted continued wide usage include Klippel-Trenaunay, Parkes Weber, and Rendu-Osler-Weber. Klippel-Trenaunay syndrome is comprised of congenital venous anomalies, cutaneous capillary malformations, and limb hypertrophy.[7] Parkes Weber syndrome is characterized by the presence of a macrofistulous congenital AV malformation and in this important feature is differentiated from Klippel-Trenaunay syndrome. An example of Parkes Weber syndrome is illustrated in Figure 9–1. Both conditions involve primarily the lower extremities, and lymphatic abnormalities also commonly occur in both. Klippel-Trenaunay syndrome is much more common and has a better prognosis because the AV fistulas with Parkes Weber syndrome create a greater hazard for limb survival.

Rendu-Osler-Weber syndrome also warrants continued recognition because of the frequency (approximately 50%) of pulmonary AV fistulas and the suitability of these lesions for embolic therapy.[8] There is an autosomal dominant pattern of inheritance of the Rendu-Osler-Weber syndrome. The characteristic lesions are discrete, bright red maculopapules, usually a few millimeters in diameter and typically located on the face, tongue, lips, and nasal and oral mucous membranes. They also can often be seen on the conjunctiva, on the palmar aspect of the fingers, and in

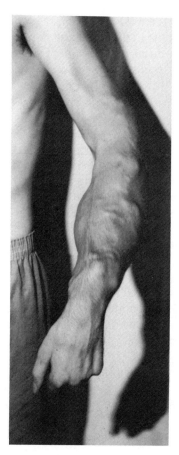

Figure 9-1. *Macrofistulous AV malformation involving the left upper extremity.* A 19-year-old male with a macrofistulous AV malformation involving the left upper extremity. Ulcer on the forearm for 2 years with recurrent bleeding and reduced exercise tolerance. Cardiac catheterization demonstrated markedly increased cardiac output (16.4 L/min) and cardiac index (8.8 L/min per square meter), decreasing by 34% with digital compression of the axillary artery. Blood flow in the left subclavian vein measured 7.41 L/min, decreasing to 1.03 L/min with digital occlusion of the left axillary artery. The left upper extremity blood flow represented 45% of the resting cardiac output. Amputation was performed at the midarm level, and elastic support applied to the stump. One year later, the cardiac output was 7.8 L/min and cardiac index 4.1 L/min per square meter, with normal and equal right and left subclavian vein flow.

the nail beds. There may be involvement of many mucosal surfaces, for example, the nasal septum, tongue, gastrointestinal tract, and bladder, and lesions also can occur in the bronchial and vaginal mucosa. Internally, lesions are also found in the liver, spleen, pancreas, kidney, and brain. The lesions are prone to ulceration and bleeding. The pulmonary AV fistula that may be seen in the Rendu-Osler-Weber syndrome may be complicated by cyanosis, clubbing of the fingers, and polycythemia if there is a marked degree of shunting.

Though present from birth, congenital vascular malformations often may not become symptomatic until later in life. Those lesions with major AV shunting have a predilection to more rapid progression during adolescence or during pregnancy.

Congenital vascular malformations can occur in virtually any region of the body. Most of the lesions are complex, drawing their arterial supply from several arteries and possibly several arterial territories. The lesions usually feed into many different veins. Congenital vascular malformations involving the brain, dura, and spinal cord pose special problems because of the potential for bleeding and neurologic deficit owing to the critical location in the central nervous system. Involvement of the vein of Galen is a special situation in the neonate or infant in whom the degree of AV shunting is large and the presentation may be dominated by high output cardiac failure.[9] The diagnosis and treatment of congenital vascular malformations involving the central nervous system continue to pose difficult problems despite advances in recent years. Because of the specialized nature of the problem, the subject will not be reviewed further for this chapter. There are several recent comprehensive reviews of central nervous system vascular malformations.[10,11]

Other unusual types of congenital AV malformations that present special problems in diagnosis and management can occur in the heart with a coronary fistula,[12] in the liver with drainage into the portal system,[13] in the kidney,[14] and in the intestine.[15] Coronary AV fistulas may present with left-to-right shunts and a continuous murmur with cardiac failure. Diagnosis requires cardiac catheterization and selective angiography, which demonstrates the anomaly and quantitates the shunt. Intrahepatic arterial-portal fistulas may present with portal hypertension and need to be differentiated from other, more common causes of this problem. Computerized tomography and magnetic resonance imaging have greatly aided the diagnosis, but final confirmation with arteriography is usually required. Embolization therapy has been successfully employed for treatment and is considered the treatment of choice for this lesion.[13] Congenital AV malformation of the kidney is a rare but correctable cause of renovascular hypertension.[14]

EXTREMITIES

Congenital AV malformations involving the extremities occur quite rarely. At the Mayo Clinic, 185 such cases were encountered in a 50-year period.[16] In this series, the lower extremity was involved in 62%, upper extremities in 22%, pelvis and buttocks in 12%, and a combination of multiple locations in 4%. Congestive heart failure occurred very rarely, developing in only 3% of the patients. When encountered, it was more likely to be found in infants and adolescents with very large shunts. Congenital AV malformation of the extremity was rarely fatal, and there was a 97.9% survival in a mean follow-up of 22.9 years in the Mayo Clinic study. Other than the cosmetic abnormality associated with the lesions, the major symptoms that occurred were pain, ulceration of the skin and subcutaneous tissues, and varicose veins.

MAGNETIC RESONANCE IMAGING

Magnetic resonance imaging (MRI) is a major development in the diagnosis of congenital vascular malformations of the extremities.[17] Examples are illustrated in Figures 9–2 and 9–3. MRI has several advantages over computerized tomographic examinations in the diagnosis of vascular malformations. MRI has the ability to determine blood flow characterization as well as to define the pathologic anatomy of the lesion in question. Transverse as well as longitudinal views are possible. Flow patterns can be characterized into high-flow vascular spaces with delineation of the feeding arteries and draining veins and slow flow patterns with laminar flow characteristics. Intravascular thrombus can be seen if present. The cellularity of the lesion in question can be appreciated and highly cellular structures differentiated from spongy lesions. Hemorrhage from an AV malformation into soft tissues can be seen, and the relationship of the malformation to adjacent muscle and bone can be clearly defined. MRI of congenital AV malformations almost always demonstrates more extensive disease than appreciated by the physical examination or angiography.

MRI has become the key test used in the management of many patients with

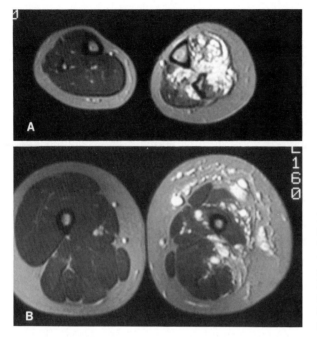

Figure 9–2. Klippel-Trenaunay syndrome in a 17-year-old woman. MRI shows an extensive venous malformation involving multiple muscle groups in the left leg (*A*) and left thigh (*B*) with extensive involvement of the anterior and lateral subcutaneous tissues of the thigh.

congenital vascular malformations and can serve as the primary imaging modality in the investigation of patients with these lesions. Often, no additional tests are necessary when the lesion in question has low flow characteristics. In high-flow malformations, arteriography is usually necessary to provide the additional information required for a decision about surgical or embolic therapy.

ARTERIOGRAPHY

The essential diagnostic information for proper management of patients with congenital vascular malformations often may be obtained without resorting to invasive diagnostic procedures, but if surgical treatment or catheter embolic therapy is being seriously considered, an arteriogram is indicated. There are several limitations to arteriography. Frequently, there are myriad tiny AV communications, only a portion of which may be visualized. There is a tendency for contrast media to shunt across the more proximal large AV communications, leaving the

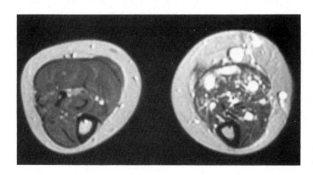

Figure 9–3. Microfistulous AV malformation in a 35-year-old woman. MRI of the right leg shows a complex vascular malformation with flow characteristics of a predominantly venous malformation. There is extensive involvement of the subcutaneous tissue and multiple muscles by the malformation.

distal fistulas unopacified. Numerous arteries may supply a lesion, and multiple veins may drain it. Rapid flow in the artery and vein proximal to the lesion is usually present. Arteriography crudely estimates the degree of AV shunting. Furthermore, it does not define the fascial planes or the muscular groups involved.

TREATMENT

There are three therapeutic alternatives for the treatment of congenital AV malformations—surgery, embolization, or conservative management. Surgical treatment that had been used in the past included ligation of the feeding vessels only, but this procedure is to be condemned. Ligation only enhances collateral flow into vessels with the least resistance, the fistulas. Furthermore, ligation eliminates the best access to the lesion if embolization is to be done. A better surgical procedure is complete excision of the AV malformation. However, this can be applied only to smaller, more localized low-flow lesions.

Embolization therapy is performed with a variety of embolic materials.[18] As yet, the ideal substance has not gained universal acceptance. Materials that have been used have included coils, balloons, and a variety of plastic substances to obstruct the vessel. Embolization therapy may in certain cases be performed as initial treatment prior to potentially surgical resectable AV malformations. In certain anatomic sites, embolization is the clear treatment of choice, for example, pulmonary AV fistulas. Repeated embolizations may be performed if necessary. The potential complications are necrosis of the tissue, ischemic damage to nerves involved in the malformation, and passage of the embolic material through the lesion resulting in pulmonary emboli.

Conservative treatment for congenital AV malformation involves the use of firm elastic support to the lesion and proper care to avoid trauma to the involved part. Elastic support is the mainstay of therapy. It has been demonstrated to reduce cardiac output by up to 20% in large congenital AV malformations of the extremities. Proper support can control pain, lessen the likelihood of bleeding from the lesions, reduce and retard the development of varices. Conservative treatment with elastic support is also an important aspect of management following either surgery or embolization therapy when remnants of the AV malformation persist.

Congenital AV malformations are rarely cured by any mode or combination of therapy that is available. The surgical treatment of all but the most localized lesions has been disappointing.[16] Recurrence of symptoms and further development of more extensive AV communications are common after surgery or embolization therapy if there are residual AV channels, as there almost always are. The residual microscopic AV fistulas increase slowly in size after any therapy, often with clinical recurrence of the lesion with the attendant signs and symptoms. For these reasons, a conservative approach to management is recommended, and embolization or surgery is reserved for patients who develop symptoms of pain or ulceration, or who have large enough AV malformations to greatly increase the cardiac output and produce congestive heart failure.

Embolization therapy is recommended for the treatment of large, unresectable AV malformations that are symptomatic with pain or ulceration, or in those rare instances in which the shunting is of such magnitude as to threaten cardiac decompensation. Repeated embolization may be necessary for large malformations. In certain anatomic sites, particularly pulmonary AV malformations and in the abdominal viscera, where surgical resection would pose special problems, embolization is the treatment of choice. Rarely, amputation of a portion of an extremity is still the treatment of choice in certain large AV malformations involving an extremity in which there is marked increase in cardiac output, with severe pain and ulceration of the extremity.

Patients who have predominantly cosmetic abnormalities from congenital vascular malformations and low flow may be successfully treated with argon laser therapy. Port-wine stains on the face are such an example. Such therapy should be delayed until the patient is past adolescence.

REFERENCES

1. Gomes, MMR and Bernatz, PE: Arteriovenous fistulas: A review and ten-year experience of the Mayo Clinic. Mayo Clin Proc 45:81, 1970.
2. Celoria, GM, Friedmann, P, Rhee, SW, and Berman, J: Fistulas between the aorta and left renal vein. J Vasc Surg 6:191, 1987.
3. McAuley, CE, Peitzman, AB, deVries, EJ, et al: The syndrome of spontaneous iliac arteriovenous fistula: a distinct clinical and pathophysiologic entity. Surgery 99:373, 1986.
4. Rozin, L and Perper, JA: Spontaneous fatal perforation of aorta and vena cava by Mobin-Uddir umbrella. Am J Forensic Med Pathol 10:149, 1989.
5. Szilagy, DE, Smith, RF, Elliott, JP, and Hageman JH: Congenital arteriovenous anomalies of the limbs. Arch Surg 111:423, 1976.
6. Bean, WB: Vascular spiders and related lesions of the skin. Charles C Thomas, Springfield, IL, 1958.
7. Gloviczki, P, Hollier, LN, Telander, RL, et al: Surgical implications of Klippel-Trenaunay syndrome. Ann Surg 197:353, 1983.
8. McCue, CM, Hartenberg, M, and Nance, WE: Pulmonary arteriovenous malformations related to Rendu-Osler-Weber syndrome. Am J Med Genet 19:19, 1984.
9. Johnston, IH, Whittle, IR, Besser, M, and Morgan, MK: Vein of Galen malformation: Diagnosis and management. Neurosurg 20:747, 1987.
10. Atlas, SW: Intracranial vascular malformations and aneurysms. Current imaging applications. Radiol Clin North Am 26:821, 1988.
11. Aminoff, MJ: Vascular malformations of the central nervous system. In Mulliken, JB and Young, AE (eds): Vascular Birthmarks. WB Saunders, Philadelphia, 1988.
12. Wellens, F, Neuvaert, F, Leclerc, JL, and Primo, G: Coronary artery fistula: An absolute surgical indication. Acta Chir Belg 84:339, 1984.
13. Redmond, PL and Kumpe, DA: Embolization of an intrahepatic arterioportal fistula: Case report and review of the literature. Cardiovasc Intervent Radiol 11:274, 1988.
14. Maldonado, JE, Sheps, SG, Bernatz PE, et al: Renal arteriovenous fistula: A reversible cause of hypertension and heart failure. Am J Med 37:499, 1964.
15. Hemingway, AP: Angiodysplasias. Postgrad Med J 64:259, 1988.
16. Schwartz, RS, Osmundson, PJ, and Hollier, LH: Treatment and prognosis in congenital arteriovenous malformation of the extremity. Phlebology 1:177, 1986.
17. Pearce, WH, Rutherford, RB, Whitehill, TA, and Davis, K: Nuclear magnetic resonance imaging: Its diagnostic value in patients with congenital vascular malformations of the limbs. J Vasc Surg 8:64, 1988.
18. Halbach, VV, Higashida, RT, and Hieshima, GB: Interventional neuroradiology. Am J Roentgenol 153:467, 1989.

CHAPTER 10

Vasospastic Disorders

Jess R. Young, M.D.

The vasospastic disorders of the extremities—Raynaud's phenomenon, livedo reticularis, and acrocyanosis—are an interesting group. Each has a primary and secondary form. The primary forms of these conditions are usually harmless, rarely resulting in ulcerations or more severe ischemia. The secondary forms can be associated with serious disorders that can result in severe ischemia, amputations, or even death. Therefore, when a patient with a vasospastic disorder is seen, the physician must make an effort to differentiate the primary from the secondary forms.

RAYNAUD'S PHENOMENON

Raynaud's phenomenon is a well-recognized clinical entity characterized by intermittent pallor or cyanosis of the fingers or toes, often followed by a third stage, rubor, secondary to vasodilatation. These episodes can be precipitated by cold or emotional stress.

Raynaud's phenomenon may be idiopathic and without apparent cause (Raynaud's disease), or it may occur as a manifestation of certain underlying conditions (secondary Raynaud's phenomenon).

PATHOPHYSIOLOGY

The pathophysiology of arteriospastic attacks in secondary Raynaud's phenomenon is understandable. The decreased blood flow may be caused by persistent vasoconstriction, by increased blood viscosity, or by normal sympathetic stimuli on digital arteries with low blood pressure distal to stenoses or obstructions. Persistent vasoconstriction may be caused by drug therapy such as β-adrenergic blocking agents or ergotamine preparations. Increased blood viscosity can occur in cryoglobulinemia and polycythemia. Digital arterial disease can occur in connective tissue disorders and in vinyl chloride disease.

In primary Raynaud's disease there is no abnormality of the blood vessels, and blood viscosity is normal. Two theories have been proposed to explain the vasospastic attacks in primary Raynaud's disease. The first theory, attributed to Maurice Raynaud,[1] proposes that there is an overactivity of the sympathetic nervous system. However, normal microelectrode recordings of skin sympathetic nerve activity at rest and with various stimuli, normal catecholamine levels, and normal vasoconstriction of the contralateral hand during cooling of one hand in patients with primary Raynaud's disease do not substantiate this theory. The second theory, proposed by Lewis,[2] suggested that there was a local fault at the digital artery level. Although recent evidence supports this theory, we still do not know the nature of this local fault.

CLINICAL FEATURES

Raynaud's phenomenon presents as episodic attacks of well-demarcated discoloration of the digits brought on by cold or emotional stress (Fig. 10–1). One or more digits are usually affected, the fingers more than the toes, except in unusual cases when the hands, feet, and even the ears and nose may be involved. The color changes are classically triphasic with pallor, cyanosis, and rubor. At times there may be only pallor or cyanosis. The rubor phase is a result of the reactive hyperemia following either pallor or cyanosis. Numbness or pain may be present during the pallor or cyanotic phase, and burning paresthesias may be present during the hyperemic phase. The Raynaud's event usually does not last longer than 15 to 30 minutes after returning to a warm environment.

Women account for 60% to 90% of patients with Raynaud's phenomenon.[3] They are more likely to have either primary Raynaud's disease or Raynaud's phenomenon in association with a connective tissue disorder. Men with Raynaud's

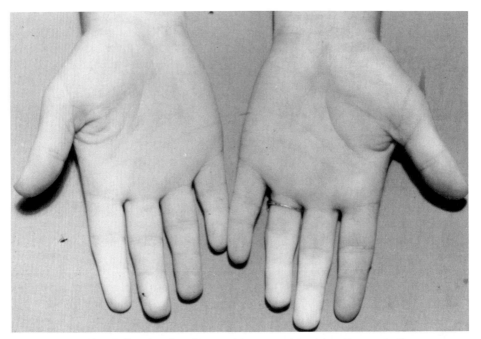

Figure 10–1. Pallor phase in a 21-year-old woman with primary Raynaud's disease.

phenomenon generally present at an older age and have a much higher incidence of atherosclerosis.

The prevalence of Raynaud's phenomenon is unknown, but one study by Maricq and coworkers[4] found that symptoms suggestive of the disorder were found in 4% of men and 5% of women interviewed. A report in 1978 by Olsen and Neilson[5] reported that 22% of 85 women between the ages of 21 and 50 had Raynaud's phenomenon. In 1987 a study of 3000 Swedish women by Leppert and associates[6] found the prevalence to be 15% to 16%.

RAYNAUD'S PHENOMENON—PRIMARY OR SECONDARY?

The differentiation between primary and secondary Raynaud's phenomenon may be difficult, but it is most important in treatment and in prognosis.

In 1932 Allen and Brown[7] proposed five criteria for the diagnosis of Raynaud's disease (primary Raynaud's phenomenon): (1) the presence of Raynaud's phenomenon; (2) bilaterality of Raynaud's phenomenon; (3) ischemic lesions limited to small areas of superficial gangrene; (4) exclusion of conditions that might cause Raynaud's phenomenon; and (5) symptoms of Raynaud's phenomenon for at least 2 years in the absence of any causal condition. These are still valid criteria and will permit a correct diagnosis of Raynaud's disease in over 95% of patients. There have been reports of cases in which Raynaud's phenomenon appeared 5 or more years before the clinical onset of a connective tissue disease, but these instances are unusual.

Some of the features which would indicate that a patient with Raynaud's phenomenon might have an underlying disorder are listed in Table 10-1. Some of the conditions that may cause secondary Raynaud's phenomenon are listed in Table 10-2. The general categories include connective tissue diseases, occupational causes, drugs, toxins, occlusive arterial diseases, neurologic conditions, and blood abnormalities. In patients with Raynaud's phenomenon, particular attention must be given to the search for one of the connective tissue disorders and to the patient's occupation, avocation, and list of medications that they are taking.

Table 10-1. Clues That Raynaud's Phenomenon May Be Secondary

1. Male sex
2. Onset after 40 years of age
3. Abrupt onset with rapid progression
4. Unilateral involvement
5. Ischemic changes
6. Absence of one or more pulses (except dorsalis pedis)
7. Positive Allen test for radial or ulnar artery occlusion
8. Fingertip ulcerations
9. Hand or finger spider telangiectasia
10. Sclerodactylia
11. Systemic symptoms (malaise, fever, weight loss, rash, etc.)
12. Arthralgias, arthritis
13. Occupation (pianist, typist, those using vibrating tools, etc.)
14. Abnormal laboratory tests (sedimentation rate elevation, anemia, positive LE, positive antinuclear factor, abnormal serum protein, etc.)

Table 10–2. Conditions That May Cause Secondary
Raynaud's Phenomenon

---

1. Connective tissue disease
   a. Scleroderma
   b. Rheumatoid arthritis
   c. Systemic lupus erythematosus
   d. Dermatomyositis
   e. Sjögren's syndrome
   f. Mixed connective tissue disease
2. Related to occupation
   a. Vibration (pneumatic hammers, chain saws, riveting machines, polishers, typewriters, pianos, etc.)
   b. Hypothenar hammer syndrome
   c. Vinyl chloride disease
3. Drug ingestion (β-adrenoceptor blockers, ergot, methysergide)
4. Intoxication (lead, arsenic)
5. Occlusive arterial disease (arteriosclerosis obliterans, thromboangiitis obliterans, etc.)
6. Blood abnormalities (cryoglobulins, cold agglutinins, macroglobulins)
7. Neurologic conditions (thoracic outlet syndrome, carpal tunnel syndrome, etc.)
8. Primary pulmonary hypertension
9. Hypothyroidism

The most common condition associated with Raynaud's phenomenon is an underlying connective tissue disease. Porter and coworkers[8] reported a series of 219 patients who were evaluated and followed for 10 years. Of these, about half developed a definite connective tissue disorder; another 18% were suspected of having a connective tissue disease, but this could not be proved; and in 29% no underlying condition could be found. Raynaud's phenomenon may be the first symptom of a connective tissue disease. This is true in up to 80% of scleroderma patients and up to 10% of those with systemic lupus erythematosus.

The presence of antinuclear antibodies in patients with Raynaud's phenomenon usually signifies that a collagen vascular disease is present or will become evident in the future. Elderly patients may have a titer as high as 1:64 without systemic disease, but in younger patients the titer rarely exceeds 1:16. A speckled pattern is often present in scleroderma. Anticentromere antibodies are present in the majority of patients with the CREST syndrome. A homogenous pattern of antinuclear antibodies with antibodies to DNA is often present in systemic lupus erythematosus. Antinuclear antibodies and rheumatoid factor may also be present in other connective tissue diseases, and these can also be induced by drugs such as procainamide.

The value of nail-fold capillary microscopy in predicting which patients may develop a connective tissue disorder has been well demonstrated.[9] Normally the capillary loops of the skin of the nail fold are regularly spaced in hairpin loops and are lined along the axis of the digit. In scleroderma, mixed connective tissue disease, and dermatomyositis, there is a decreased number of capillaries. The capillaries that are present are enlarged and deformed, and avascular areas are present. Patients with primary Raynaud's disease usually have a normal nail-fold capillary pattern. In systemic lupus erythematosus, tortuous capillary loops may be present and the subpapillary venous plexus is more prominent than in normal subjects. The value of the nail-fold test is that an abnormal capillary pattern indicates a secondary cause for the Raynaud's phenomenon, whereas a normal pattern would favor the diagnosis of primary Raynaud's disease.

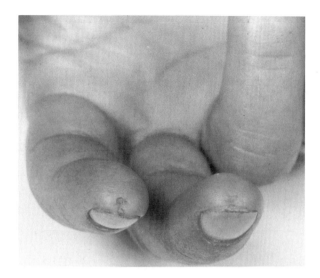

Figure 10–2. These small, healed fingertip ulcerations are almost pathognomonic of scleroderma.

CLINICAL EVALUATION

The clinical evaluation of a patient with Raynaud's phenomenon should begin with a detailed history of the complaints. The diagnosis of Raynaud's phenomenon cannot be made unless either pallor or cyanosis, or both, are present. Reactive hyperemia may or may not be noted.

If the patient has bilateral and symmetric involvement of multiple digits, he or she is more likely to have primary Raynaud's disease. If only one hand is involved, especially if the condition has been present for several months, this would be stronger evidence for secondary Raynaud's phenomenon.

In taking a history and doing the physical examination, special emphasis should be placed on the signs and symptoms of connective tissue diseases such as arthralgias, edema, fingertip ulcerations (Fig. 10–2), telangiectasias (Fig. 10–3), periungual infections, pigmentary changes, skin eruptions, history of photosensitivity, sicca symptoms, fever, weight loss, or dysphagia. Questions should be directed

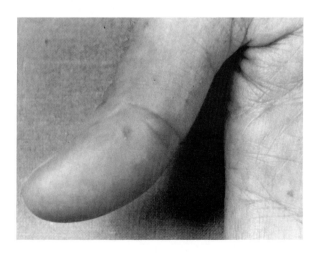

Figure 10–3. Spider telangiectasias of the thumb and at the base of the index finger in a patient with scleroderma and Raynaud's phenomenon.

at the patient's medications, occupation, hobbies, sports, and history of prior arterial disease. Pulses should be checked and thoracic outlet maneuvers carried out. A baseline laboratory workup should include a complete blood count, erythrocyte sedimentation rate, chemistry profile, ANA test, and urinalysis. If scleroderma is suspected, radiographs of the hand, pulmonary function testing, and an esophageal study should be included. If an underlying disorder is suspected, further immunologic tests that may be helpful include serum protein electrophoresis, immunoglobulins, complement levels, rheumatoid factor, anti-DNA antibody, and antiextractable nuclear antigens (ENA). Cryoglobulins and cold agglutinins can be checked for.

Both ultrasound and plethysmography may be helpful in providing the location and degree of blockage in the digital vessels. Arteriography is seldom needed to establish the diagnosis of Raynaud's phenomenon.

PROGNOSIS

In a long-term study of 307 women with primary Raynaud's phenomenon,[10] 38% had stable disease, 36% improved, 16% became worse, and the symptoms disappeared in 10%. Only 0.4% (two patients) had digital amputations.

Connective tissue disease does not frequently develop over the ensuing years in patients with primary Raynaud's disease. Of 87 patients followed for an average of 5 years after the onset of symptoms, only 5% developed scleroderma of the CREST variety, although 17% of those patients had antinuclear antibodies.[11]

TREATMENT

The fact that so many types of treatment have been proposed for Raynaud's phenomenon emphasizes the point that no one treatment has been outstandingly successful. One problem in selecting therapy is that there are few objective, randomized, double-blind studies demonstrating the effectiveness of one medication or form of therapy over another.

Treatment must be tailored to the needs of the patient. The frequency and severity of symptoms, the presence of ischemic lesions, the risk-benefit ratio of the various therapeutic measures, and patient compliance should all be considered.

General Measures

EDUCATION AND REASSURANCE. Most patients are anxious about the possibility of serious complications, especially amputations. If no secondary cause for the Raynaud's phenomenon is found, reassurance is a major step in treatment. The patient should be told that the pallor and cyanosis are merely exaggerations of a normal reaction to cold exposure or to stress and that no serious circulatory disorder is present.

STOP SMOKING. All patients with Raynaud's phenomenon should stop smoking because smoking increases the tendency toward arterial spasm. If patients cannot stop, advise at the least that they smoke only in a warm environment for minimal impact on the Raynaud's phenomenon.

AVOIDANCE OF COLD AND STRESS. All patients must understand the effects of stress and cold on their vascular disease. They should try to avoid stressful situations and the time of exposure to cold weather should be minimized. The entire body—the head and feet as well as the hands—must be kept warm.

AVOIDANCE OF MEDICATIONS THAT AGGRAVATE RAYNAUD'S PHENOMENON. The patient should be cautioned against taking vasoconstrictive medications such as β-blockers, ergotamine preparations, and oral contraceptives.

Medications

Most patients with Raynaud's phenomenon will have only mild to moderate symptoms and will respond favorably to the aforementioned general measures. Certainly fewer than half will have symptoms severe enough to justify medication. When medication is prescribed, it should be used only in cold months and should be stopped during warm weather.

SYMPATHETIC BLOCKING AGENTS. Reserpine, both orally and parenterally, has been used in the past, but the parenteral preparation is no longer available. We rarely use reserpine now because of the side effects. Other medications are more effective and have fewer complications.

Other medications that have been used include methyldopa, tolazoline, guanethidine, phenoxybenzamine, and prazosin. Because the use of these medications may be limited by their side effects, combinations of medications, using lower doses of each, may reduce the severity of the reactions.

DIRECT VASODILATORS. The calcium channel blocking agents act as vasodilators by inhibiting calcium entry into the cells. Nifedipine is the preferred drug[12] with regard to patient satisfaction and side effects. The dosage depends on the severity of the symptoms. Some patients will have sufficient improvement on 10 mg once or twice daily. If this is not effective, the dosage can be slowly increased to 10 to 20 mg three to four times daily, titrating the drug according to its effectiveness and its side reactions. The sustained release form also can be used.

Other direct vasodilators have been tried with varying success in the past including isosuprine, nylidrin, and isoproterenol. Griseofulvin, an antifungal agent, is also a direct vasodilator that has been reported by some[13] to be effective in Raynaud's phenomenon. This is an expensive medication that does not seem to have any advantages over other agents. Nitroglycerin also has been used, both topically and sublingually.[14]

OTHER MEDICATIONS. Pentoxifylline does not seem to be effective in Raynaud's phenomenon, although it might help some patients with digital artery obstruction. Ketanserin, a serotonin antagonist, has been reported[15] to be effective in the treatment of Raynaud's phenomenon.

Surgery

The role of surgical cervicothoracic sympathectomy is limited in Raynaud's phenomenon. Its use should be reserved for patients with severely ischemic digits, rest pain, or nonhealing ulcers that are not responding to conservative measures. These latter conditions are usually encountered in Raynaud's phenomenon associated with one of the connective tissue diseases. Unfortunately, sympathectomy does not usually affect the long-term course of the disease.

Other Measures

When Raynaud's phenomenon occurs secondary to a connective tissue disease, treatment of the disease should improve the Raynaud's phenomenon.

In tense patients, behavior modification techniques may be helpful in relieving tension; a tranquilizer may be prescribed to minimize the reults of stress.

Temperature biofeedback techniques[16] may help in patients with the time and inclination to get involved in this type of program.

Plasmapheresis has been used by some[17] in the treatment of severe Raynaud's phenomenon but is probably most beneficial to those who have increased viscosity or abnormal serum protein such as cryoglobulins.

LIVEDO RETICULARIS

Livedo reticularis is characterized by a violet or blue mottling of the skin in a reticular, lacelike, fishnet pattern (Fig. 10–4). It is intensified by cold exposure and improved or relieved by warming.

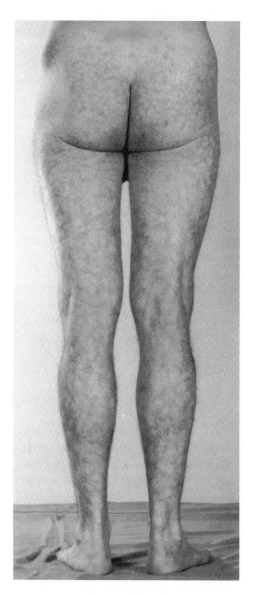

Figure 10–4. Reticular mottling of legs and buttocks in a 35-year-old man with primary livedo reticularis.

Like Raynaud's phenomenon, livedo reticularis may be either primary or secondary to some other disease. The primary form is usually a benign mottled discoloration of the extremities and sometimes the trunk, which may be relieved completely by warming. This idiopathic form of livedo also has been called cutis marmorata, livedo racemosa, and livedo annularis. Rarely does this idiopathic form cause ulceration, and when it does, the ulcers usually occur in the winter and clear in the summer. Most ulcers occur on the calves, ankles, and feet.

Benign livedo reticularis is common in women during the second to fifth decades. Primary livedo reticularis with ulceration is rare, but it is also more common in women in the third to fifth decades.

Except for the reticular discoloration of the extremities and sometimes the trunk, the physical examination in benign livedo reticularis is normal. The pulses are excellent and no evidence of any underlying disease is present.

Secondary livedo reticularis can occur with connective tissue diseases (Fig. 10–5), cryoglobulinemia, atheromatous emboli (Fig. 10–6), hyperviscosity states, and hypercoagulable disorders. In recent years the occurrence of anticardiolipin antibodies with livedo reticularis has been reported with increasing frequency.[18] These antibodies may be encountered in patients with recurring arterial or venous thrombi and spontaneous abortions. Anticardiolipin antibodies may be the cause of these syndromes and may precede other clinical manifestations by several years.

Sneddon's syndrome[19] is characterized by livedo reticularis associated with cerebrovascular lesions causing transient ischemic attacks or strokes. Many of these patients also have been found to have anticardiolipin antibodies.

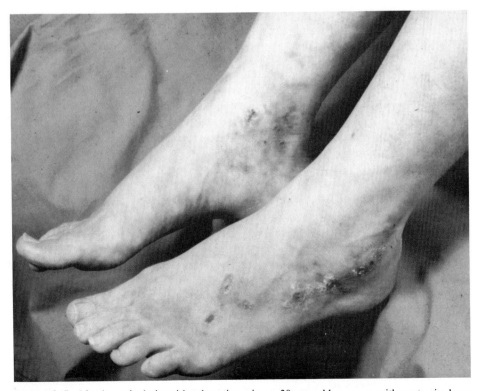

Figure 10–5. Livedo reticularis with ulcerations in a 30-year-old woman with systemic lupus erythematosus.

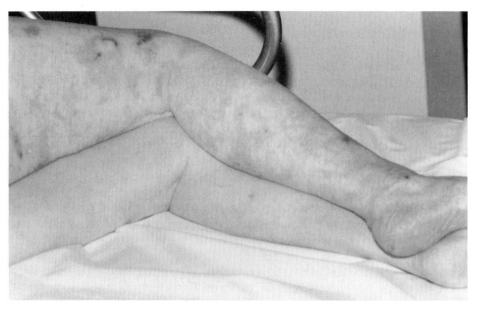

Figure 10–6. Livedo reticularis with ulcerations of right leg and foot in a 62-year-old man with a shower of atheromatous emboli from an atherosclerotic plaque in his left common iliac artery.

Amantadine hydrochloride (Symmetrel), a medication used for parkinsonism, can cause livedo reticularis. This is usually a benign form of livedo and does not cause ulceration or ischemia. It usually disappears within weeks of stopping the medication.

No treatment is usually necessary for the benign, idiopathic form of livedo reticularis. If the patient objects to the unsightly appearance of the skin, a trial of vasodilating drugs as was outlined in the treatment of Raynaud's phenomenon can be given. For the rare patient with livedo reticularis complicated by ischemic ulcers, the treatment follows the same steps as the treatment of Raynaud's phenomenon. When livedo reticularis occurs secondary to some other disorder, treatment is that of the associated disease.

ACROCYANOSIS

Acrocyanosis is the rarest of the vasospastic disorders. In a large, busy vascular medicine department at the Cleveland Clinic only one patient has been encountered with this problem over the last 30 years.

Acrocyanosis is a constant, persistent cyanotic discoloration of the fingers and usually of the hands, toes, and feet (Fig. 10–7). The face and ears are sometimes involved. There is usually a coldness associated with the cyanosis, and the coldness and discoloration are aggravated by exposure to cold temperature.

In the past, it was thought that unlike Raynaud's phenomenon and livedo reticularis, there was only one form of acrocyanosis and not a secondary form. However, recently there has been a report of the association of acrocyanosis with Asperger's syndrome, an autistic disorder.[20] Patients with autism frequently have raised levels of serotonin in their blood,[21] and serotonin is known to cause vasoconstriction. It was thought that a stagnation of blood flow in the skin resulted from arterial and venous vasoconstriction.

With this one exception, the patient with acrocyanosis does not need to be concerned about some serious underlying disease. It is almost always a benign disorder with an excellent prognosis. Ischemic lesions never occur.

With the exception of Asperger's syndrome, the etiology of the arterial spasm is unknown. This constant spasm in the small arteries, arterioles, and venules of the skin leads to a slowing of blood flow and increased extraction of oxygen from the blood, resulting in cyanosis.

Acrocyanosis is usually seen in women. A typical patient is a young woman who has noted a persistent cyanosis of her hands, and usually the feet, for as long as she can remember. Although the discoloration improves in warm weather or in a warm room, it never disappears completely. Physical examination is usually normal except for the cyanosis. In some patients, edema and increased sweating of the hands and feet may occur. Laboratory studies are normal.

The striking cyanosis may suggest a central cyanosis secondary to cardiac or pulmonary disease or to an arteriovenous fistula. This possibility can be eliminated by finding a normal arterial oxygen saturation. Raynaud's phenomenon can be excluded inasmuch as the color changes in this disorder are episodic and not persistent. Cyanosis secondary to arterial occlusive disease can be eliminated by the fact that no pain is present in acrocyanosis and the color changes have been present for the patient's lifetime.

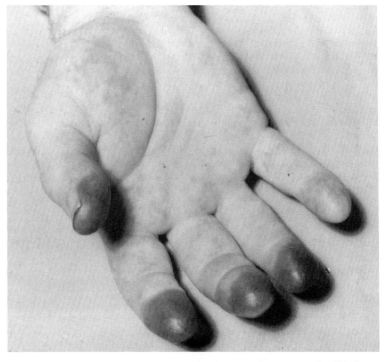

Figure 10–7. Acrocyanosis in a 45-year-old man who has had persistent cyanosis of his fingers, and less in his hands since birth.

No treatment is needed other than an explanation of the disorder and a reassurance regarding the prognosis. Most patients have already learned to avoid cold exposure as much as possible. If the patient is embarrassed by the appearance of the blue hands, the use of vasodilating drugs such as phenoxybenzamine or calcium channel blockers may be of benefit. Sympathectomy for such a benign disorder does not seem appropriate; moreover, a return of sympathetic tone after dorsal sympathectomy frequently occurs.

REFERENCES

1. Raynaud, M: On local asphyxia and symmetrical gangrene of the extremities. Translated by T. Barlow. The Syndenham Society, London, 1888.
2. Lewis, T: Experiments relating to the peripheral mechanism involved in spasmodic arrest of the circulation in the fingers, a variety of Raynaud's disease. Heart 15:7, 1929.
3. Kleinsmith, D: Raynaud's syndrome: An overview. Semin Dermatol 4:104, 1985.
4. Maricq, HR, Weinrich, MC, Keil, JE, et al: Prevalence of Raynaud phenomenon in the general population. J Chronic Dis 39:423, 1986.
5. Olsen, N and Nielsen, SL: Prevalence of primary Raynaud phenomena in young females. Scand J Clin Invest 37:761, 1978.
6. Leppert, J, Aberg, H, and Ringqvist, I: Raynaud's phenomenon in a female population: Prevalence and association with other conditions. Angiology 38:871, 1987.
7. Allen, EV and Brown, GE: Raynaud's disease: A critical review of minimal requisites for diagnosis. Am J Med Sci 183:187, 1932.
8. Porter, JM, Rivers, SP, Anderson, CJ, et al: Evaluation and management of patients with Raynaud's syndrome. Am J Surg 142:183, 1981.
9. Harper, FE, Maricq, HR, Turner, RE, et al: A prospective study of Raynaud phenomenon and early connective tissue disease. Am J Med 72:883, 1982.
10. Gifford, RW, Jr, and Hines, EA, Jr: Raynaud's disease among women and girls. Circulation 16:1012, 1957.
11. Gerbracht, DD, Steen, VD, Ziegler, GL, et al: Evolution of primary Raynaud's phenomenon (Raynaud's disease) to connective tissue disease. Arthritis Rheum 28:87, 1985.
12. White, CJ, Phillips, WA, Abrahams, LA, et al: Objective benefit of nifedipine in the treatment of Raynaud's phenomenon: Double-blind controlled study. Am J Med 80:623, 1986.
13. Charles, CR and Carmick, ES: Skin temperature changes in Raynaud's disease after griseofulvin. Arch Dermatol 101:331, 1970.
14. Peterson, LL and Vorhies, C: Raynaud's syndrome: Treatment with sublingual administration of nitroglycerin, swinging arm maneuver, and biofeedback training. Arch Dermatol 119:396, 1983.
15. Arneklo-Nobin, B, Elmer, O, and Akesson, A: Effect of long-term ketanserin treatment on 5-HT levels, platelet aggregation and peripheral circulation in patients with Raynaud's phenomenon. Int Angiol 7:19, 1988.
16. From the NIH: Biofeedback for patients with Raynaud's phenomenon. JAMA 242:509, 1979.
17. O'Reilly, MJG, Talpos, G, Roberts, VC, et al: Controlled trial of plasma exchange in treatment of Raynaud's syndrome. BMJ 1:1113, 1979.
18. Asherson, RA, Mayou, SC, Merry, P, et al: The spectrum of livedo reticularis and anticardiolipin antibodies. Br J Dermatol 120:215, 1989.
19. Sneddon, IB: Cerebrovascular lesions and livedo reticularis. Br J Dermatol 77:180, 1965.
20. Morris, PK and Morris, D: Association of acrocyanosis with Asperger's syndrome. J Ment Defic Res 34:87, 1990.
21. Anderson, GM: Monoamines in autism: An update of neurochemical research on a pervasive developmental disorder. Med Biol 65:67, 1987.

CHAPTER 11

Occlusive Arterial Disease of the Upper Extremity

John W. Joyce, M.D.

Diagnosis of upper extremity arterial lesions poses a challenge for three reasons: experiences are infrequent; etiology is quite diverse; and presentations overlap with vasospastic, neurogenic, orthopedic, and the microcirculatory syndromes of numerous systemic diseases. This chapter presents an overview of arterial problems of the upper extremity with the thesis that, given the natural history of these disorders, the diagnosis can be defined by a directed history, sensitized examination, and selective testing.

It is noteworthy that the major sources of upper extremity arterial disease are confined to three anatomic locations. These are the origins of the brachiocephalic arteries in the chest, the subclavian-brachial-axillary zone, and the hand. Lesions occurring in the forearm and above the elbow are far less frequent and usually represent direct trauma (including interventional diagnostic and therapeutic procedures), infection, or embolism. Disabling claudication is quite uncommon with occlusive lesions at the takeoff of the brachiocephalic arteries, owing to the excellent collateral flow about the shoulder and the intermittent use of the upper extremity in tasks, in contrast to the sustained metabolic demands walking makes in the lower extremity. Systemic symptoms, both generalized such as fever, weight loss, and malaise, or specific, such as myalgia, cutaneous manifestations, and cardiac findings, are not infrequent and reflect the increased incidence of vasculitis, hematologic disorders, and cardiac disease that is more common in a population with upper extremity arterial disease. In practice, diagnosis of these diverse lesions yields to competent examination, selective testing, and quality angiography that must include all three zones from the arch of the aorta down to the hand. Indeed, with the evolution of hematologic and immune testing, and the advances of arteriography, knowledge of upper extremity arterial disease has become most cohesive, and both therapy and prognosis better directed. The reader is referred to several, excellent, contemporary reviews.[1-3]

EXAMINATION SKILLS

The physical assessment of a patient with upper extremity arterial disease requires examination of the heart, appreciation of the body habitus, careful examination of the skin, and examination of the pulses. The cardiac examination may define embolic sources or coexistent disease that explain the limb symptoms (most commonly, atherosclerotic coronary disease, but also Marfan's syndrome and Ehlers-Danlos syndrome). The skin manifests the temperature and color changes of ischemia, lesions typical of embolism and infarction, or changes reflecting systemic disease including scleroderma, lupus erythematosus, or vasculitis. The arteries themselves provide three basic and essential observations: the presence or absence of the pulses, aneurysms, and/or bruits.

PULSES

The radial, ulnar, brachial, subclavian, and carotid pulses are assessed to determine whether normal, reduced, or absent. The patient is usually examined in the upright position, utilizing gentle pressure with two or three fingers, and controlling the wrist joint with the contralateral hand, in the case of the radial and ulnar pulse. There are numerous variations of the ulnar pulse and palmar arch, and the ulnar pulse may be absent for congenital or acquired reasons, or quite frequently obscured by heavy musculotendinous structures.[4]

The Allen test is an essential extension of the basic pulse examination when there is an absent radial or ulnar pulse or arterial disease of the hand. The examiner occludes the patient's radial or ulnar pulse with the firm pressure of one or two fingers, has the patient exsanguinate the hand by making a fist or two, and then instructs the patient to relax both hand and wrist. When the noncompressed artery is patent, then the hand will flush to normal color in less than 3 seconds. When refilling is delayed, stenosis or occlusion of the noncompressed vessel is diagnosed. The maneuver can be repeated on the opposite artery. When only part of the palm or given digits fails to flush after release of the proximal occlusion, palmar arch or digital occlusive disease is confirmed. It is critical that the wrist be relaxed; the patient will often hyperextend the wrist on release of the arterial pressure, and tense ligamentous structures in the wrist can compress the artery, giving a false-positive test.[5] This can be avoided by controlling the wrist with the nonexamining hand and repeating the maneuver until satisfied the test is valid (Fig. 11–1).

BRUITS

The presence of a bruit indicates turbulent flow. This may be the result of stenosis, aneurysm, or high output states. When the bruit is continuous throughout systole and diastole, it is diagnostic of an arterial-venous fistula. The author routinely auscults the supraclavicular space and the carotid artery from the base of the neck to the mandibular angle. When a bruit is defined, its proximal or distal extent is noted. Auscultation is also performed selectively at other sites when a pulse is abnormal or an aneurysm is found. Auscultation over the neurovascular bundle in an area of scar from prior direct or interventional trauma can be productive, detecting either stenosis or fistula formation.

ANEURYSMS

When the examiner routinely checks the pulses as listed, aneurysms will be detected when present. Those rare lesions of the forearm and upper arm are usually brought to one's attention by the patient himself or herself.

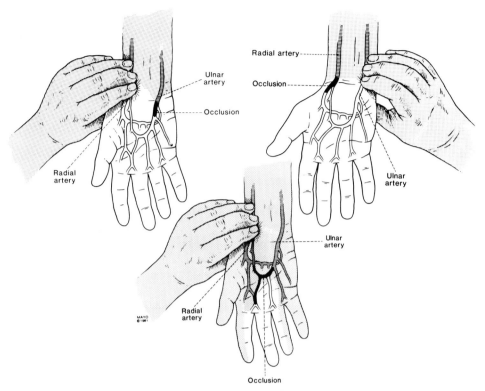

Figure 11-1. The Allen test. In all instances, an artery is occluded; the hand has been exsanguinated and subsequently released and relaxed. In the upper left, there is occlusion of the ulnar artery with distal pallor during compression, confirming ulnar occlusion. In the upper right, an occluded radial artery is documented by distal pallor after exsanguination. Note the lower picture: The ulnar artery is patent, but there is distal ischemia after release of the wrist because of incompetence of the palmar arch and digital arteries. (Courtesy Dr. J. A. Spittell, Jr., Mayo Foundation, Rochester, Minnesota.)

EXTENSIONS OF EXAMINATION

The aforementioned Allen sign is the most common extension of the arterial examination. When there is occlusive arterial disease of a major artery in the limb or hand, ischemia can be estimated by instructing patients to bring their arms up to a 90° position at their sides, as though being held up by a robber. There should be no pallor at 1 minute. When pallor occurs at lesser intervals of time, this should be recorded in seconds, which correlates with the degree of ischemia. In addition, the thoracic outlet maneuvers are important adjuncts when assessing the various outlet syndromes and will be discussed later.

ACUTE OCCLUSION

The manifestations of acute arterial occlusions of the upper extremity will depend upon the location and extent of the clot, and pre-existing status of the vascular bed, and the collateral flow. The presentation therefore is variable. Patients with occlusion of the ulnar artery but with an intact radial and palmar arch circulation may be unaware that a pulse has been lost. In contrast, occlusion of the axillary artery before the bifurcation of the brachial and profunda brachial deprives the arm of collateral flow, and the distal findings will be those of severe ischemia: marked pallor, pain, paresthesias, and eventually paralysis and tenderness of the muscles. As in acute arterial occlusion of the lower extremity, establishing an etiology is essential both for definitive treatment and, more importantly, for the prognosis of the patient.

The major sources of acute occlusion are emboli, trauma, and thrombosis in situ. In the case of the upper extremity, embolism from the heart is the most common cause of acute occlusion. The majority of emboli arise in the left atrium, predominantly from atrial fibrillation, with or without associated valvular disease. The left ventricle is the second most common source of clot, usually in association with acute myocardial infarction, but also in the setting of ventricular aneurysm, cardiomyopathy, or severe congestive heart failure. As in all acute arterial occlusions, it is essential therefore to establish the etiology and treat the primary underlying disease as well as to relieve the ischemic obstruction. Interventional procedures are probably the second most frequent cause of acute occlusion in the upper extremity. Pathology can be local occlusion owing to local arterial laceration or dissection with secondary thrombosis, arterial-venous fistula, and, on occasion, distal embolization. Proximal arterial disease is the third major cause of acute occlusion. The most common sources would be atherosclerotic occlusive disease of the origins of the brachiocephalic vessels, aneurysms of these vessels, and the thoracic outlet syndrome.[6,7]

It is desirable to restore all acutely occluded arteries to their prior status, but this is not always feasible owing to technical factors or to concomitant serious cardiac or systemic disease. Embolic lesions from cardiac sources can be treated by balloon embolectomy with a high degree of success. Both atrial and ventricular thrombus can be suppressed by anticoagulants to prevent further emboli. When the embolus is an infected fragment from valvular endocarditis, initial sterilization of the blood and subsequent repair of the valve are usually required. Arterial occlusion secondary to direct trauma by accident or intervention should be carefully defined by arteriography. Techniques of local repair by direct suture, patch grafts, and interposition grafts are successful, but long-term patency rates drop off. Repair is always indicated in the face of significant ischemia, local hematoma, concomitant nerve compression, or distal embolus.[7-9]

CHRONIC OCCLUSIVE DISEASE

Atherosclerotic occlusive disease of the upper extremities is confined predominantly to the orifices and first few centimeters of the innominate, left subclavian, and occasionally right subclavian artery. The lesions may be stenotic or complete occlusions, and that of the left subclavian is the most frequent. The majority manifest simply as a reduced blood pressure in the involved limb and are asymptomatic. Even in the face of total occlusion, few patients experience claudication. Occlusive disease of the left subclavian artery at its origin has its importance as an embolic source, the debris usually being of modest size and causing digital and occasionally palmar artery occlusions. This is an infrequent event, but once embolism occurs, it tends to be repetitive, and surgical exclusion of the proximal subclavian with bypass grafting to the adjacent left carotid or the aorta is a treatment of choice (Fig. 11–2). Unrecognized significant stenosis of the subclavian may jeopardize a left internal thoracic (mammary) artery bypass graft to the heart either by subsequent

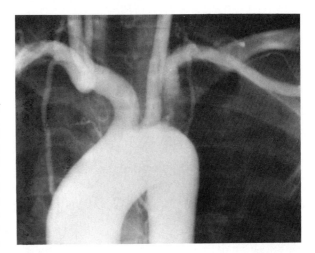

Figure 11–2. Significant stenosis of left subclavian artery at its takeoff. This 42-year-old woman presented with infarction of digits 2, 3, and 4 of the left hand and had been treated as vasculitis with high-dose prednisone. The contralateral right hand had no findings. The left subclavian artery was transected and reimplanted on the left carotid. Amputation of several digits was required.

occlusion or embolization. This can be avoided usually by screening with bilateral blood pressure readings, though some prefer an additional injection of contrast material at the time of coronary catheterization to assess patency of the left subclavian artery.

It is common for neuroradiologists to observe reverse flow in the left vertebral artery coming from the cerebral circulation to the left arm in the face of proximal stenosis of the left subclavian artery. This is frequently termed the *subclavian steal syndrome.* Indeed, there is a steal in terms of flow, yet the word "syndrome" is usually not justified in that there are no symptoms related to this altered collateral flow in the majority of instances. Furthermore, when neurologic symptoms are associated with this flow pattern, in the majority of instances they are attributable to occlusive disease in the extracranial carotid or intercranial vessels rather than in the vertebral artery itself. In an evaluation of 156 patients with stenosis of the left subclavian artery, 61 demonstrated reverse flow in the vertebral-left subclavian system. Neurologic symptoms occurred in 112 patients with subclavian artery stenosis, but the symptoms were explained by other extracranial occlusive disease in 98 of these patients. This particular study identified only 9 patients whose neurologic symptoms were presumptively related to the steal itself.[9] There remains, however, a group of patients with primary proximal subclavian artery ulcerative and stenotic lesions who can embolize through the ipsilateral vertebral artery and thereby exhibit transient vertebrobasilar insufficiency. Such patients can be successfully treated by surgical removal or exclusion of the proximal subclavian site.[10]

Stenotic or occlusive disease of the innominate artery is less frequent than that of the left subclavian artery but far less innocuous. The actual incidence of the process and its rate of complication are unknown. However, when complications do occur, they are typically embolic episodes to the brain causing transient ischemic attack, fixed stroke, amaurosis fugax or vertebrobasilar insufficiency, and, to a lesser degree, upper extremity ischemia. When identified, direct repair by endarterectomy, bypass grafting with exclusion of the lesion, or interposition grafting is successful, durable, and of low mortality[11] (Fig. 11–3).

The internal carotid artery remains the major source in the brachiocephalic system of emboli causing transient ischemic attacks or stroke. The author, however,

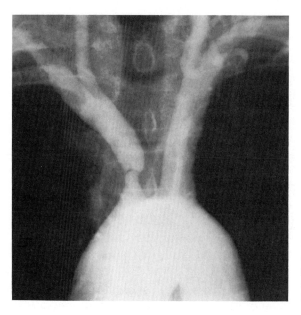

Figure 11–3. This 52-year-old male had three episodes of amaurosis fugax in the antecedent 6 months; carotid angiography that did not include the arch was "normal." The innominate artery lesion was treated by endarterectomy.

makes a plea that the proximal innominate and subclavian arteries not be forgotten at the time of angiography inasmuch as the lesions are quite amenable to repair, and they explain some embolic episodes that are overlooked when attention is drawn to the carotid arteries alone.

ANEURYSMS

Upper extremity aneurysmal disease is uncommon. Only 73 patients with brachiocephalic aneurysms were noted over a 40-year period at a large referral center for vascular disease.[13] During that same period, 300–400 operations were done annually for occlusive arterial disease of the lower extremities and a similar number for aneurysmal disease of the abdominal aorta. In this experience, 41 patients had subclavian artery aneurysms, 25 patients had carotid artery aneurysms, and only 6 patients had innominate artery aneurysms. Atherosclerosis was the most common etiologic factor followed by a few instances of trauma. Fibromuscular dysplasia was responsible for about a quarter of the carotid artery aneurysms. Other less common causes included local dissection, infection, prior endarterectomy or anastomosis, cystic medial disease, and radiation. All carotid aneurysms were palpable, and about half of those of the subclavian and innominate arteries could be felt in the supraclavicular space. At the time of presentation, 64% of the carotid aneurysms had already embolized, causing transient ischemic attacks or a stroke. Neurologic complications were present at presentation in approximately 10% of the subclavian artery aneurysms and a third of those with innominate lesions. Almost half of those patients with subclavian artery aneurysms had embolized also to the arm causing pulse deficits and claudication, and in two patients causing tissue loss. Rupture is rare in all limb aneurysms and occurred in only 3 of the 41 patients with subclavian artery lesions; infection was responsible for 2 of these. Proximal brachiocephalic aneurysms warrant repair to prevent embolic complications in the cerebral and limb circulations (Fig. 11–4).

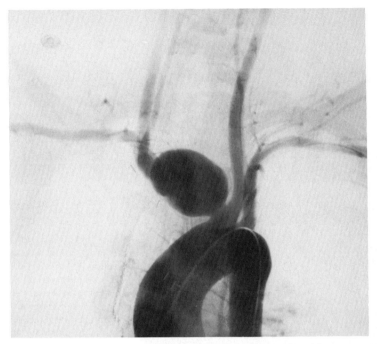

Figure 11–4. Right subclavian artery aneurysm was defined by arteriography, after abnormal shadow was noted on chest roentgenogram for "general examination." The patient was a 74-year-old male without symptoms. In retrospect, aneurysm was palpable above the clavicle when searched for. There had been no embolic complications, and the lesion was removed prophylactically and an interposition synthetic graft placed.

Aneurysms in the axillary space may represent an extension of the poststenotic dilation of a thoracic outlet syndrome, or on rare occasion the Ehlers-Danlos syndrome. Aneurysms of the hand, wrist, forearm, and upper arm distal to the axilla are predominantly explained by direct trauma or infection that is usually embolic from endocarditis (Fig. 11–5). Aneurysms of the intrathoracic vessels, brachiocephalic vessels, and upper extremities are amenable to resection and direct grafting.[12,13]

SELECTED UNCOMMON PROBLEMS

Acute and chronic occlusive lesions and aneurysmal disease of the upper extremity parallel the examination, diagnostic, and therapeutic information of the lower extremity. There are an additional six entities that are an intrinsic part of the differential diagnosis of upper extremity arterial syndromes. A profile of each follows.

THROMBOANGIITIS OBLITERANS

Buerger's disease is characterized by occlusive arterial disease in youthful users of tobacco, predominantly males, which begins in the toes and feet and then progresses over a few years to involve all of the vessels of the calves and occasionally higher. Disease is always bilateral, and in 30% to 70% the upper extremity will be

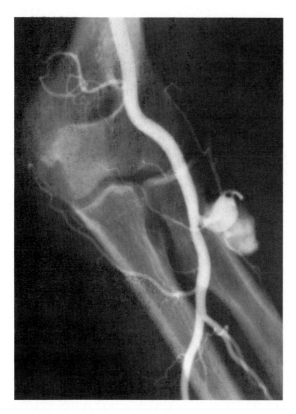

Figure 11–5. This 39-year-old male had fever of 100 to 102° F for approximately 6 months. Pulsatile mass in the left forearm prompted medical opinion. Similar, larger mass was present in the right inguinal area. Diagnosis of bacterial endocarditis was established by cardiac examination and blood cultures, which were positive for *Streptococcus viridans.* Both aneurysms were excised and local repair accomplished after sterilization of the blood.

involved and on occasion will be the presenting complaint. Patients usually initially experience periungual infarcts or slow healing of minor hand wounds, Raynaud's phenomenon on cold exposure, and then gradually develop ischemic ulcers following trauma or infection, with loss of phalanges. Progress of the disease inevitably stops when tobacco use is aborted, but progression is almost inevitable if tobacco is continued even in small amounts. Ischemic lesions are treated with gentle debridement and local amputation. On rare occasions, reconstructive surgery has been feasible in the lower extremity but not in the arm or hand. Vasodilating drugs such as prazosin or nifedipine sometimes reduce pain and promote healing, but only if tobacco has been stopped. Sympathectomy plays a similar, supportive role.[14,15]

VIBRATION SYNDROME

High-frequency, vibratory tools such as chain saws, jackhammers, grinders, and riveting devices can induce a characteristic clinical problem after several years of use. This is called the vibration syndrome. In their first few years, the patients will experience dysesthesias of the involved hand, occasionally with Raynaud's phenomenon, but only during the time of the use of the instrument. Subsequently they will develop dysesthesias and cold sensitivity that is persistent outside the environment of the vibratory tool, and eventually they may have reduced appreciation of touch and temperature in the involved hand. After several years a late stage can be frank digital artery occlusion with cyanosis, ulceration, and gangrene. This syndrome is recognized by careful attention to the occupational history.[16]

PALMAR OCCLUSIVE DISEASE OF OCCUPATIONAL ORIGIN

In the author's experience, the most common source of occlusive disease in the hands and digits in males results from the use of the palm of the hand as a hammer. Most commonly, the patient utilizes the hypothenar eminence either at work or at home as a hammer, striking wrenches, levers, milk can covers, and so on, in a repetitive fashion. This results in intimal injury to the ulnar artery as it crosses the hamate bone at its hook, and eventually the artery either becomes aneurysmal and embolizes or occludes. This may result in Raynaud's phenomenon, but more commonly, repetitive episodes of occlusive disease of the digital arteries of various fingers of the hand. The usual distribution of lesions is on the ulnar side, but because of variations in the arch, the lesions may be on fingers two or three, or even the thumb. Occupational occlusive disease occurs commonly in the dominant hand, but many occupations require the use of the contralateral, less dominant hand, so the occupational history must be careful and thorough. In early episodes the lesions will heal spontaneously, but with repetitive episodes, local amputation, with or without sympathectomy, is required for healing. Most importantly, the primary lesions in the palm must be identified by arteriography. If aneurysmal disease is present, the aneurysm can be removed, and in the presence of an intact deep or superficial palmar arch, healing will take place. Direct excision and graft repairing of ulnar artery lesions has had a low patency, but direct microsurgical repair of ulnar and palmar lesions is feasible with a high degree of immediate success in selected cases. The durability of such repairs remains to be defined.[17,18]

It should be added that on two occasions the author has observed occupational occlusive disease of the thenar eminence. In both instances the symptoms occurred after only a few days of direct trauma to the thenar eminence, and both patients experienced cyanosis, pain, and sensitivity of the distal phalanx of the thumb and index finger. Arteriography demonstrated occlusion of the arteries supplying the base of the thumb and first finger, with distal embolization. Both patients healed without sequelae save minor sensitivity to cold, in that the syndrome was recognized early and there were no repetitive episodes. The trauma was identified in one patient as repetitive stapling utilizing the thenar eminence, and in the second, holding a heavy sharp-edged bound volume for several hours in the grasp of the index and thumb.

THORACIC OUTLET SYNDROME

The majority of patients having compression of the neurovascular bundle in the thoracic outlet present with various syndromes of pain of the upper extremity, shoulder, face, and neck. Approximately 5% to 20% of patients, however, will impinge predominantly the artery, causing a focal stenosis at the level of the clavicle. This eventually occludes in a few patients, but more commonly forms a poststenotic dilation. This can frequently be felt either above or below the clavicle. Subsequently, the arterial lesions can induce (1) Raynaud's phenomenon, (2) microembolization with repetitive episodes of digital ischemia, or (3) macroembolization with acute occlusion of the named arteries of the forearm, causing acute

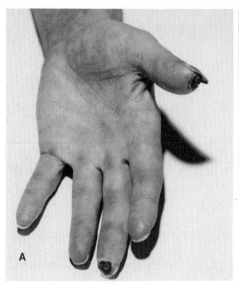
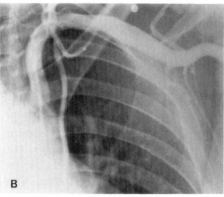

Figure 11–6. (*A*) Digital infarct in a 26-year-old male house painter. For approximately 4 years he reported Raynaud's phenomenon of fingers 2 to 5 on cold exposure. Finger ulcer following minor trauma developed 3 weeks before assessment. Previous diagnosis had been thromboangiitis obliterans. (*B*) Arch arteriogram of the patient in Fig. 11–6*A*. Note poststenotic dilation at clavicle in fine shadow in this area. At surgery this represented the focus for multiple microemboli. Repair consisted of resection of cervical and first ribs, and saphenous vein interposition graft of the axillosubclavian artery.

ischemia and subsequent claudication. In several cases all of these components will be present in the same patient. In a carefully recorded experience, Kieffer[19] delineated 38 patients with vascular symptoms requiring decompression of the thoracic outlet during a time frame in which 187 similar operations were performed for patients with neurologic symptoms only. It was noteworthy that aneurysmal lesions predominated and that all except three of the patients had an abnormal osseous structure on the involved side, predominantly cervical ribs, and an occasional abnormal first rib or injured clavicle. Of note, cervical ribs are best defined by cervical spine roentgenograms and are often easily missed on the standard chest roentgenogram. Once defined, the treatment is surgical with three goals: first, removal of the osseous defect and creation of more space in the outlet by removal of the first rib; second, repair of the proximal arterial aneurysm or stenosis; and, third, relief of any distal ischemia by means of embolectomy and/or sympathectomy. The patients should be observed. Approximately half will have a similar osseous deficit on the other side and a small number of these will develop an arterial lesion (Figs. 11–6*A* and 11–6*B*)

TEMPORAL ARTERITIS

Approximately 10% of patients with temporal arteritis will experience extracranial occlusive arterial disease. In its typical setting, the syndrome is easily diagnosed by the sequential occurrence of systemic symptoms such as fever, malaise, or weight loss, followed by significant headaches and a visible, tender, inflamed temporal or occipital artery. A sedimentation rate exceeding 60 mm/h (often greater than 100 mm/h) and a normochromic, normocytic anemia almost invariably accompany the disease. However, diagnosis may be subtle because any one of the aforementioned symptoms may predominate, suggesting a systemic disease, or because aged patients sometimes fail to remember the series of events that occurred prior to their presentation. Finally, as the appreciation of this diagnosis has become established, it has been recognized that fewer than 50% of the patients will have an identifiable abnormal temporal artery.

The extracranial arterial manifestations of temporal arteritis occur between the third and the sixth month in patients who have not been treated or who have not been treated adequately. The most commonly involved arteries are the brachioaxillary, profunda femoris, and superficial femoral, with lesser frequencies of involvement of the vessels of the upper arm, visceral arteries, and coronary and cerebral vessels. On rare occasions, the process can cause aneurysmal disease of the ascending, descending, or abdominal aorta. On rare occasions, involvement of the ascending aorta will result in acute dissection and death by pericardial tamponade.

The arterial lesions are characterized by multiple, focal, long taperings, often with poststenotic dilations, and generous collateral formation. The process will lead to occlusion of the involved artery over a period of 2 to 4 months. Limb involvement is almost always bilateral. Presentation of simultaneous onset of bilateral symmetric claudication of the arms or legs progressing over a period of just a few weeks or 2 or 3 months is pathognomonic of temporal arteritis when symptoms involve the upper extremity and very strongly suggestive of it when symptoms occur in the lower extremity. This presentation warrants diagnostic arteriography. The films are typical (Fig. 11–7). Ischemic complications are extremely rare and

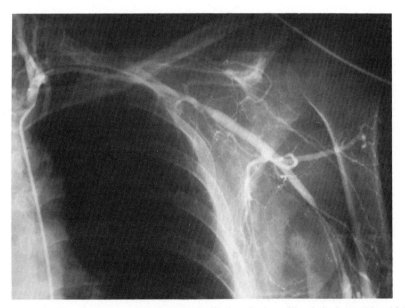

Figure 11–7. Typical focal taperings with poststenotic dilations in the axillosubclavian and brachial portions of the left upper extremity. Similar lesions occurred on the right side. The patient was a 62-year-old housewife who in the antecedent 3 months lost detectable blood pressure and pulses in the upper extremity, and experienced claudication with three or four brushes of her hair and while cleaning her teeth. ESR was 118 mm/h, and she gave a history of "flu-like illness" 4 months earlier. Temporal artery biopsy was positive.

usually result because of trauma distal to a long-standing occlusion. Of signal importance, suppressive steroid therapy can reverse the process and return pulsatile flow and blood pressure if initiated before the lesions occlude completely. Even when complete occlusion has taken place, steroid therapy is valuable inasmuch as some improvement in peripheral flow, documented by Doppler indices, can be expected.[20]

TAKAYASU'S ARTERITIS

Takayasu's arteritis, a chronic inflammatory arteriopathy presumed to be of autoimmune origin, occurs predominantly in females in the second, third, and fourth decades. Although the major descriptions have come from the Orient, it is clear the disease has its distribution in most racial and ethnic groups throughout the world. Because of its low incidence and random appearance in time and place, over 30 eponyms have been assigned to this disease process. Perhaps the most correct is nonspecific aortoarteritis, a term preferred by the Japanese Ministry of Health. Sixty to seventy percent of the patients will experience a few weeks or months of subtle or dramatic systemic symptoms similar to temporal arteritis: fever, malaise, myalgias, frank arthritis, and cutaneous disease. However, the remainder of patients may first present with occlusive disease of the brachiocephalic arteries and, to a lesser degree, those of the leg. The aorta is involved pathologically in almost all patients with focal irregularities, stenosis, and occasionally aneurysms of a modest degree. Branch vessel involvement occurs predominantly where the vessel leaves the aorta (Fig. 11–8A), but additional distal lesions are also encountered and in the upper extremity may mimic temporal arteritis, both in

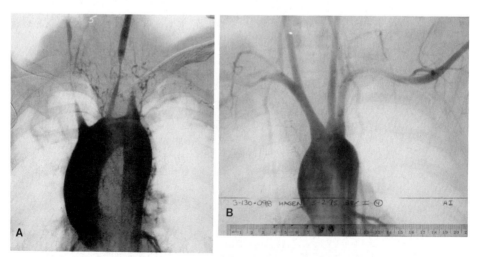

Figure 11–8. (*A*) Classic tapered lesions of the proximal innominate, left common carotid, and left subclavian arteries with slight irregularities of the thoracic aorta are typical of Takayasu's arteritis. Note sparring of the internal carotid artery. This 32-year-old female had no cerebral symptoms. (*B*) This 34-year-old woman presented with abdominal angina. Arteriography confirmed complete occlusion of the superior mesenteric and celiac arteries at their origin, and significant stenosis of both renal arteries at their origin. Note focal taperings of the subclavian arteries bilaterally, identical in appearance to those seen with temporal arteritis.

appearance and behavior (Fig. 11–8*B*). The most critical lesions are those producing stenosis of the renal vasculature, causing severe renal vascular hypertension. The most common cause of death is from the complications of renal vascular hypertension. A less frequent but highly dramatic pattern of presentation occurs in the patients with severe stenosis of the common carotid arteries, resulting in hypoperfusion and occasionally visual symptoms (Fig. 11–8*B*).

When the disease is encountered in the active phase, it has been established that steroid therapy will suppress progression of the arteritis and allow healing of stenotic vessels. There is recognized, however, a late phase in which the arteritis is inactive, but gradual fibrosis can cause late occlusion. Steroid therapy, and sometimes cytotoxic therapy, is indicated to control the acute phase. The principles of reconstructive surgery have been widely applied to this disease, with renal artery stenosis the most frequent surgical indication, followed by bypass grafting from the aorta to the internal carotids for some patients with hypoperfusion, and occasional operations for aneurysmal disease or limb claudication. It is important that surgery not be undertaken when the disease is active, at which time there is a propensity for stenosis at the suture line.[21]

SUMMARY

Occlusive and aneurysmal diseases of the large vessels of the upper extremity are uncommon experiences in most practices. Yet, by utilizing basic principles learned in the lower extremity that emphasize proper historic and physical examination, and by the selective use of angiography, these problems can be delineated and effectively treated. Some of the variations in anatomic location and the natural histories of some conditions more prevalent in the upper extremity have been emphasized.

REFERENCES

1. Machleder, HI (ed): Vascular Disorders of the Upper Extremity. Future Publishing, Mt. Kisco, New York, 1990.
2. Pearce, WH and Yao, JST (eds): Upper extremity ischemia. Seminars on Vascular Surgery. WB Saunders, Philadelphia, 1990.
3. Spittell, JA, Jr: Occlusive arterial disease of the upper extremities. Cardiovasc Clin 13(2):59, 1983.
4. Colemann, SS and Ansun, BJ: Arterial patterns in the hand based upon a study of 650 specimens. Surg Gynecol Obstet 113:409, 1961.
5. Kamienski, RW and Barnes, RW: Critique of the Allen test for continuity of the palmar arch assessed by Doppler ultrasound. Surg Gynecol Obstet 142:861, 1976.
6. Sachatello, CR, Ernst, CB, and Griffen, WO, Jr: The acutely ischemic upper extremity: Selective management. Surgery 76:1002, 1974.
7. Davies, MG, O'Malley, K, Feeley, M, et al: Upper limb embolus: A timely diagnosis. Ann Vasc Surg 5:85, 1991.
8. McCarthy, WJ, Flinn, WR, Yao, JST, et al: Results of grafting for upper limb ischemia. J Vasc Surg 3:741, 1986.
9. McCready, RA, Procter, CD, and Hyde, GL: Subclavian-axillary vascular trauma. J Vasc Surg 3:24, 1986.
10. Walker, PM, Paley, D, Harris, KA, et al: What determines the symptoms associated with subclavian artery occlusive disease. J Vasc Surg 2:154, 1985.
11. Ricotta, JJ, Ouriel, K, Green, RM, et al: Embolic lesions from the subclavian artery causing transient vertebrobasilar insufficiency. J Vasc Surg 4:372, 1986.
12. Brewster, DC, Moncure, AC, Darling, C, et al: Innominate artery lesions: Problems encountered and lessons learned. J Vasc Surg 2:99, 1985.

13. Bower, TC, Pairolero, PC, Hallett, JW, Jr, et al: Brachiocephalic aneurysms: The case for early recognition and repair. Ann Vasc Surg 5:125, 1991.
14. Lie, JT: The rise and fall and resurgence of thromboangiitis obliterans (Buerger's disease). Acta Pathol Jpn 39:153, 1989.
15. Hirai, M and Shionoya, S: Arterial obstruction of the upper limb in Buerger's disease: Its incidence and primary lesion. Br J Surg 66:124, 1979.
16. Vibration Syndrome: Current Intelligence Bulletin 38. National Institute Occupational Safety and Health, 1982.
17. Conn, J, Jr, Buerger, JJ, and Bell, JL: Hypothenar hammer syndrome: Posttraumatic digital ischemia. Surgery 68:1122, 1970.
18. Mehlhoff, TL and Wood, MB: Ulnar artery thrombosis and the role of interposition vein grafting: patency with microsurgical technique. J Hand Surg 16:274, 1991.
19. Kieffer, E: Arterial complications of thoracic outlet syndrome. In Bergen, JJ and Yao, JST (eds): Evaluation and Treatment of Upper and Lower Extremity Circulatory Disorders. Grune & Stratton, New York, 1984.
20. Klein, RG, Hunder, GG, Stanson, AW, et al: Large artery involvement in giant cell (temporal) arteritis. Ann Intern Med 83:806, 1975.
21. Hall, S, Barr, W, Lie, JT, et al: Takayasu arteritis: A study of 32 North American patients. Medicine (Baltimore) 63:89, 1985.

CHAPTER 12

Vascular Diseases
of the Cervical Carotid Artery

Irene Meissner, M.D.
Bahram Mokri, M.D.

The cervical carotid artery provides the anatomic substrate of rather limited categories of vascular pathology, including atherosclerotic occlusive disease, dissection, and fibromuscular disease. Nonetheless, it boasts one of the most controversial reputations in regard to natural history and treatment options concerning, in particular, pressure-significant carotid occlusive disease.

This chapter reviews the main categories of vascular disease of the carotid artery. Pathophysiology and pathology, clinical presentation and diagnostic studies, prognosis, and management issues are discussed.

ATHEROSCLEROTIC DISEASE OF THE CERVICAL CAROTID ARTERY

PATHOPHYSIOLOGY

Atherosclerosis is the most common cause of occlusive disease of the extracranial cervical carotid artery. The pathogenesis of atherosclerosis is still incompletely understood, although the pathologic features of advancing stages of the arteriosclerotic process in response to vessel injury have been described. This process includes platelet adhesion and aggregation in areas of endothelial damage, intimal hyperplasia secondary to smooth muscle proliferation, formation of connective tissue matrix elastin and collagen, and the deposition of intracellular and extracellular lipids.

Although the progression of atherosclerosis is clearly age-related, other risk factors including hypertension, diabetes, hyperlipidemia, and coagulation abnormalities also have been implicated in acceleration of the atherosclerotic process.[1-4] Interacting effects of these variables make the independent contribution of any single marker or risk factor for atherosclerosis difficult to assess. Adding to the complexity of the pathophysiology are recent observations of interactions between lipid and lipoprotein atherogenic properties and procoagulant factors within blood.[5] The balance between fibrinolysis and thrombosis is regulated by various coagulation factors: factors VII and VIII, von Willebrand's factor, and plasma proteins, including protein C, protein S, tissue plasminogen activator, and fibrinogen.[6–13] Platelets have been implicated increasingly in the pathogenesis of atherosclerosis by several mechanisms, including their attachment to subendothelium after vascular or endothelial injury. Platelets may subsequently release growth factor and stimulate the proliferation of smooth muscle cells in the intima.[14,15]

Exogenous effects such as radiation to the cervical region also may accelerate the atherosclerotic process.

VASCULAR PATHOLOGY

The anatomic substrate of carotid stenosis has been extensively analyzed, including the classic studies by Fisher and colleagues[16] and Torvik and Jörgensen.[17]

The natural history of carotid occlusive disease reflects a dynamic phenomenon. The so-called fatty streak refers to histologically identified, intimal lesions consisting of lipid deposits within subendothelial smooth muscle cells that do not cause vessel obstruction. Stenosis and occlusion are caused by arteriosclerotic plaque, with or without associated hemorrhage or thrombosis (Fig. 12–1). The histologic composition of advanced atherosclerosis includes a core of lipid deposits and atheromatous debris surrounded by smooth muscle cells, collagen, elastic fibers, and proteoglycans. Plaques may become ulcerated and give rise to arterial emboli consisting of either atheromatous debris or superimposed bland thrombus, common in the extracranial carotid artery but rarely encountered in intracranial arteries (Figs. 12–2 and 12–3). Postulated mechanisms for producing occluding arteriothrombosis include an endothelial surface damaged by an ulcerated plaque or intramural hemorrhage into a plaque.[18] These processes are accelerated by systemic factors such as hypertension and diabetes. Other stages of arteriosclerosis include

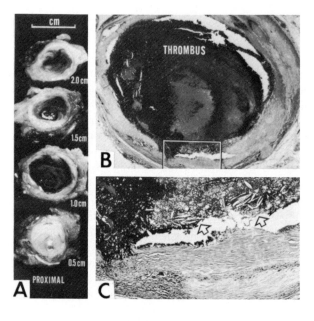

Figure 12–1. (*A*) Serial, equal-thickness cross sections of internal carotid artery demonstrating near occlusion at most proximal segment (0.5 cm) due to atherosclerotic disease, with acute thrombosis in distal three sections. (*B*) Cross section of occluded artery at 1.0 cm from its origin. (Hematoxylin and eosin.) (*C*) Enlarged view of boxed area in *B*, revealing plaque rupture and extruded atheromatous debris mixed with thrombus. (From Lie,[62] by permission of Mayo Foundation.)

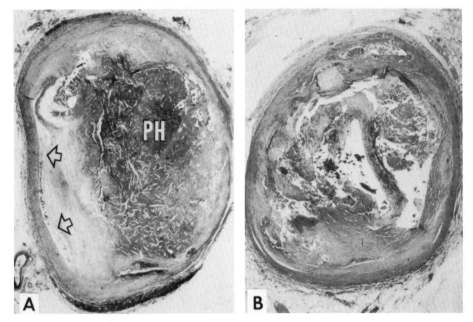

Figure 12-2. Cross section of advanced atherosclerosis of internal carotid artery. (*A*) Plaque hemorrage *(PH)* in large eccentric intimal plaque results in compression of lumen *(arrows)*. (*B*) Plaque ulceration and rupture, the nidus for distal embolization of atheromatous material. (From Lie,[62] by permission of Mayo Foundation.)

antegrade thrombus extension, usually to the first sizable collateral branch and thrombus-plaque organization with eventual lumen recanalization.

Dolichoectasia or fusiform dilatation reflecting an atherosclerotically weakened vessel is a relatively common finding of little clinical significance in the extracranial carotid artery, usually occurring in the vicinity of the carotid bifurcation. In contrast, arteriosclerotic dilatation of intracranial vessels may cause symptoms via mass effect or by acting as a nidus for thromboembolic phenomena.

THE "PRESSURE-SIGNIFICANT" LESION

The commonly referred to "hemodynamically significant" or "pressure-significant" arterial stenosis is the degree of luminal narrowing beyond which further small decrements in luminal area would result in an abrupt reduction in pressure and flow rate distal to the stenosis, the so-called critical stenosis.[19,20] Hemodynamically significant stenosis varies directly with the effective cross-sectional area of an artery and inversely with velocity of blood flow. Hemodynamic studies have shown that a reduction in pressure may be observed when the vessel luminal diameter is decreased by 50%, corresponding to a cross-sectional decrease of 75%. Under routine conditions, normal blood flow still may be present; however, under conditions requiring augmentation of blood flow, this degree of narrowing may act as a critical stenosis. Significant compromise in blood flow may occur when the luminal stenosis approaches 75%. Information regarding the presence or absence of pressure-significant carotid occlusive disease is useful in guiding patient management and selecting appropriate potential surgical candidates.

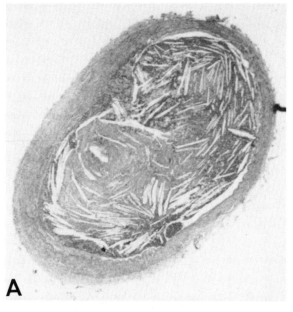

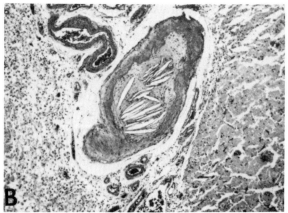

Figure 12–3. (*A*) Cross section of recent atheromatous embolus in middle cerebral artery. Note typical needle-shaped cholesterol–fatty acid crystals in embolus. (Hematoxylin and eosin.) (*B*) Organized atheromatous embolus within branch of middle cerebral artery. (Hematoxylin and eosin.) (From Okazaki, H.: *Fundamentals of Neuropathology.* Igaku-Shoin Limited, Tokyo, p. 25, 1983, by permission of the publisher.)

CLINICAL FEATURES

The clinical syndromes reflect ischemia in the territory of the cervical carotid artery branches, namely the ophthalmic, middle cerebral, and anterior cerebral arteries. The events may be transient as in amaurosis fugax or cerebral transient ischemic attack (TIA) or last more than 24 hours and cause retinal or cerebral infarction in the aforementioned vascular territories. Involvement of the dominant hemisphere may cause different combinations of aphasia, apraxia, hemiparesis, or hemisensory deficit as well as cognitive or behavioral changes with frontal lobe involvement.

A clear, uniform definition of a clinical hemodynamic event has, however, eluded clinicians, and correlation of the clinical event with the underlying vascular abnormality is a challenging task.

THE ASYMPTOMATIC PATIENT: BRUIT OR STENOSIS—WHO CARES?

The identification of patients with asymptomatic, hemodynamically significant internal carotid system lesions has increased dramatically with the development of reliable noninvasive diagnostic studies such as carotid ultrasonography and oculoplethysmography (OPG).[21] The carotid bruit often becomes the focal point when discussing cerebrovascular disease in the asymptomatic patient. However, although carotid bruits are well-recognized markers for generalized atherosclerotic disease, they are not necessarily predictive of the degree of underlying carotid stenosis, having been found in the absence of, or in association with, various degrees of carotid stenosis.

Despite a plethora of literature devoted to the asymptomatic localized carotid bruit, its prognostic importance is still poorly understood.[22-24] This stems in part from the inclusion of heterogeneous patient pools consisting of those with strokes contralateral to the carotid with the bruit, lacunar infarcts, and intracranial hemorrhage as well as cardioembolic events.[25]

In a prospective study of 1004 patients who had undergone carotid arteriography for all causes, Ingall and associates[26] assessed the predictive value of carotid bruit for moderate to severe atherosclerosis. Diffuse or localized bruits were equally predictive of moderate to severe extracranial carotid occlusive disease but were poor predictors of intracranial carotid system pathology. It is likely that the natural history of asymptomatic patients is different from that of asymptomatic vessels within patients who have had previous ischemic events in other vascular territories.

Wiebers and coworkers[27] studied the predictive value of diffuse and localized carotid bruits with regard to TIA, ischemic and hemorrhagic stroke, and death in a sample of patients with a bruit compared with a population-based control group known not to have a carotid bruit. Patients with an asymptomatic carotid bruit were approximately three times more likely to have an ischemic stroke than the bruit-free control group, with an actuarial stroke rate of 1.5% per year or 7.5% at 5 years.

In a retrospective study of patients with and without OPG-determined pressure-significant carotid system lesions, Meissner and associates[28] observed an actuarial stroke rate of 3.4% per year during a 4-year period, irrespective of the existence of an underlying bruit. These results suggest that the presence of a pressure-significant lesion, as defined by OPG, may be a better predictor of future cerebral ischemic events than the presence of a bruit alone.

DIAGNOSTIC EVALUATION

Noninvasive Studies

The advent and technologic advancements within the noninvasive vascular laboratory have enhanced the accuracy of detection and quantification of extracranial carotid occlusive disease.

These studies can be subdivided best into two groups—indirect and direct techniques. The indirect techniques use physiologic hemodynamic measurements within distal ophthalmic and external carotid arterial systems to provide data about the more proximal internal carotid system. The direct techniques focus on the carotid bifurcation area, providing physiologic information and vessel wall imaging data. Limitations of these techniques include the inability to reliably distinguish high-grade stenosis from occlusion, to identify intraplaque hemorrhage, and to detect ulceration.

INDIRECT TECHNIQUES

Ophthalmodynamometry (Retinal Artery Pressures). A calibrated hand-held ophthalmodynamometer is used to compare relative and absolute abnormalities in retinal systolic arterial pressures. These values reflect pressure-significant disease in the ipsilateral internal carotid system, proximal to and including the central retinal artery. The results of this study are not easily reproduced, and although it is used as a quick bedside screening test of retinal or carotid vascular disease, it generally has been superseded by the techniques mentioned below.

Oculoplethysmography. OPG[21,29] measures the ocular systolic pressure in relation to the brachial systolic pressure via the gradual reduction of a preselected vacuum administered via scleral eye cups. Abnormal values are suggestive of an internal carotid system pressure-significant lesion. Portability, easy reproducibility, low cost, and rapid administration make this a useful study, particularly for sequential testing such as before and after endarterectomy.

Periorbital Directional Doppler Ultrasonography. This technique assesses the direction and quality of periorbital Doppler flow at rest and after digital arterial compression maneuvers; it is an indirect measure of compensatory collateral supply via the external carotid circulation.

DIRECT TECHNIQUES—ULTRASOUND IMAGING TECHNIQUES. These techniques include frequency spectral analysis, real-time B-mode ultrasonography (B scanning), and duplex sonography combining Doppler and B-scan studies. Direction of flow determinations can be made; however, this information has only limited value in the study of the cervical carotid artery. Velocity profiles are defined; the frequency shift is proportional to the velocity and produces a velocity spectrum in which widths generally parallel the degree of turbulence of flow through the artery at the site sampled. The Doppler spectrum from a normal vessel with laminar flow has a peak frequency below 4 kHz. Widening of the frequency range during systole, the so-called spectral broadening, and high peak frequencies occur with tighter stenoses. Real-time B-mode ultrasonography, with ever-improving image resolution, allows for the identification of arterial walls by the reflected signal, which can be distinguished from veins by the pulsatility characteristics. Plaques within the carotid artery have been found to vary considerably in sonic qualities, ranging from echolucent to echo-dense, representing the so-called soft plaque versus hard plaque, respectively.[30]

SUMMARY. Overall, invasive and noninvasive studies are directed toward the detection of hemodynamically significant carotid occlusive disease—approximately 75% cross-sectional area stenosis.[31] Limitations of the indirect studies include the inability to quantitate the degree of occlusive disease or to visualize the bifurcation region; direct techniques are confounded by nonarteriosclerotic arterial kinking, high carotid bifurcations, body habitus (stout, short necks), or acoustic shadowing of calcific plaques.

Tremendous advances in magnetic resonance technology have led to magnetic resonance angiography as an exciting new noninvasive modality uniquely adapted to the evaluation of vascular structures, including the cervical carotid artery.[32] Once the limitations in spatial resolution, volume imaging, and motion-related signal loss of preliminary studies are overcome, this technique may ultimately decrease the need for invasive screening angiography.

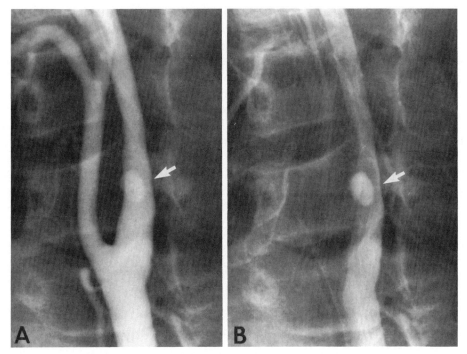

Figure 12–4. (*A*) Right carotid angiogram demonstrating 1-cm deep ulcer in right internal carotid artery *(arrow)*. (*B*) Note that with dye washout, ulcer crater remains filled *(arrow)*.

Invasive Studies

Cerebral angiography is currently the standard imaging technique for the detection of extracranial and intracranial carotid occlusive disease. Digital subtraction angiography is limited by often poor visualization of the intracranial circulation. Although angiography cannot define plaque pathology, it is helpful in estimating the presence or absence of large mural thrombi and in identifying ulceration (Fig. 12–4), even though it may not accurately predict intraplaque hemorrhage or the rostrocaudal extent of the plaque. The carotid slim sign[33] is caused by the apparent diffuse narrowing of the entire internal carotid artery (ICA) distal to a high-grade stenosis, due to a decrease in the intraluminal perfusion pressure of the vessel. This finding usually reflects ipsilateral marginal cerebral perfusion and may identify patients at higher risk for cerebral ischemic events as well as complications of postoperative cerebral hyperperfusion.[34]

THERAPEUTIC MODALITIES

At the basis of all forms of management is preventive therapy. No treatment focused on mitigating the ischemic insult itself will alter the natural history of the underlying disease process, particularly in regard to the progression of atherosclerosis. In this regard, emphasis on risk factor management—i.e., treatment of hypertension, hyperlipidemia, and concomitant cardiac disease—must not be overlooked. An understanding of the mechanisms underlying focal ischemia is crucial to planning rational treatment options. For example, the management of a presumed hypertensive lacunar event is significantly different from that of a presumed large vessel thrombotic event related to cervical carotid artery stenosis. Therefore, a careful history by an experienced clinical interpreter is essential and facilitates selection of appropriate diagnostic tests and subsequent therapeutic interventions.

Medical Treatment

The medical therapeutic modalities may be divided into two major categories: agents that increase cerebral blood flow (CBF) and thereby cerebral perfusion, and those affording cytoprotection by decreasing neuronal energy requirements and attenuating degradative metabolic cascade reactions.[35]

In the first category (increased CBF), existing and potential future treatment options include

1. Antithrombotic agents
   a. Anticoagulant therapy to prevent the formation of fibrin, which maintains stability of the early platelet thrombus
   b. Antiplatelet agents for prevention of platelet aggregation and adherence to a region of endothelial injury
2. Calcium channel blockers
3. Serotonin antagonists
4. Thrombolytic therapy, including streptokinase and tissue plasminogen activator (t-PA)

The controversy about the use of aspirin in carotid occlusive disease has not been resolved. There have been more than 30 trials of antiplatelet therapy for patients with a history of TIA, minor stroke, unstable angina, or myocardial infarction that involved close to 30,000 patients. A recent meta-analysis of these data revealed that allocation to antiplatelet treatment had no apparent effect on nonvascular mortality; however, the vascular mortality rate decreased by 15% and nonfatal vascular events (stroke or myocardial infarction) by 30%.[36] There still are controversies regarding the comparative efficacy of low- versus high-dose aspirin therapy[37,38] and the sex predilection of effect.[39,40] Ticlopidine hydrochloride, a recently developed antiplatelet agent, produced an approximately 30% reduction of relative risk of recurrent stroke compared with placebo[41] and a 20% reduction of risk of initial or recurrent stroke after ischemic symptoms compared with aspirin.[42] Although approval by the Food and Drug Administration is still pending, this drug may become a future treatment option, particularly for patients who are failures on or intolerant of aspirin therapy.

Calcium channel blockers and serotonin antagonists are appealing therapeutic candidates in that their potential use is based on known mechanisms of ischemic injury. They may, therefore, provide a rational intervention in future treatment of acute stroke. Preliminary safety, tolerability, and efficacy studies of t-PA are in progress.[43,44]

Surgical Treatment

THE SYMPTOMATIC PATIENT. Population-based studies and clinical trials of patients with symptomatic carotid occlusive disease have yielded stroke rate estimates of 10% in the first month after the initial TIA and 5% to 6% per year thereafter with antiplatelet or anticoagulant therapy.[45,46]

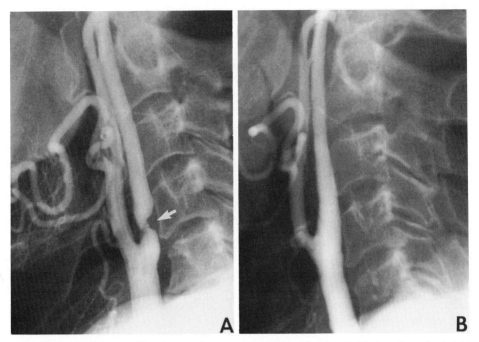

Figure 12–5. (*A*) Right carotid angiogram demonstrating high-grade, ulcerated lesion of proximal right internal carotid artery just above bifurcation *(arrow)*. (*B*) Right carotid angiogram after right carotid endarterectomy and saphenous vein patch graft. Note smooth reconstitution of vascular lumen.

A recent review of the effectiveness and durability of carotid endarterectomy in a series of 252 consecutive patients undergoing 282 carotid endarterectomies revealed an overall 1% operative minor morbidity, no major morbidity, and a 0.7% mortality. The actuarial cumulative probability of ipsilateral stroke was 1.5% at 1 month and 2% at 5 years.[47] After the initial report of carotid endarterectomy in 1954, the procedure was performed with increasing frequency, reaching a peak of 107,000 in 1985 and decreasing dramatically thereafter to an estimated 81,000 in 1987.[48,49] The decline paralleled the increased recent scrutiny of this procedure within the medical community and the subsequent initiation of several randomized clinical trials to address the risk/benefit ratio of carotid endarterectomy in patients with symptomatic carotid occlusive disease. Published operative risks have ranged from approximately 3% to 21%.[50–53] The variability probably reflects a combination of reporting bias, the medical and radiographic risk grade of the patient,[54,55] the technical skill of the surgeon, anesthetic issues, and possibly the type of repair (vein patch graft versus primary closure) (Fig. 12–5).

A recent study examining the risk of carotid endarterectomy in patients more than 70 years of age demonstrated an overall combined operative morbidity and mortality rate of 4.4%, which correlated well with preoperative arteriographic and clinical risk grading categories.[56] An earlier series[57] identified an actuarial incidence of all strokes after successful endarterectomy of approximately 2% per year in the symptomatic patient, which, when taken with the aforementioned promising surgical results, suggests that with a low perioperative morbidity and mortality, carotid endarterectomy has the potential to decrease the long-term risk of stroke. The ongoing clinical trials may shed more light on this important controversy.

Another carotid system revascularization procedure, the superficial temporal artery–to–middle cerebral artery anastomosis or extracranial-intracranial (EC-IC) bypass procedure, was, in years past, a rather frequently performed procedure in symptomatic patients with internal carotid artery occlusion or stenosis of the surgically inaccessible ICA and in patients with stenosis or occlusion of major middle cerebral artery branches. After a much publicized multicenter international trial failed to reveal a benefit of this procedure in decreasing stroke rates in patients with the aforementioned atherosclerotic disease of the ICA system, the frequency of performing the EC-IC bypass procedure decreased dramatically.[58] The conclusions reached by the trial revealed no improvement in stroke morbidity during a 5-year period within the population examined. To further identify subgroups of patients that may benefit from this procedure, such as patients with medically refractory profound hemodynamic cerebral ischemic events or those with progressive venous stasis retinopathy, would be methodologically challenging and require further controlled studies with substantial sample sizes.

THE ASYMPTOMATIC PATIENT. Currently, antiplatelet therapy along with risk factor regulation is the mainstay of medical management for the patient with asymptomatic carotid occlusive disease. The risk-to-benefit ratio of carotid endarterectomy in the asymptomatic patient has not been clearly elucidated and awaits the results of ongoing clinical trials.[59]

NONATHEROSCLEROTIC DISEASE OF THE EXTRACRANIAL CAROTID ARTERY

ANATOMIC VARIANTS

Kinking and coils of extracranial carotid arteries may occur in isolation or associated with atherosclerotic aneurysms or fibromuscular dysplasia (FMD).[60,61] Symptoms may occur on the basis of flow reduction or stasis with associated plaque formation and distal embolism. Kinking usually occurs in association with pre-existing tortuosity, particularly in the elderly. The independent contribution of these anatomic changes to the pathophysiology of cerebral ischemia is uncertain.

FIBROMUSCULAR DYSPLASIA

Dysplasia of the cervical carotid artery is often an incidental finding on angiograms performed for unrelated reasons. This entity, a segmental, nonatheromatous angiopathy of indeterminate origin, is thought to represent a developmental abnormality that affects primarily intermediate-size muscular arteries.[62] Autosomal dominant inheritance with reduced penetrance in males has been postulated[63] as well as the occurrence of FMD in association with intracranial aneurysms.[64]

Although distinguishing histologic types of FMD have been reported, the categories of medial fibroplasia and perimedial dysplasia account for at least 95% of known cases of FMD. Histopathologic hallmarks of FMD include the characteristic irregular, undulating segments of constriction, caused by abnormal hyperplastic and fibrotic media, and dilatation representing hypoplastic or absent media. Angiographically, this is seen as the typical "string of beads" or "corkscrew" appearance (Fig. 12–6).[65,66]

The symptomatic presentation generally involves a focal cerebral ischemic event in a young or middle-aged woman, typically in the absence of atherosclerotic

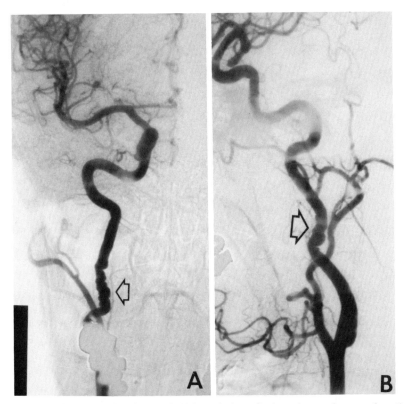

Figure 12–6. (*A*) Anteroposterior view, and (*B*) lateral view of subtraction angiogram of medial fibroplasia involving cervical carotid artery. Note typical "string of beads" appearance reflecting concentric narrowing and dilatation typical of this condition *(arrowheads).*

risk factors other than hypertension. Although fibromuscular disease can present with a clinical stroke picture similar to that of carotid occlusive disease, this disorder tends to spare the proximal 1- to 2-cm portions of the ICA reserved for atherosclerotic lesions. The frequency of subsequent cerebral ischemic events after diagnosis is rare, reflecting a benign process in most cases. However, reported complications include aneurysm formation, rupture, and arterial dissection. Medical and surgical therapeutic intervention should be guided by the presence of progressive cerebral ischemic symptoms.[67] Surgical techniques have included excision of the affected segments by using autogenous vein graft replacement, repair by patch angioplasty, transluminal balloon angioplasty, and graduated internal dilatation.

Dissection of the Cervical Internal Carotid Artery

Dissections of the ICAs occur when circulating blood penetrates into the arterial wall, splits the media, and forms a false lumen.[68] The true lumen of the ICA is often compressed by the intramural hematoma and is narrowed. Sometimes, the false lumen may expand toward the adventitia and form an aneurysmal dilatation. These are called *dissecting aneurysms* (Fig. 12–7). Use of terms such as "pseudoaneurysm" or "false aneurysm" in these situations is inappropriate. False or pseudoaneurysms are paravascular encapsulated hematomas. Although they are con-

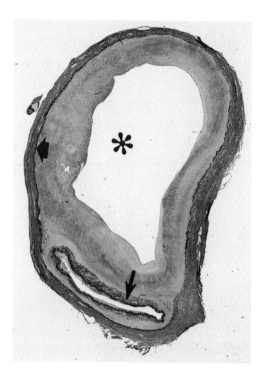

Figure 12–7. Cross section through dissecting aneurysm of extracranial internal carotid artery. True lumen is surrounded by internal elastic lamina *(arrow).* Dilated false lumen *(asterisk),* which is sac of dissecting aneurysm, has compressed true lumen. Both true lumen and false lumen are surrounded by external elastic lamina and adventitia *(arrowhead).* One can clearly see that the dissecting aneurysm is formed within layers of the media.

nected with the lumen of the artery, they are not formed from elements of blood vessel wall. Dissections may involve the cervical or intracranial segments of the ICA. The cervical (or extracranial) dissections are much more common. Dissections of the common carotid artery or external carotid artery are quite rare. ICA dissections are called *spontaneous* when no overt trauma is reported, although a trivial trauma cannot be entirely excluded in all cases.[69] They are called *traumatic* when there is a history of a definite head or neck injury.

Spontaneous and traumatic dissections of ICA will be discussed. These dissections are uncommon but not rare.

Spontaneous Dissections of the Internal Carotid Arteries

The first case was reported in 1954.[70] There were subsequent sporadic reports. As clinicians and radiologists have become increasingly familiar with the clinical and angiographic features of this entity, it has been reported with increased frequency in the past two decades and several large series have been published.[71-74] More than 120 cases of spontaneous ICA dissection were seen at the Mayo Clinic prior to 1990.

ETIOLOGY AND PATHOGENESIS. A primary arterial disease has been documented in at least some of these patients. Angiographic evidence of FMD is found in the renal artery, nondissected opposite ICA, or vertebral artery of about 15% of the patients.[71,72] Cystic medial necrosis has been described, especially in the earlier autopsy reports.[75-77] ICA dissection also has been observed in association with Marfan's syndrome.[78] A contributory role of trivial trauma cannot be excluded in some cases. Of interest is the simultaneous occurrence of dissections of both ICAs, with or without additional vertebral artery dissections in the absence of any trauma,

Table 12–1. Frequency of Symptoms and Signs in 80 Patients with Spontaneous Internal Carotid Artery Dissections

	Patients	
Symptom or Sign	No.	%
Headache	66	83
Focal cerebral ischemic symptoms	48	60
TIA*	27	
Stroke	14	
TIA and stroke	7	
Oculosympathetic paresis	40	50
Bruits	34	43
Neck pain	17	21
Lightheadedness	17	21
Syncope	8	10
Amaurosis fugax	11	14
Scalp tenderness	6	8
Neck swelling	3	4
Dysgeusia	3	4
Lower cranial nerve palsies	3	4
Asymptomatic	1	1

*TIA, transient ischemic attack.

From Meissner, I: Carotid artery disease: Medical management. In Dzau, VJ, and Cook, JP (eds): Current Management of Hypertension and Vascular Disease. BC Decker, Philadelphia (in press). By permission of Mosby—Year Book.

major or trivial. Whether there are other unknown underlying arteriopathies that subject the vessel to dissection is not clear at this time. Rare cases of familial occurrence of spontaneous ICA dissections have been reported.[79]

CLINICAL MANIFESTATIONS

Age at Onset and Gender. Some series report a higher incidence in males. We have encountered more female patients with spontaneous ICA dissection. In a review of 80 patients, 46 were women and 34 were men.[80] The mean age was 44 years, and more than 40% of the patients were between 40 and 50 years old. Therefore, in terms of stroke age, these are fairly young patients. ICA dissection is one of the important causes of stroke in younger patients.

Symptoms and Signs. Symptoms and signs in 80 patients with spontaneous ICA dissections are listed in decreasing order of frequency in Table 12–1. Headache was by far the most common manifestation, and in more than 75% of the patients, it was the initial manifestation. The headaches often are unilateral and focal and frequently occur in the frontal, orbital, and periorbital regions. Other locations include deep in the ear, mastoid region, angle of the mandible, or temporal and occipital regions. In contrast to what one might expect, neck pain is far less frequent than headache. Focal cerebral ischemic symptoms may occur in the form of TIAs (most common), stroke, or both. They often, although not always, follow a unilateral headache after a period of delay ranging from a few minutes to several days.

Oculosympathetic palsy (incomplete Horner's syndrome) is encountered in about half of the patients. This is manifested by ptosis and miosis but not by change in the sweating of the face. Sympathetic fibers that subserve the sweat glands of the face accompany the external carotid artery and therefore are not affected, whereas sympathetic fibers for the eyes follow the ICA and therefore may be affected with ICA dissections.[81]

Bruits are detected or reported in more than 40% of the patients. These can be subjective (heard by the patient but not by the examiner), objective (heard by the examiner but not by the patient), or both.

Some patients present only with lower cranial nerve palsies. Cranial nerves IX, X, XI, and XII may be affected.[82] Some patients may present only with a hemilingual weakness.[83]

At times, ICA is asymptomatic and is detected incidentally during workup for a symptomatic spontaneous vertebral artery dissection.

Although various combinations of the symptoms and signs listed in Table 12–1 may occur, the most common manifestation of the disease is unilateral headache followed after a delay by cerebral ischemic symptoms.[72] The second most common presentation is unilateral headache and oculosympathetic palsy ipsilateral to the headache.[81] These syndromes may or may not be associated with subjective or objective bruits. Sometimes, a combination of the aforementioned two syndromes may be seen.

DIAGNOSIS

Noninvasive Studies. Measurement of retinal artery pressures or OPG shows decreased pressure when there is significant stenosis or occlusion. These simple techniques could be particularly helpful in follow-up of patients when an occluded artery recanalizes or when a stenosis becomes less significant or resolves.

Magnetic resonance imaging shows absence of flow void when there is occlusion. It may show a hyperintense signal related to intraluminal hemorrhage. Sometimes the hyperintense signal is seen as a bright crescent surrounding the narrowed lumen, which is seen as a small area of flow void.[84] Carotid duplex sonography is another noninvasive technique. Although sonographic abnormalities have been described in carotid dissection, ICA dissections usually, although not invariably, occur quite distal to the bifurcation and beyond the range of carotid ultrasound. The Doppler signal may indicate significant reduction in blood flow.

Any of the noninvasive tests or combinations of them as well as intravenous digital subtraction angiography and magnetic resonance imaging angiography are helpful in the follow-up of these patients. However, at this time, conventional angiography remains the main test to document presence of carotid dissection, extent and degree of stenosis, associated dissecting aneurysms, presence of occlusion, and presence of any abnormalities in the nondissected cervicocephalic vessels.

Angiographic Findings. The major angiographic findings in spontaneous ICA dissections are listed in Table 12–2 in decreasing order of frequency.[69,85]

Luminal stenosis is the most common finding. This is usually an elongated and irregular and frequently tapered stenosis that often extends to the carotid canal (Fig. 12–8). It usually involves the cervical segment but may involve cervical and intracanalicular segments or even may extend to the cavernous segment.

Fairly abrupt reconstitution of the lumen is the second most common angiographic finding. This usually occurs at the level of entrance of the ICA into the carotid canal (Fig. 12–8).

Dissecting aneurysms occur in more than one-third of these patients (Fig. 12–

Table 12–2. Angiographic Findings in 104 Internal Carotid Arteries (of 80 Patients) Involved by Spontaneous Dissection

Finding	Arteries	
	No.	%
Luminal stenosis	81	78
Abrupt reconstitution of lumen, often at carotid canal	42	40
Aneurysms associated with dissecting vessel	41	39
Intimal flaps	30	29
Slow ICA-MCA* flow	26	25
Occlusion	17	16
Distal branch occlusions (emboli)	12	12

*ICA, internal carotid artery; MCA, middle cerebral artery.

9). They are usually, but not always, subcranial or in the upper third of the cervical segment of the ICA. They may be saccular or elongated and fingerlike.

Intimal flaps can be of various lengths (Figs. 12–9 and 12–10). Slow internal carotid-middle cerebral artery flow is observed in connection with marked luminal stenosis. Occlusions of the ICA secondary to ICA dissections often occur distal to

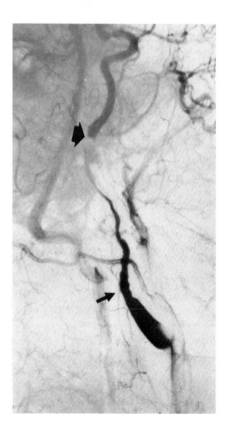

Figure 12–8. Right brachial arteriogram, lateral view, showing severe, elongated, tapered, and irregular stenosis of lumen of extracranial internal carotid artery *(arrow),* extending into intracanalicular portion of vessel. Note fairly abrupt reconstitution of lumen distal to stenosis *(arrowhead).* (From Mokri et al,[81] by permission of Mayo Foundation.)

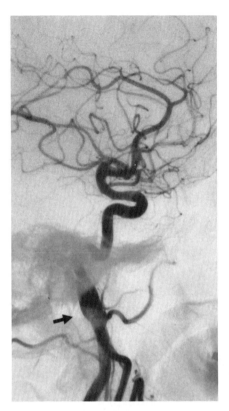

Figure 12–9. Left carotid arteriogram demonstrating dissecting aneurysm of extracranial internal carotid artery (ICA) *(arrow).* Note intimal flap between dissecting aneurysm and narrowed lumen of ICA.

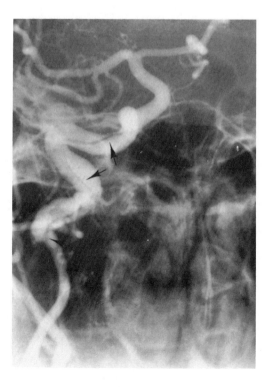

Figure 12–10. Dissection of right internal carotid artery. Note long intimal flap *(arrows).* Double-barrel lumen is formed. (From Houser et al,[85] by permission of the American Roentgen Ray Society.)

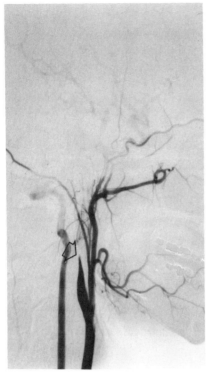

Fig. 12-11

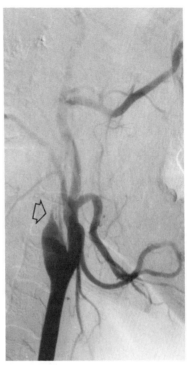

Fig. 12-12

Figures 12-11 and 12-12. Right carotid angiograms demonstrating occlusion of right internal carotid artery as result of dissection. Occlusion often occurs 1 or 2 cm distal to bifurcation and usually tapers to point, resembling configuration of flame (Figure 12-11, *arrowhead*) or radish tail (Figure 12-12, *arrowhead*).

the carotid bulb and usually taper to a point and resemble the appearance of a candle flame or radish tail (Figs. 12-11 and 12-12).

Occlusion of the distal cerebral branches (angiographic evidence of distal embolization) is found in more than 10% of the patients.

SPONTANEOUS MULTIVESSEL DISSECTIONS. Spontaneous ICA dissections are bilateral in about 30% of these patients (Fig. 12-13). Concomitant or simultaneous spontaneous vertebral artery dissections are encountered in about 6% of the patients. Additional renal artery dissection is observed in 5% of the patients (Fig. 12-14).[80,86]

TREATMENT. This is an uncommon disease. There are no collaborative or controlled studies, and no infallible method of management has emerged. Immediate mortality from massive cerebral infarction has been reported but is uncommon. Several surgical approaches have been tried. In decreasing order of enthusiasm for the results, these have included removal of intramural hematoma, arterial resection with vein graft replacement, graduated dilatation, ligation, and superficial temporal artery–middle cerebral artery bypass. One common practice is to use anticoagulant therapy for 3 to 4 months followed by antiplatelet therapy for a similar period. The patient can be followed by noninvasive techniques. One cannot make a strong argument for a definite need for repeat follow-up angiography in all patients because the majority of these patients do well regardless of the method of treatment. However, the point should be made that noninvasive tests do not reach the

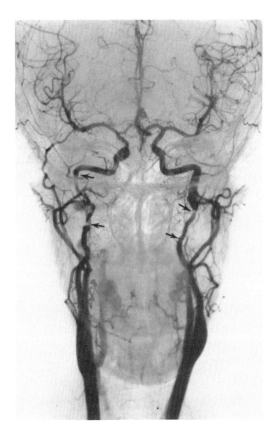

Figure 12-13. Bilateral internal carotid artery dissection manifested by elongated, irregular, narrowed segments *(arrows)* and fairly abrupt reconstitution of lumen at distal end of stenosed segments (subtracted left and right carotid angiograms, superimposed and photographed).

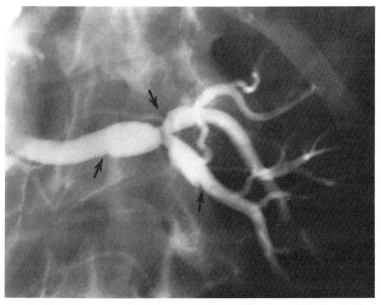

Figure 12-14. Spontaneous dissection of left renal artery in patient with bilateral spontaneous dissections of carotid arteries. Left renal arteriogram shows dissection of main and lower primary branches *(bottom arrows).* Note stenosis of bifurcation of primary branches *(top arrow).* (From Mokri,[69] by permission of Mayo Foundation.)

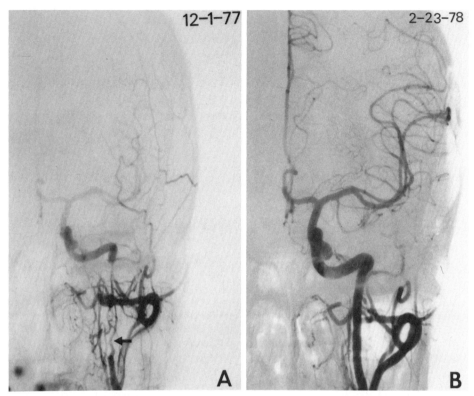

Figure 12–15. (*A*) Left carotid angiogram on December 1, 1977, shows left internal carotid artery dissection manifested by elongated stenosis *(arrow)* and abrupt reconstitution of lumen at distal end of stenotic segment. (*B*) Repeat angiography on February 23, 1978, shows almost complete resolution of stenosis.

accuracy of conventional angiography for demonstrating the shape of the lumen, configuration and degree of any residual stenosis, presence of residual dissecting aneurysms, or intimal irregularities. Surgical treatment of a residual dissecting aneurysm that has been a source of embolization should be carried out when technically possible.

PROGNOSIS. Despite the disconcerting angiographic features, most patients do quite well.[70,71,80] In our experience, up to 90% of the stenoses completely or partially resolve (Fig. 12–15); more than 60% of the aneurysms resolve angiographically (obliterate) or become smaller (Fig. 12–16). Recanalization of a completely occluded ICA by spontaneous dissection is quite uncommon. Clinically, more than 85% of these patients make excellent or complete clinical recovery. We have not yet encountered an instance of rupture of an extracranial ICA dissecting aneurysm or recurrence of dissection in the same vessel. However, in fewer than 10% of the patients, further dissections may occur in the opposite carotid artery, vertebral artery, or renal arteries.

Traumatic Dissections of Extracranial Internal Carotid Artery

Despite the relatively high frequency of cervical trauma, trauma to the cervical ICA is uncommon. Dissection of the extracranial ICA may occur in connection with penetrating or blunt trauma. Blunt injuries are usually related to motor vehicle

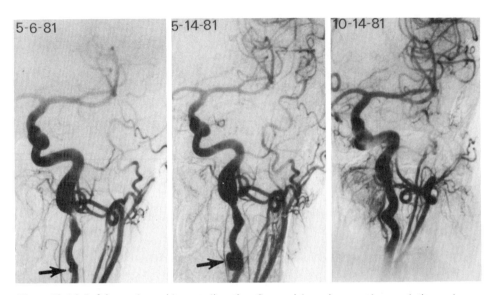

Figure 12–16. Left internal carotid artery dissection. Sequential arteriograms show evolution and resolution of dissecting aneurysm and resolution of stenosis. On arteriogram of May 6, 1981, narrowed segment is noted. A tiny aneurysm *(arrow)* can be identified. On May 14, 1981, size of aneurysm has significantly increased *(arrow),* although there is no significant change in stenosis. Arteriogram on October 14, 1981, shows complete resolution of stenosis and disappearance of aneurysm. (From Mokri,[69] by permission of Mayo Foundation.)

accidents, although other causes such as falls, blows, fist fights, sports injuries, carotid artery compression, hanging by the neck, local surgical procedures, and manipulative therapy have been reported.[71,87–89] ICA dissection also may occur in connection with blunt intraoral trauma. In particular, this may occur in children who fall on their face while carrying an elongated object (such as a pencil) in their mouth.[90] Carotid artery dissection also may occur in connection with needle puncture angiography but much less commonly from arterial catheterization.

Penetrating injuries may puncture the arterial wall and cause paravascular hematoma (which may encapsulate and lead to formation of a false aneurysm), arteriole-venous connections, arterial dissections, or thrombosis. Blunt carotid injuries may lead to dissection, thrombosis, or both. Abrupt neck flexion may lead to compression of the ICA between the upper cervical vertebral column and the angle of the mandible (Fig. 12–17A). Hyperextension or rotations of the neck may cause ICA injury[91] by stretching the vessel against the transverse process of C-2 and C-3 (Fig. 12–17B). Flexion and extension injuries are commonly encountered in association with motor vehicle accidents, which, in our experience, are the most common cause of traumatic ICA dissections due to blunt injuries. Direct signs of injury are absent in about half of these patients.[89] Even in the remaining half, such signs are often minor (such as mild bruises or skin abrasions). Fractures of the mandible, neck, and base of the skull, however, may be present in some of these patients. Although reported, evidence of primary arterial disease (such as FMD) in traumatic ICA dissections is rare.[92]

Clinical manifestations of traumatic ICA dissections may vary. In severe accidents, particularly when the patient is comatose or if multiple organ injuries have occurred, traumatic ICA dissections may go undiagnosed. Suspicion of traumatic ICA dissection should arise when after trauma, lateralizing signs develop that can-

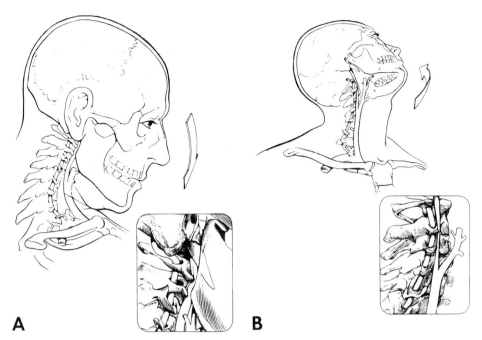

Figure 12-17. (*A*) Severe neck flexion may lead to compression of internal carotid artery (ICA) between angle of mandible and upper cervical spine (impingement injury). (*B*) Hyperextension and rotation of neck may lead to stretching of cervical segment of ICA against transverse processes of second and third vertebral bones (stretch injury). (From Zelenock et al,[91] by permission of the American Medical Association.)

not be explained by imaging findings as direct cerebral posttraumatic events. Cerebral angiography should be performed when possible. Patients who survive severe injuries and in whom ICA dissections go undiagnosed may be neurologically intact or may have neurologic deficits that are often attributed to "head injury." Some of these patients may be left with residual posttraumatic dissecting aneurysms, which, at a later date (even months or years later), may become symptomatic by causing cerebral ischemic events (TIAs or strokes) as the result of embolization from a thrombus within the aneurysm (Fig. 12–18).

Posttraumatic ICA dissection is more likely to be detected in patients who are not comatose or who have not suffered multiple organ injury. Patients with posttraumatic dissections most commonly present with cerebral ischemic symptoms delayed from the accident by a variable time. Development of Horner's syndrome, amaurosis fugax, TIAs, or bruits (particularly in younger patients) may help to draw attention to ICA dissection. Although some of the patients may die as the result of massive cerebral infarction and edema and some are left with significant neurologic deficits, most make a good recovery. Angiographic findings in traumatic ICA dissections are essentially similar to those in spontaneous ICA dissections. However, in our experience, dissecting aneurysms occur more frequently with the traumatic dissections, fewer aneurysms resolve or become smaller, and fewer stenoses resolve or improve, whereas more stenoses progress to occlusion. Traumatic dissections appear more likely to leave the patients with neurologic deficits.[87]

TREATMENT. During the acute phase of the disease, anticoagulant therapy should be considered when there are suggestions of progression of neurologic defi-

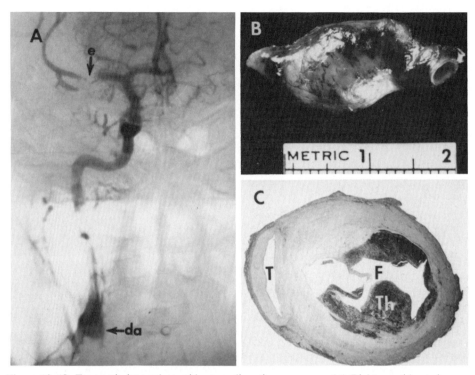

Figure 12–18. Traumatic internal carotid artery dissecting aneurysm. (*A*) Right carotid arteriogram demonstrates dissecting aneurysm (*da*) of extracranial internal carotid artery at level of C-2 and presumed embolus (*e*) lodged at proximal part of right middle cerebral artery. (*B*) Gross appearance of aneurysm after its resection. (*C*) Cross section of specimen demonstrates true lumen of internal carotid artery (*T*) as well as false lumen of aneurysm (*F*) and appearance of thrombus (*Th*) within aneurysmal sac. (*A* and *C* from Mokri et al,[96] by permission of Mayo Foundation.)

cits related to focal cerebral ischemia, thromboembolism, and distal embolization.[93–95] However, anticoagulation therapy may not be possible or may be contraindicated when there is evidence of cerebral or visceral trauma. In the absence of symptoms of cerebral ischemia in these posttraumatic patients, one might have difficulty justifying anticoagulant therapy. There might be a rationale for using antiplatelet agents. When dissection is confined to the proximal portion of the ICA, surgical repair may be possible in some cases. In more distal dissections, sometimes superficial temporal–middle cerebral artery bypass may be beneficial. In acute cases, the decision for operation must be made cautiously. In long-standing cases with residual dissecting aneurysms that cause embolization, resection of the aneurysm should be done when technically possible.[96,97]

NONDISSECTING ANEURYSMS OF THE CERVICAL INTERNAL CAROTID ARTERY

These aneurysms are quite rare. They are often atherosclerotic in origin, although in the earlier literature, infectious causes—including syphilis and contiguous infection originating in the pharynx or mastoid—were reported. These aneurysms may be fusiform or saccular. In contrast to the dissecting aneurysms, they may grow continuously and may rupture and bleed[61,96,98,99] (Figs. 12–19 and 12–20).

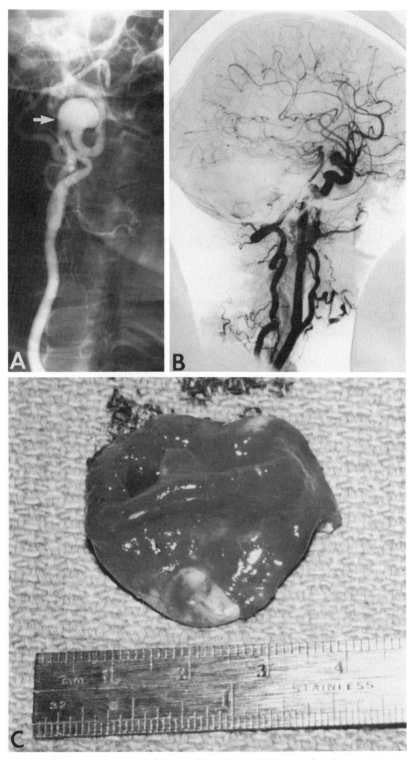

Figure 12–19. (*A*) Preoperative lateral right carotid angiogram demonstrating giant aneurysm over cervical internal carotid artery *(arrow),* of apparently spontaneous development. (*B*) Postoperative subtraction angiogram reviewing excision of aneurysm. The vessel was repaired with a saphenous vein patch graft. (*C*) Pathologic appearance of excised aneurysm, approximately 2.5 cm.

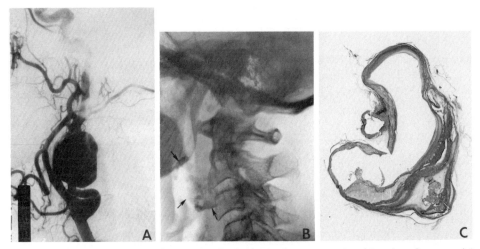

Figure 12–20. (*A*) Left carotid angiogram showing large saccular aneurysm in midportion of extracranial internal carotid artery. (*B*) Calcifed shell of aneurysm can be seen in plain radiograph *(arrows)*. (*C*) Section through wall of aneurysm demonstrating atherosclerotic changes with large deposits of lipid and calcium. (*A* and *B* from Mokri, B and Piepgras, DG: *Cervical internal carotid artery aneurysm with calcific embolism to the retina.* Neurology 31:211, 1981. By permission of Edgell Communications. *C* from Mokri et al,[96] by permission of Mayo Foundation.)

Clinical Manifestations

These aneurysms may present with cerebral or retinal ischemic symptoms. However, not infrequently they may present as pulsating, tender, or nontender masses externally at about the angle of the mandible, or internally in the lateral pharyngeal wall at about the tonsillar fossa.[80] Dysphagia may develop as the result of the local mass effect or as the result of compression of the nerves supplying the pharyngeal muscles or the tongue. Ipsilateral oculosympathetic palsy or headaches may occur. If these aneurysms are left untreated, they may cause complications related to the rupture of the aneurysm (bleeding from mouth, ear, or nose), or complications resulting from the local mass effect (dysphagia, stridor, cranial nerve palsies, oculosympathetic palsy), or complications resulting from embolization (TIAs, stroke, amaurosis fugax, visual field defect).

Treatment

When possible, the resection of the aneurysm is the treatment of choice, particularly in view of moderate advances in neurodiagnostic and surgical techniques. Redundant tortuosity of the ICA, especially in association with saccular aneurysms, may allow end-to-end anastomosis after resection. Otherwise, an autogenous vein graft or prosthetic graft can be used.[97]

ARTERITIS

Takayasu's arteritis, a panarteritis of unknown origin,[100] and giant cell (temporal) arteritis[101–103] may affect brachiocephalic vessels as well as the intracranial vasculature. Either may produce cerebral ischemic symptoms mimicking those of atherosclerotic cerebrovascular disease.

REFERENCES

1. Tell, GS, Crouse, JR, and Furberg, CD: Relation between blood lipids, lipoproteins, and cerebrovascular atherosclerosis: A review. Stroke 19:423, 1988.

2. Salonen, R, Seppänen, K, Rauramaa, R, and Salonen, JT: Prevalence of carotid atherosclerosis and serum cholesterol levels in Eastern Finland. Arteriosclerosis 8:788, 1988.

3. Holme, I, Enger, SC, Helgeland, A, et al: Risk factors and raised atherosclerotic lesions in coronary and cerebral arteries: Statistical analysis from the Oslo Study. Arteriosclerosis 1:250, 1981.

4. Kannel, WB, Dawber, TR, Sorlie, P, and Wolf, PA: Components of blood pressure and risk of atherothrombotic brain infarction: The Framingham Study. Stroke 7:327, 1976.

5. Seed, M, Hoppichler, F, Reaveley, D, et al: Relation of serum lipoprotein(a) concentration and apolipoprotein(a) phenotype to coronary heart disease in patients with familial hypercholesterolemia. N Engl J Med 322:1494, 1990.

6. Grotta, JC, Yatsu, FM, Pettigrew, LC, et al: Prediction of carotid stenosis progression by lipid and hematologic measurements. Neurology 39:1325, 1989.

7. Meade, TW: The epidemiology of hemostatic and other variables in coronary artery disease. In Verstraete, M, Vermylen, J, Linjnen, HR, and Arnout, J (eds): Thrombosis and Haemostasis. International Society on Thrombosis and Haemostasis and Leuven University Press, Leuven, 1987.

8. Dalaker, K, Hjermann, I, and Prydz, H: A novel form of factor VII in plasma from men at risk for cardiovascular disease. Br J Haematol 61:315, 1985.

9. Meade, TW, North, WRS, Chakrabarti, R, et al: Haemostatic function and cardiovascular death: Early results of a prospective study. Lancet 1:1050, 1980.

10. Kannel, WB, Castelli, WD, and Meeks, SL: Fibrinogen and cardiovascular disease. Abstract of paper for 34th Annual Scientific Session of the American College of Cardiology, Anaheim, CA, March 1985.

11. Stone, MC and Thorp, JM: Plasma fibrinogen—a major coronary risk factor. J R Coll Gen Pract 35:565, 1985.

12. Miletich, JP and Broze, GJ, Jr: Age and gender dependence of total protein S antigen in the normal adult population (abstract). Blood 72:371a, 1988.

13. Horellou, MH, Conard, J, Bertina, RM, and Samama, M: Congenital protein C deficiency and thrombotic disease in nine French families. Br Med J 289:1285, 1984.

14. Fuster, V and Griggs, TR: Porcine von Willebrand disease: Implications for the pathophysiology of atherosclerosis and thrombosis. Prog Hemost Thromb 8:159, 1986.

15. Myreng, Y, Aursnes, I, Hjermann, I, et al: Von Willebrand factor and cardiovascular risk. Thromb Res 41:867, 1986.

16. Fisher, CM, Gore, I, Okabe, N, and White, PD: Atherosclerosis of the carotid and vertebral arteries—extracranial and intracranial. J Neuropathol Exp Neurol 24:455, 1965.

17. Torvik, A and Jörgensen L: Thrombotic and embolic occlusions of the carotid arteries in an autopsy material. Part 1. Prevalence, location and associated diseases. J Neurol Sci 1:24, 1964.

18. Imparato, AM, Riles, TS, and Gorstein, F: The carotid bifurcation plaque: Pathologic findings associated with cerebral ischemia. Stroke 10:238, 1979.

19. Mann, FC, Herrick, JF, Essex, HE, and Baldes, EJ: The effect on the blood flow of decreasing the lumen of a blood vessel. Surgery 4:249, 1938.

20. Moore, WS, and Malone, JM: Effect of flow rate and vessel calibre on critical arterial stenosis. J Surg Res 26:1, 1979.

21. Wiebers, DO, Folger, WN, Forbes, GS, Younge, BR, and O'Fallon, WM: Ophthalmodynamometry and ocular pneumoplethysmography for detection of carotid occlusive disease. Arch Neurol 39:690, 1982.

22. Yatsu, FM and Hart, RG: Asymptomatic carotid bruit and stenosis: A reappraisal. Stroke 14:301, 1983.

23. Chambers, BR and Norris, JW: Outcome in patients with asymptomatic neck bruits. N Engl J Med 315:860, 1986.

24. Roederer, GO, Langlois, YE, Jager, KA, et al: The natural history of carotid arterial disease in asymptomatic patients with cervical bruits. Stroke 15:605, 1984.

25. Wolf, PA, Kannel, WB, Sorlie, P, and McNamara, P: Asymptomatic carotid bruit and risk of stroke: The Framingham Study. JAMA 245:1442, 1981.

26. Ingall, TJ, Homer, D, Whisnant, JP, et al: Predictive value of carotid bruit for carotid atherosclerosis. Arch Neurol 46:418, 1989.

27. Wiebers, DO, Whisnant, JP, Sandok, BA, and O'Fallon, WM: Prospective comparison of a cohort

with asymptomatic carotid bruit and a population-based cohort without carotid bruit. Stroke 21:984, 1990.

28. Meissner, I, Wiebers, DO, Whisnant, JP, and O'Fallon, WM: The natural history of asymptomatic carotid artery occlusive lesions. JAMA 258:2704, 1987.

29. Gee, W, Oller, DW, Amundsen, DG, and Goodreau, JJ: The asymptomatic carotid bruit and the ocular pneumoplethysmography. Arch Surg 112:1381, 1977.

30. Mohr, JP, Petty, GW, Duterte, DI, and Oropeza, L: Doppler vascular ultrasonography in neurology, update 2. In Rowland, LP (ed): Merritt's Textbook of Neurology, ed 8. Lea & Febiger, Philadelphia, 1989, pp 3–16.

31. Castaldo, JE, Nicholas, GG, Gee, W, and Reed, JF: Duplex ultrasound and ocular pneumoplethysmography concordance in detecting severe carotid stenosis. Arch Neurol 46:518, 1989.

32. Ross, JS, Masaryk, TJ, Modic, MT, et al: Magnetic resonance angiography of the extracranial carotid arteries and intracranial vessels: A review. Neurology 39:1369, 1989.

33. Lippman, HH, Sundt, TM, Jr, and Holman, CB: The poststenotic carotid slim sign: Spurious internal carotid hypoplasia. Mayo Clin Proc 45:762, 1970.

34. Houser, OW and Sundt, TM, Jr: Correlation of angiographic flow patterns with syndromes of ischemic stroke. In Sundt, TM, Jr (ed): Occlusive Cerebrovascular Disease: Diagnosis and Surgical Management. WB Saunders, Philadelphia, 1987, p 101.

35. Meyer, FB: Ischemic neuronal protection. Prosp Neurol Surg 1:57, 1990.

36. Antiplatelet Trialists' Collaboration: Secondary prevention of vascular disease by prolonged antiplatelet treatment. Br Med J 296:320, 1988.

37. UK-TIA Study Group: United Kingdom transient ischaemic attack (UK-TIA) aspirin trial: Interim results. Br Med J 296:316, 1988.

38. Boysen, G, Sørensen, PS, Juhler, M, et al: Danish very-low-dose aspirin after carotid endarterectomy trial. Stroke 19:1211, 1988.

39. The ESPS Group: The European Stroke Prevention Study (ESPS): Principal end-points. Lancet 2:1351, 1987.

40. Escolar, G, Bastida, E, Garrido, M, et al: Sex-related differences in the effects of aspirin on the interaction of platelets with subendothelium. Thromb Res 44:837, 1986.

41. Gent, M, Blakely, JA, Easton, JD, et al: The Canadian American ticlopidine study (CATS) in thromboembolic stroke. Lancet 1:1215, 1989.

42. Hass, WK, Easton, JD, Adams, HP, Jr, et al, for the Ticlopidine Aspirin Stroke Study Group: A randomized trial comparing ticlopidine hydrochloride with aspirin for the prevention of stroke in high-risk patients. N Engl J Med 321:501, 1989.

43. The tPA Acute Stroke Study Group: An open multicenter study of the safety and efficacy of various doses of tPA in patients with acute stroke: A progress report (abstract). Stroke 21:181, 1990.

44. Brott, T, Haley, C, Levy, D, et al: Safety and potential efficacy of tissue plasminogen activator (tPA) for stroke (abstract). Stroke 21:181, 1990.

45. The Canadian Cooperative Study Group: A randomized trial of aspirin and sulfinpyrazone in threatened stroke. N Engl J Med 299:53, 1978.

46. Whisnant, JP and Wiebers, DO: Clinical epidemiology of transient cerebral ischemic attacks (TIA) in the anterior and posterior cerebral circulation. In Sundt, TM, Jr (ed): Occlusive Cerebrovascular Disease: Diagnosis and Surgical Management. WB Saunders, Philadelphia, 1987, p 60.

47. Sundt, TM, Jr, Whisnant, JP, Houser, OW, and Fode, NC: Prospective study of the effectiveness and durability of carotid endarterectomy. Mayo Clin Proc 65:625, 1990.

48. Pokras, R and Dyken, ML: Dramatic changes in the performance of endarterectomy for diseases of the extracranial arteries of the head. Stroke 19:1289, 1988.

49. Dyken, ML: Dramatic changes in the performance of endarterectomy for diseases of the extracranial arteries of the head (letter to the editor). Stroke 20:129, 1989.

50. Kirshner, DL, O'Brien, MS, and Ricotta, JJ: Risk factors in a community experience with carotid endarterectomy. J Vasc Surg 10:178, 1989.

51. Toronto Cerebrovascular Study Group: Risks of carotid endarterectomy. Stroke 17:848, 1986.

52. Fode, NC, Sundt, TM, Jr, Robertson, JT, et al: Multicenter retrospective review of results and complications of carotid endarterectomy in 1981. Stroke 17:370, 1986.

53. Easton, JD and Sherman, DG: Stroke and mortality rate in carotid endarterectomy: 228 consecutive operations. Stroke 8:565, 1977.

54. Sundt, TM, Jr, Sandok, BA, and Whisnant, JP: Carotid endarterectomy: Complications and pre-operative assessment of risk. Mayo Clin Proc 50:301, 1975.

55. Beebe, HG, Clagett, GP, DeWeese, JA, et al: Assessing risk associated with carotid endarterectomy: A statement for health professionals by an Ad Hoc Committee on Carotid Surgery Standards of the Stroke Council, American Heart Association. Stroke 20:314, 1989.

56. Meyer, FB, Meissner, I, Fode, NC, and Losasso, TJ: Carotid endarterectomy in elderly patients. Mayo Clin Proc 66:464, 1990.

57. Whisnant, JP, Sandok, BA, and Sundt, TM, Jr: Carotid endarterectomy for unilateral carotid system transient cerebral ischemia. Mayo Clin Proc 58:171, 1983.

58. The EC/IC Bypass Study Group: Failure of extracranial-intracranial arterial bypass to reduce the risk of ischemic stroke: Results of an international randomized trial. N Engl J Med 313:1191, 1985.

59. Mayo Asymptomatic Carotid Endarterectomy Study Group: Effectiveness of carotid endarterectomy for asymptomatic carotid stenosis: Design of a clinical trial. Mayo Clin Proc 64:897, 1989.

60. Effeney, DJ, Ehrenfeld, WK, Stoney, RJ, and Wylie, EJ: Fibromuscular dysplasia of the internal carotid artery. World J Surg 3:179, 1979.

61. Schecter, DC: Cervical carotid aneurysms, parts I and II. NY State J Med 79:892;1042, 1979.

62. Lie, JT: Pathology of occlusive disease of the extracranial arteries. In Sundt, TM, Jr (ed): Occlusive Cerebrovascular Disease: Diagnosis and Surgical Management. WB Saunders, Philadelphia, 1987, p 19.

63. Mettinger, KL: Fibromuscular dysplasia of the brain. II. Current concept of the disease. Stroke 13:53, 1982.

64. Lie, JT, and Kim, H-S: Fibromuscular dysplasia of the superior mesenteric artery and coexisting cerebral berry aneurysms. Angiology 28:256, 1977.

65. Osborn, AG and Anderson, RE: Angiographic spectrum of cervical and intracranial fibromuscular dysplasia. Stroke 8:617, 1977.

66. Mettinger, KL and Ericson, K: Fibromuscular dysplasia of the brain: Observations on angiographic, clinical and genetic characteristics. Stroke 13:46, 1982.

67. Corrin, LS, Sandok, BA, and Houser, OW: Cerebral ischemic events in patients with carotid artery fibromuscular dysplasia. Arch Neurol 38:616, 1981.

68. Anderson, WAD and Scotti, TM: Synopsis of Pathology, ed 10. CV Mosby, St. Louis, 1980, p 290.

69. Mokri, B: Dissections of cervical and cephalic arteries. In Sundt, TM, Jr (ed): Occlusive Cerebrovascular Disease: Diagnosis and Surgical Management. WB Saunders, Philadelphia, 1987, p 38.

70. Jentzer, A: Dissecting aneurysm of the left internal carotid artery. Angiology 5:232, 1954.

71. Hart, RG and Easton JD: Dissections of cervical and cerebral arteries. Neurol Clin 1:155, 1983.

72. Mokri, B, Sundt, TM, Jr, Houser, OW, and Piepgras, DG: Spontaneous dissection of the cervical internal carotid artery. Ann Neurol 19:126, 1986.

73. Biller, J, Hingtgen, WL, Adams, HP, Jr, et al: Cervicocephalic arterial dissections: A ten-year experience. Arch Neurol 43:1234, 1986.

74. Fisher, CM, Ojemann, RG, and Robertson, GH: Spontaneous dissection of cervico-cerebral arteries. Can J Neurol Sci 5:9, 1978.

75. Anderson, RMcD and Schechter, MM: A case of spontaneous dissecting aneurysm of the internal carotid artery. J Neurol Neurosurg Psychiatry 22:195, 1959.

76. Boström, K and Liliequist, B: Primary dissecting aneurysm of the extracranial part of the internal carotid and vertebral arteries: A report of three cases. Neurology 17:179, 1967.

77. Brice, JG and Crompton, MR: Spontaneous dissecting aneurysms of the cervical internal carotid artery. BMJ 2:790, 1964.

78. Austin, MG and Schaefer, RF: Marfan's syndrome, with unusual blood vessel manifestations: Primary medionecrosis dissection of right innominate, right carotid, and left carotid arteries. Arch Pathol 64:205, 1957.

79. Mokri, B, Piepgras, DG, Wiebers, DO, and Houser, OW: Familial occurrence of spontaneous dissection of the internal carotid artery. Stroke 18:246, 1987.

80. Mokri, B: Spontaneous extracranial internal carotid artery dissections (ICAD) (abstract). J Neurol 237(suppl 1):S11, 1990.

81. Mokri, B, Sundt, TM, Jr, and Houser, OW: Spontaneous internal carotid dissection, hemicrania, and Horner's syndrome. Arch Neurol 36:677, 1979.

82. Waespe, W, Niesper, J, Imhof, H-G, and Valavanis, A: Lower cranial nerve palsies due to internal carotid dissection. Stroke 19:1561, 1988.

83. Lieschke, GJ, Davis, S, Tress, BM, and Ebeling, P: Spontaneous internal carotid artery dissection presenting as hypoglossal nerve palsy. Stroke 19:1151, 1988.

84. Rothrock, JF, Lim, V, Press, G, and Gosink, B: Serial magnetic resonance and carotid duplex examinations in the management of carotid dissection. Neurology 39:686, 1989.

85. Houser, OW, Mokri, B, Sundt, TM, Jr, et al: Spontaneous cervical cephalic arterial dissection and its residuum: Angiographic spectrum. AJNR 5:27, 1984.

86. Mokri, B, Stanson, AW, and Houser, OW: Spontaneous dissections of the renal arteries in a patient with previous spontaneous dissections of the internal carotid arteries. Stroke 16:959, 1985.

87. Mokri, B, Piepgras, DG, and Houser, OW: Traumatic dissections of the extracranial internal carotid artery. J Neurosurg 68:189, 1988.

88. Chandler, WF: Carotid Artery Injuries. Futura Publishing, Mount Kisco, New York, 1982.

89. Yamada, S, Kindt, GW, and Youmans, JR: Carotid artery occlusion due to nonpenetrating injury. J Trauma 7:333, 1967.

90. Pitner, SE: Carotid thrombosis due to intraoral trauma: An unusual complication of a common childhood accident. N Engl J Med 274:764, 1966.

91. Zelenock, GB, Kazmers, A, Whitehouse, WM, Jr, et al: Extracranial internal carotid artery dissections: Noniatrogenic traumatic lesions. Arch Surg 117:425, 1982.

92. Young, PH, Smith, KR, Jr, Crafts, DC, and Barner, HB: Traumatic occlusion in fibromuscular dysplasia of the carotid artery. Surg Neurol 16:432, 1981.

93. Batzdorf, U, Bentson, JR, and Machleder, HI: Blunt trauma to the high cervical carotid artery. Neurosurgery 5:195, 1979.

94. Dragon, R, Saranchak, H, Lakin, P, and Strauch, G: Blunt injuries to the carotid and vertebral arteries. Am J Surg 141:497, 1981.

95. Stringer, WL and Kelly, DL, Jr: Traumatic dissection of the extracranial internal carotid artery. Neurosurgery 6:123, 1980.

96. Mokri, B, Piepgras, DG, Sundt, TM, Jr, and Pearson, BW: Extracranial internal carotid artery aneurysms. Mayo Clin Proc 57:310, 1982.

97. Sundt, TM, Jr, Pearson, BW, Piepgras, DG, et al: Surgical management of aneurysms of the distal extracranial internal carotid artery. J Neurosurg 64:169, 1986.

98. Shipley, AM, Winslow, N, and Walker, WW: Aneurysm in the cervical portion of the internal carotid artery: An analytical study of the cases recorded in the literature between August 1, 1925, and July 31, 1936; report of two new cases. Ann Surg 105:673, 1937.

99. Winslow, N: Extracranial aneurysm of the internal carotid artery: History and analysis of the cases registered up to Aug. 1, 1925. Arch Surg 13:689, 1926.

100. Hunder, GG and Lie, JT: The vasculitides. Cardiovasc Clin 13:261, 1983.

101. Caselli, RJ, Hunder, GG, and Whisnant, JP: Neurologic disease in biopsy-proven giant cell (temporal) arteritis. Neurology 38:352, 1988.

102. Howard, GF, III, Ho, SU, Kim, KS, and Wallach, J: Bilateral carotid artery occlusion resulting from giant cell arteritis. Ann Neurol 15:204, 1984.

103. Fortner, GS and Thiele, BL: Giant cell arteritis involving the carotid artery. Surgery 95:759, 1984.

CHAPTER 13

Aneurysmal Disease

William M. Morre, Jr., M.D.
Larry H. Hollier, M.D.

Accounts of the clinical recognition of aneurysms may be found in some of the earliest records of medical practice, documented by great physicians such as Galen. However, it was not until this century that significant progress was made in the areas of diagnosis and management of aneurysmal disease. Technological advances and an aggressive approach by insightful physicians have facilitated that progress. Improved understanding of the risk factors, etiology, pathogenesis, and distribution patterns of aneurysmal disease now permits a more objective approach in the management of these patients.

An aneurysm may occur anywhere in the arterial system and is defined as a localized dilation of an artery that is 1½ times the normal diameter of the affected artery.[1] The management of an aneurysm in a given patient is dictated by a myriad of factors including size, location, extent, symptoms, etiology, and coexistent pathology. A detailed discussion of the current recommendations for the management of aneurysms, considering all combinations of these factors, is beyond the scope of this chapter. However, it is the intent of the authors to provide an overview of risk factors, causes, distribution patterns, preferred methods of diagnosis, and general guidelines for managing the patient with aneurysmal disease.

The development of aneurysms can be attributed to multiple factors; however, there are two basic features that are consistently present: congenital or acquired arterial wall weakness and the mechanical stresses produced by systemic arterial flow.[2] Discoveries of abnormal intercellular and intracellular interactions within the arterial wall of patients with aneurysmal disease have taken investigative research to the molecular and biochemical levels. This research eventually should provide the information to account for the cellular abnormalities observed in aneurysmal arterial tissues. A genetic predisposition toward the development of abdominal aortic aneurysms (AAAs) has been confirmed in laboratory and clinical analyses.[3-6] Based on his elaborate genetic and biochemical studies, Tilson[3] proposed a unifying hypothesis that is best summarized in his own words: "The concept of allelic variation of the x-linked gene for a connective tissue antiprotease is a hypothesis that unified the two mainstreams of AAA research over the last several years. It brings the concept of x-linkage to account for the obvious with the empirical observations of proteolytic activity in AAA tissue." Further analysis of large kindreds and additional laboratory studies should advance our understanding of the contribution of heredity to this disease process.

The natural history of an untreated aneurysm is expansion, rupture, thrombosis, and/or distal embolization, and the result of these complications can be hemorrhage, death, or end-organ ischemia with resultant tissue loss and impairment or loss of function. Considering these potentially devastating consequences of nontreatment and the improved results of perioperative medical, anesthetic, and surgical management techniques, it is both safe and prudent to assume an aggressive approach toward the management of aneurysms in most anatomic locations, in most patients.

CLASSIFICATION OF ANEURYSMS

Although many elaborate laboratory and clinical investigations have been and are being conducted in an effort to identify etiologic and pathologic features of aneurysmal disease, the diversity of the disease process and its clinical presentation warrant a clinical classification. Rutherford[2] presents the traditionally accepted clinical classification scheme, which includes four categories of etiologies: degenerative, inflammatory, mechanical, and congenital; as well as the form (saccular, fusiform, or dissecting), structure (true or false), size, and location, which serve to further classify aneurysms. Rutherford suggests that a revision of these categories could provide a more practical scheme for clinical purposes. A recent article defines such a revised classification system that serves as the current standards for reporting on arterial aneurysms.[1] These recommendations are the result of the extensive evaluation of the classification of aneurysms by a subcommittee established by the Society of Vascular Surgeons and the North American Chapter of the International Society for Cardiovascular Surgery. It is recommended that aneurysms be classified with a combination of the following factors: (1) site, (2) origin, (3) histologic features, and (4) clinicopathologic manifestations. This classification scheme is both inclusive and exhaustive and should serve as the foundation for classification in the future. Regardless of the classification used by an individual physician, it should be consistent, and as the concept of a national vascular registry materializes, we should search for classification uniformity.

INCIDENCE

The incidence of aneurysms varies with regard to anatomic location and the population being assessed, among several other features. In general, the frequency of the diagnosis of aneurysms is increasing. This is due to an increased average age of the general population, increased awareness of the existence of aneurysmal disease and the association with other cardiovascular diseases such as hypertension and coronary artery disease, improved diagnostic capabilities and availability, improved access to medical care, and an absolute increase in the incidence of aneurysms as an independent variable. An epidemiologic study, spanning 30 years, revealed a significant increase in the occurrence of abdominal aortic aneurysms from 8.7 new aneurysms diagnosed per 100,000 person-years from 1950 to 1960, to 36.5 per 100,000 person-years from 1971 to 1980.[7]

There also has been an obvious increase in traumatic aneurysms following invasive, nonoperative procedures owing to the increased utilization of cardiac and peripheral angiography, atherectomy, balloon and laser angioplasty, and thrombolytic therapy. The field of endovascular surgery has recently witnessed tremendous technologic advances that require cannulation of the femoral, brachial, or axillary arteries with relatively large bore percutaneous introducers that facilitate these endovascular procedures. Potential catheter-related complications, in addition to pseudoaneurysm formation, include arteriovenous fistula, uncontrolled hemorrhage, arterial thrombosis, and peripheral embolization.[8,9]

There has also been an increased incidence of femoral pseudoaneurysms due to chronic parenteral drug abuse over the past several decades.[10] This generally occurs following repeated injections resulting in infection of the arterial wall and surrounding tissues.

CLINICAL PRESENTATION

Most central aneurysms are asymptomatic (75%) at the time of the diagnosis and are discovered on routine physical or radiologic examinations, during laparotomy or postmortem examination, or by the patient. Peripheral aneurysms are also usually asymptomatic but are most frequently discovered by the patient or on physical examination.

Symptomatic aneurysms may present with pain due to expansion, leak, or frank rupture. The pain is usually sharp, sudden in onset, and frequently described by the patient as "tearing" in nature. The pain from an abdominal aortic aneurysm is usually localized to the back, in the region of the upper lumbar or lower thoracic vertebrae. Pain from thoracic aortic aneurysms is experienced in the interscapular region. Either abdominal or thoracic aneurysms may cause abdominal pain. Rapidly progressing hypotension, tachycardia, and shock follow a significant leak or rupture, and expeditious evaluation and emergency surgical intervention is indicated. The pain experienced with periperhal aneurysms is localized to the area of involvement and is less likely to be related to rapid expansion, leak, or rupture, but rather to compression of adjacent structures or to thrombosis or embolization.

The symptoms following embolization from an aneurysm will vary depending on the end organs affected and whether there is macroembolization or microembolization, and may range from stroke to renal failure or lower extremity ischemia. Aneurysm thrombosis may be symptomatic or asymptomatic depending on location, the rate of progression of thrombosis, and the presence or absence of adequate collateral circulation.

The risk of a patient experiencing one of these three complications (leak or rupture, distal embolization, or thrombosis) is dependent upon a variety of factors that serve as the basis for the previously discussed classification scheme, that is, location, size, etiology, and so on. For example, an AAA is more prone to rupture than to thrombose or emit distal emboli, whereas thrombosis is the most common complication of a popliteal artery aneurysm, followed by distal embolization and rupture, respectively. It is for this reason that we have developed a section, later in this chapter, devoted to summarizing the unique characteristics of aneurysms in different anatomic locations and how this information affects management.

DIAGNOSTIC EVALUATION

Physical examination continues to be the most valuable tool in diagnosing aneurysms. The exceptions to this statement are small aneurysms and those con-

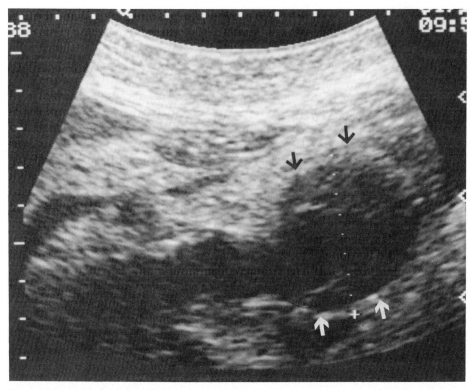

Figure 13–1. Abdominal ultrasound demonstrating abdominal aortic aneurysm with moderate amount of intramural thrombus.

fined to the chest cavity. Most experienced clinicians can estimate the diameter of an aneurysm within 10% to 20% of the actual diameter, solely on the basis of careful palpation.

Plain radiographs are valuable in ruling out other pathology, which is critically important in the acute setting. With regard to the specific evaluation of an aneurysm, these studies provide little information. Calcium deposition within the aneurysm wall (medial calcinosis) is frequently revealed on plain radiographs but is not usually an accurate means of assessing aneurysm size or extent.

B-mode ultrasound is an excellent, inexpensive screening tool and provides relatively accurate information regarding aneurysm size and extent, except within the thoracic cavity (Fig. 13–1). Coupled with color-flow Doppler, ultrasonographic evaluation of peripheral aneurysms has taken on a new dimension and provides detailed information, which is especially useful in the assessment of peripheral pseudoaneurysms.

Contrast-enhanced computed tomography (CT) is somewhat more accurate than ultrasound in assessing the size and extent of central aneurysms (Fig. 13–2), especially if there is suprarenal, intrathoracic, or deep pelvic extension. This technique is seldom required for examination of peripheral aneurysms. Dynamic CT scanning appears to be helpful in evaluating a hemodynamically stable patient when the differential diagnosis includes acute or chronic aortic dissection or leaking aneurysm. In our limited experience with this technique, we have been impressed

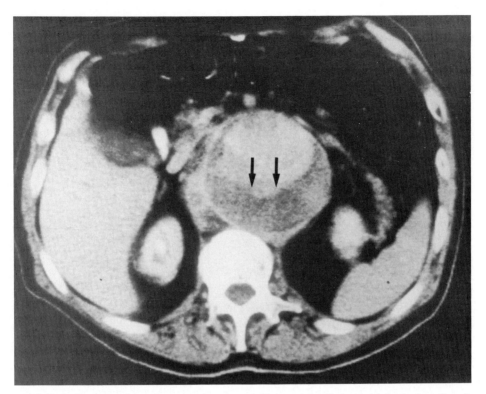

Figure 13–2. Contrast-enhanced computed tomogram demonstrating the upper abdominal portion of a large thoracoabdominal aortic aneurysm. *Arrows* indicate a moderately large volume of intramural thrombus.

with the capability of differentiating between the true and false lumen of an aortic dissection and identifying the delayed filling of a periadventitial collection of contrast of a leaking aneurysm. A recent study suggests that most patients (81%) with aortic aneurysms can be adequately evaluated by CT scan alone.[11]

Magnetic resonance imaging (MRI) of central aneurysms provides essentially the same information as the CT scan with about the same accuracy (Fig. 13–3); however, the vascular MRI may prove to reveal significantly more information. These techniques are more expensive than CT scanning and frequently more difficult to interpret; therefore, we utilize MRI only if the CT scan fails to provide enough information or if there is an indication for MRI to assess other pathology. The potential benefit of obtaining coronal, sagittal, and cross-sectional views with MRI may prove to be useful (Fig. 13–4).

Angiography is being utilized more selectively in central and peripheral aneurysms. We obtain an angiogram in all patients with thoracoabdominal, suprarenal aortic, mesenteric, carotid, and popliteal aneurysms to search for coexistent aneurysmal or occlusive disease. Angiography frequently can identify critical intercostal arteries in patients with thoracoabdominal aortic aneurysms,[12,13] which may guide intercostal reimplantation at the time of surgical repair. Other indications for angiography in the patient with an AAA include horseshoe kidney, clinical suggestion of renal artery stenosis, mesenteric insufficiency, aortoiliac occlusive disease, or lower extremity aneurysmal disease.[11] Patients with pseudoaneurysms at the site of

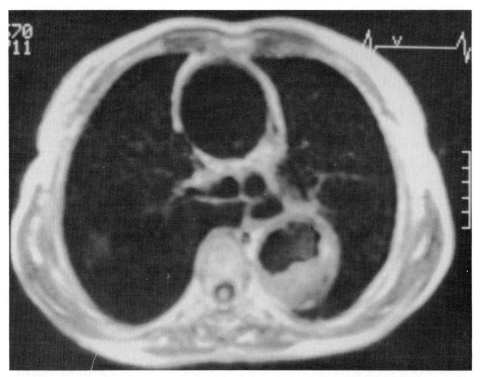

Figure 13-3. Magnetic resonance image demonstrating a large thoracoabdominal aortic aneurysm, involving the ascending and descending aorta in transverse section.

catheter placement frequently will have angiograms that were obtained at the time of catheterization, and these studies should be reviewed prior to operative repair of the ultrasonographically diagnosed pseudoaneurysm.

Angiograms serve as a poor reference for aneurysm size assessment because of the unpredictable amount of intramural thrombus lining the aneurysm. However, examination of multiple views—anterior-posterior, lateral, and oblique—is helpful in delineating the extent of the aneurysm.

MANAGEMENT OF ANEURYSMS

ABDOMINAL AORTIC ANEURYSMS

In a classic article in 1950, Estes[14] reported significantly lower survival rates for patients with AAA as compared with age-matched controls from the normal population. DeBakey and coworkers in 1964[15] and Szilagyi and associates in 1966[16] demonstrated that patients undergoing surgical treatment of AAA survived longer than patients managed nonoperatively. Since those studies, advances in technology have led to improvements in diagnosis, pharmacologic and anesthetic management, perioperative monitoring, and surgical technique, resulting in lower perioperative morbidity and mortality rates and improved long-term survival. These clinical factors permit an aggressive approach toward operative intervention, even in the elderly and high-risk patient populations.[17] There is a significantly increased risk

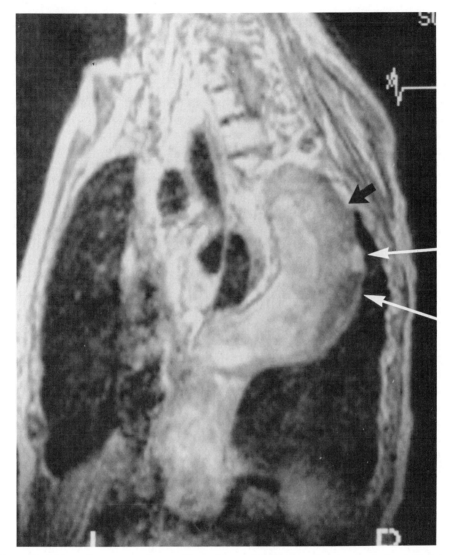

Figure 13–4. Magnetic resonance image of large thoracoabdominal aortic aneurysm in the sagittal view.

of rupture of AAAs greater than 5 cm in diameter and in those with documented expansion of greater than 10% per year. We therefore encourage elective operative repair in most of the patients falling into these categories, even if the aneurysm is 4 to 5 cm in diameter.

The most commonly used method of AAA repair is transabdominal endoaneurysmorrhaphy with graft replacement of the affected segment, which frequently requires a bifurcated graft that extends to the iliac arteries. This is accomplished under general endotracheal anesthesia, through a xiphoid-to-pubis midline incision. The anastomoses are sewn to nonaneurysmal vessel, but the proximal anastomosis always should be placed at least as high as the immediate infrarenal aortic segment. A retroperitoneal approach is preferred by some surgeons and may decrease the incidence of pulmonary complications. Aneurysm wrapping with various materials and intentional thrombosis of the aneurysm with concomitant extra-anatomic bypass are other historical methods of operative management, but have few, if any, indications. These latter two methods appear to fall short of optimal management and have no obvious impact on decreasing perioperative morbidity or mortality.[17]

The elective perioperative mortality is less than 3% in the low and moderate risk patient population with a perioperative morbidity rate of less than 10%, in most reported series. The most common perioperative complications include myocardial infarction, pulmonary or renal dysfunction, hemorrhage, stroke, and infection. If there is a requirement for suprarenal cross-clamping, there is a dramatic increase in the incidence of renal dysfunction. The perioperative mortality and morbidity rates for repairing ruptured AAAs are substantially higher, that is, 30% to 50% and 50% to 80%, respectively. Therefore, early diagnosis and concerted management by the referring physician and the vascular surgeon, careful follow-up, and timely operative intervention are essential elements in the successful management of the patient with an abdominal aortic aneurysm.

THORACOABDOMINAL AORTIC ANEURYSMS

Thoracoabdominal aortic aneurysms (THAAA) involve the descending thoracic and abdominal aorta, usually including the visceral and renal segments. Large type II THAAAs may involve the aorta from the left subclavian artery to the iliacs (Fig. 13–5). Rupture of a THAAA poses the greatest threat to life, and the risk of this complication appears to be related to size and extent. Detailed evaluation with CT scan or MRI and angiography is indicated. All patients with THAAAs greater than 5 cm should be evaluated for possible aneurysm repair. Remarkable progress

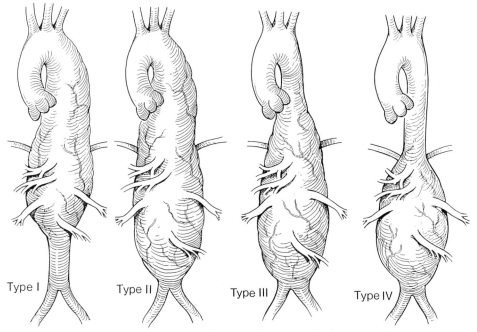

Figure 13–5. Artist's rendition of the four types of thoracoabdominal aortic aneurysms.

Table 13–1

Aneurysm type	I	II	III	IV	Total
Number of patients	26	22	32	50	130
Paraparesis	1	1	2	0	4 (3.1%)
Paraplegia	1	1	0	0	2 (1.5%)
Total neurologic deficit	2 (7.7%)	2 (9.9%)	2 (6.3%)	0	6 (4.6%)

8.3%*

7.5%*

*Combined neurologic deficit.

has been made in the successful operative management of these patients over the past 20 years. The previously formidably high morbidity and mortality rates have been reduced to acceptable levels that now permit routine elective operative repair, even in high-risk patients.[18] The morbidity and mortality of emergency repair remains quite high. The major complications following THAAA repair include death, myocardial infarction, renal failure, paralysis or paraplegia, pulmonary insufficiency, and stroke. Specific perioperative measures may be taken to reduce the rate of these complications. A significant reduction of the incidence of myocardial infarction has been noted following detailed preoperative cardiac evaluation[18,19] and optimization of cardiac function by pharmacologic manipulation, and myocardial revascularization via percutaneous transluminal angioplasty, atherectomy, or coronary artery bypass grafting prior to THAAA repair. Renal dysfunction is reduced by perfusion techniques.[20–24] Cerebrospinal fluid drainage, free-radical scavenger administration, intercostal artery reimplantation, glucose-load restriction, relative hypothermia, and barbiturate administration are all methods that appear to decrease the risk of neurologic complications following cross-clamp–induced spinal cord ischemia (Table 13–1).[23–26]

The presence of a suprarenal or thoracoabdominal aortic aneurysm should be suspected in any patient in whom the aneurysm appears to extend to or beyond the costal margin. Current recommendations include elective repair of all THAAAs greater than 5 cm. Early referral to a vascular surgeon experienced in managing THAAAs should be sought upon discovery of such a lesion.

ISOLATED ILIAC ARTERY ANEURYSMS

Isolated iliac artery aneurysms are uncommon and comprise 2% to 3% of all true arterial aneurysms. Most of these lesions are asymptomatic (78%) and are discovered incidentally on physical exam.[27] One-third of the patients have multiple aneurysms. Nearly 90% of these aneurysms are located in the common iliac artery. Symptoms usually involve pain, and rarely patients present with symptoms from other organ systems secondary to compression, such as ureteral obstruction or bowel complaints. There is a high incidence of rupture as these lesions enlarge and a high mortality in patients who experience rupture; therefore, prompt operative intervention is indicated. Repair may be performed via the retroperitoneal or transperitoneal route and is accomplished by graft replacement of the involved arterial segment and ligation or reimplantation of the internal iliac artery.

CAROTID ARTERY ANEURYSMS

Aneurysms of the extracranial carotid artery may be fusiform or saccular. The more common fusiform aneurysms are usually secondary to atherosclerotic degeneration and are frequently bilateral and associated with aneurysms in other locations. Saccular aneurysms are usually unilateral and occasionally related to atherosclerotic degeneration, but more frequently they are related to a traumatic or congenital cause. Atherosclerotic aneurysms of either type are almost always associated with hypertension.[28] Rare causes of carotid aneurysms include arteritis, carotid dissection, and infection (syphilitic or bacterial).

Carotid aneurysms may cause neurologic symptoms following thrombosis or rupture but are most commonly due to distal embolization.[28] Rapid expansion or carotid dissection may cause symptoms related to compression of adjacent structures, particularly the cranial nerves. Compression of the cervical sympathetics may cause a Horner's syndrome.

The treatment of choice for extracranial carotid aneurysms is interposition graft replacement of the affected segment with saphenous vein; however, Dacron and PTFE also serve as acceptable conduits. Pseudoaneurysms following trauma or previous carotid artery surgery rarely require interposition grafting and can usually be safely managed by direct suture repair or patch angioplasty. Care must be taken not to injure attenuated adjacent structures during the course of the operative dissection. We routinely use an intraluminal shunt during the repair of carotid aneurysms. The devastating, permanent neurologic complications resulting from embolization, thrombosis, or rupture mandate timely repair of these lesions.

FEMORAL AND POPLITEAL ARTERIAL ANEURYSMS

Aneurysms occurring in the femoral or popliteal arteries are almost always caused by atherosclerotic degeneration and are frequently bilateral and associated with a high incidence of aneurysms at other sites. There is a high incidence of thromboembolic complications that may jeopardize limb viability. Rupture is less common at these sites. Conservative management of these aneurysms results in complications in 40% to 70% of these patients over 5 years.[29,30] The treatment of choice is interposition graft replacement of the affected segment with prosthetic or autologous vein. Ligation and bypass of popliteal artery aneurysms is an acceptable but less optimal alternative. The long-term results of interposition graft replacement are excellent. The unusual case of graft thrombosis is generally related to the development of distal occlusive disease and poor runoff.

SUBCLAVIAN AND AXILLARY ARTERY ANEURYSMS

Aneurysms of the subclavian and axillary arteries are quite rare, and most (90%) are symptomatic.[31] Distal embolization is the most common complication; thrombosis and rupture are extremely rare. Clinical manifestations are usually related to embolization, but nerve compression, claudication, and pain also may occur. The knowledge of the presence of a subclavian or axillary aneurysm is an indication for operative intervention. Angiography is useful in planning the operation. Aneurysm repair may require concomitant first rib resection and scalenectomy if the cause is related to thoracic outlet syndrome. Exlusion and interposition grafting with saphenous vein or prosthetic material is the treatment of choice.

Aneurysm ligation and axilloaxillary bypass graft placement is a valuable alternative when the aneurysm is extremely large or the fragility of the vessel at the proposed site of anastomosis prevents safe placement of an interposition graft.

ARTERIAL PSEUDOANEURYSMS

Pseudoaneurysms generally occur as a direct result of arterial trauma. The most common causes are (1) iatrogenic incidents secondary to arterial cannulization or following a surgical procedure and (2) traumatic accidents resulting in blunt or penetrating arterial injury. Most small, central pseudoaneurysms are asymptomatic; however, as enlargement occurs, symptoms frequently arise as the result of compression of adjacent structures. Peripheral pseudoaneurysms usually present as an enlarging palpable, pulsatile mass, frequently with pain or discomfort or with symptoms of distal embolization. Angiography is usually required to diagnose central pseudoaneurysms, but duplex scanning is an accurate method of diagnosing peripheral pseudoaneurysms. All patients with suspected or known pseudoaneurysms should be considered for operative repair. Direct repair is performed with nonabsorbable monofilament suture in most cases. Anastomotic aneurysms occasionally require patch angioplasty or anastomotic revision. Catheter-related pseudoaneurysms of a severely diseased atherosclerotic vessel frequently require patch angioplasty.

SUMMARY

The frequency of the diagnosis of arterial aneurysms is increasing. Aneurysms in many locations remain asymptomatic and require careful evaluation of at-risk patient populations. Screening of first-degree relatives of patients with known AAA now appears to be indicated. A high index of suspicion of the possible presence or the existence of known aneurysms should prompt timely referral for evaluation by a vascular surgeon. Consideration of a patient's candidacy for surgical intervention should involve the evaluation of a myriad of factors, some of which have been elucidated in this overview. The saftey of surgical intervention for aneurysm repair has continued to improve, and most patients can be surgically managed with an acceptably low rate of morbidity and mortality.[17]

REFERENCES

1. Johnston, KW, Rutherford, RB, Tilson, MD, et al: Suggested standards for reporting on arterial aneurysms. J Vasc Surg 13:452, 1991.
2. Rutherford, RB: Arterial aneurysms. In Rutherford, RB (ed): Vascular Surgery, ed 3. WB Saunders, Philadelphia, 1989.
3. Tilson, MD: A perspective on research in abdominal aortic aneurysm disease, with a unifying hypothesis. In Bergan, JJ and Yao, JST (eds): Aortic Surgery. WB Saunders, Philadelphia, 1989.
4. Johansen, K and Koepsell, T: Familial tendency for abdominal aortic aneurysms. JAMA 256:1934, 1986.
5. Webster, MW, St Jean, PL, Steed, DL, et al: Abdominal aortic aneurysm: Results of a family study. J Vasc Surg 13:366, 1991.
6. Webster, MW, Ferrell, RE, St Jean, PL, et al: Ultrasound screening of first-degree relatives of patients with an abdominal aortic aneurysm. J Vasc Surg 13:9, 1991.
7. Bickerstaff, LK, Hollier, LH, Van Peenen, HJ, et al: Abdominal aortic aneurysms: The changing natural history. J Vasc Surg 1:6, 1984.

8. Oweida, SW, Roubin, GS, Smith, RB, et al: Post-catheterization vascular complications associated with percutaneous transluminal coronary angioplasty. J Vasc Surg 12:310, 1990.

9. Dorros, G, Cowley, MJ, Simpson, J, et al: Percutaneous transluminal coronary angioplasty: Report of complications from the National Heart, Lung, and Blood Institute Percutaneous Transluminal Coronary Angioplasty Registry. Circulation 67:723, 1983.

10. Rush, DS and Morre, WM: Peripheral arterial infection and infected pseudoaneurysm. In Nichols, RL, Hyslop, NE, and Bartlett, JG (eds): Decision Making in Surgical Sepsis. BC Decker, Philadelphia, 1991.

11. Todd, GJ, Nowygrod, R, Benvenisty, A, et al: The accuracy of CT scanning in the diagnosis of abdominal and thoracoabdominal aortic aneurysms. J Vasc Surg 13:302, 1991.

12. Keiffer, E, Richard, T, Chiras, J, et al: Preoperative spinal cord arteriography in aneurysmal disease of the descending and thoracoabdominal aorta: Preliminary results in 45 patients. Ann Vasc Surg 3:34, 1986.

13. Williams, GM, Perler, BA, Burdick, JF, et al: Angiographic localization of spinal cord blood supply and its relationship to postoperative paraplegia. J Vasc Surg 13:23, 1991.

14. Estes, JE: Abdominal aortic aneurysm: A study of one hundred and two cases. Circulation 2:258, 1950.

15. DeBakey, ME, Crawford, ES, Cooley, DA, et al: Aneurysm of the abdominal aorta: Analysis of results of graft replacement therapy one to eleven years after operation. Ann Surg 160:622, 1964.

16. Szilagyi, DE, Smith, RF, DeRusso, FJ, et al: Contribution of abdominal aortic aneurysmectomy to prolongation of life. Ann Surg 164:678, 1966.

17. Hollier, LH, Reigel, MM, Kazmier, FJ, et al: Conventional repair of abdominal aortic aneurysm in the high risk patient. J Vasc Surg 3:712, 1986.

18. Hollier, LH, Symmonds, JB, Pairolero, PC, et al: Thoracoabdominal aortic aneurysm repair: Analysis of postoperative morbidity. Arch Surg 123:871, 1988.

19. Brewster, DC, Okada, RD, Strauss, HW, et al: Selection of patients for preoperative coronary angiography: Use of dipyridamole-stress-thallium myocardial imaging. J Vasc Surg 2:504, 1985.

20. Luft, FC, Hamburg, RJ, Dyer, JK, et al: Acute renal failure following operation for aortic aneurysm. Gynecol Obstet 141:374, 1975.

21. Ochsner, JL, Mills, NL, and Gardner, PA: A technique for renal preservation during suprarenal abdominal aortic operations. Surg Gynecol Obstet 159:388, 1984.

22. Ochsner, JL and Ancalmo, N: Renal preservation during thoracoabdominal aortic surgery. In Bergan, JJ and Yao, JST (eds): Aortic Surgery. WB Saunders, Philadelphia, 1989.

23. Hollier, LH and Moore, WM: Avoidance of renal and neurologic complications following thoracoabdominal aortic aneurysm repair. Acta Chir Scand Suppl 555:129, 1990.

24. Hollier, LH: Causes and prevention of spinal cord ischemia. In Veith, FJ (ed): Current Critical Problems in Vascular Surgery, vol 2. Quality Medical Publishing, St Louis, 1990.

25. Hollier, LH: Protecting the brain and spinal cord. J Vasc Surg 5:524, 1987.

26. Granke, K, Hollier, LH, Moore, WM, et al: Longitudinal study of cerebrospinal fluid drainage in polyethylene glycol-conjugated superoxide dismutase in paraplegia associated with thoracic aortic cross-clamping. J Vasc Surg 13:615, 1991.

27. McCready, RA, Pairolero, PC, Gilmore, JC, et al: Isolated iliac artery aneurysms. Surgery 93:688, 1983.

28. Rhodes, EL: Aneurysms of the extracranial carotid arteries. Arch Surg 111:339, 1976.

29. Szilagyi, DE, Schwartz, RL, and Reddy, DJ: Popliteal artery aneurysms. Their natural history and management. Arch Surg 116:724, 1981.

30. Cutler, BS and Darling, RC: Surgical management of femoral aneurysms. Surgery 74:764, 1973.

31. Hobson, RW II, Isreal, MR, and Lynch, TG: Axillosubclavian arterial aneurysms. In Bergan, JJ and Yao, JST (eds): Aneurysms. Grune & Stratton, New York, 1982.

CHAPTER 14

Penetrating Aortic Ulcer

Francis J. Kazmier, M.D.

The descriptive phrase *penetrating aortic ulcer* signifies that an atheroma with ulceration has penetrated the internal elastic lamina deeply into the media, producing hematoma formation within the medial layer of the aortic wall.

DESCRIPTION OF CASES

Interest in studying this entity was precipitated by a patient with hypertension and the abrupt onset of back pain, leading to a working diagnosis of aortic dissection.[1] Initial aortography did not demonstrate either a radiolucent intimal flap or contrast in a false lumen (Fig. 14–1A). There was, however, penetrating ulceration in the wall of the lower descending thoracic aorta and the suggestion of an extra-luminal soft tissue density along the left posterior border of the descending thoracic aorta (Fig. 14–1B). Recurrence of the back pain several days later led to a repeat aortogram with the ulcer now larger (Fig. 14–1C). Confirmation of the pathology was obtained at surgery. There was a large periaortic hematoma in the area of the angiographically defined ulcerated aortic atheroma. Tissue examination showed an ulcer with a 1-cm crater penetrating the media and in communication with the medial hematoma. At several areas, the hematoma had ruptured the media and was contained only by the adventitial layer of the aortic wall. Sixteen patients from a total of 684 thoracic aortograms met criteria for both penetrating ulceration and the presence of wall hematoma. The index case and this initial experience have been reviewed in detail previously, as well as an additional case of penetrating aortic ulceration in which magnetic resonance imaging played a role in defining the patient's problem.[1,2]

A summary of the salient points gained from these studies and experience is pertinent to this discussion. The characteristic presentation for these patients is that of an older person with both hypertension and atherosclerosis, who presents with abrupt back or chest pain, without any deficit in arterial pulses, without symptoms of cerebrovascular insufficiency, and usually without aortic valve involvement or compromise of any visceral vessels (Table 14–1). Aortic dissection was the initial clinical impression in 10 of our original 16 patients.[1] Pulse deficits were not noted

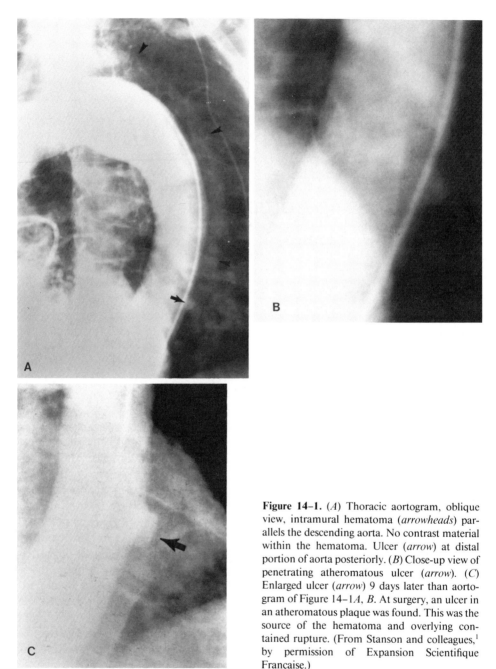

Figure 14-1. (*A*) Thoracic aortogram, oblique view, intramural hematoma (*arrowheads*) parallels the descending aorta. No contrast material within the hematoma. Ulcer (*arrow*) at distal portion of aorta posteriorly. (*B*) Close-up view of penetrating atheromatous ulcer (*arrow*). (*C*) Enlarged ulcer (*arrow*) 9 days later than aortogram of Figure 14–1*A*, *B*. At surgery, an ulcer in an atheromatous plaque was found. This was the source of the hematoma and overlying contained rupture. (From Stanson and colleagues,[1] by permission of Expansion Scientifique Française.)

in any patients. None presented with cerebrovascular insufficiency and aortography was done for pain in 13 of 16 patients. Seven of the 16 were treated conservatively initially, only to have persistent or recurrent pain lead to consideration of surgery.

In the index case, as well as in the additional cases in that series in which adequate surgical tissue was available for review, there was aortic hematoma and an

Table 14–1. Characteristics Distinguishing Aortic Dissection
From Penetrating Aortic Ulcer

Characteristic	Aortic Dissection	Penetrating Aortic Ulcer
Patient profile	Preexisting hypertension; occasionally bicuspid aortic valve, Marfan's syndrome	Elderly; hypertension; severe atherosclerosis
Symptoms	Severe chest or back pain, which may be migratory	Similar
Signs	Pulse inequality; compromise of flow in visceral vessels; neurologic deficits; aortic valve insufficiency	Absent
Diagnostic studies	Intimal flap in proximal aorta or isthmus; contrast medium fills false lumen. Displacement of intimal calcium	Localized ulceration into wall of descending thoracic aorta; creation of intramural hematoma. No false lumen visible. Displacement of intimal calcium
Treatment	Surgical approach for types I and II; uncompolicated type III may be managed medically	Surgical approach

Source: From Cooke and associates,[2] by permission of Mayo Foundation.

entry site from an ulcerated atherosclerotic plaque. The fate of a penetrating ulcer (Fig. 14–2) may include medial hematoma formation, which in turn may remain localized or dissect proximally, distally or both for variable length. A false aneurysm supported only by adventitia is a possibility and transmural rupture is still another possible outcome. In our initial experience medial dissection with wall hematoma was the most common end result for these symptomatic ulcers.[1]

Patients with ulcers limited only to the intima and ulcers not associated with thickening of the aortic wall were excluded from consideration. Most ulcers of the aorta that are small, not associated with intramural hematoma, and asymptomatic are not important clinically.

Angiographic findings with penetrating ulcers are particularly subtle and in sharp contrast to those of classic aortic dissection beginning in the usual sites in either the ascending thoracic aorta or just distal to the ligamentum arteriosum in the descending thoracic aorta. Penetrating ulcers involve the descending thoracic aorta almost exclusively in our experience. Contrast filling of the hematoma is uncommon with an aortic ulcer.[1] An intimal flap is rarely seen, and if noted, rather than being smooth and thin as in classic dissection, it is irregular and thickened. The entry site for a penetrating ulcer is variable, and though the site may be anywhere in the descending thoracic aorta, mid to distal sites are common. Intimal calcification, which is often better seen with CT scanning, is inwardly displaced with both penetrating ulcers and classic dissections, reflecting the presence of intramural hematoma. In addition to its help in identifying wall hematoma, chest CT may actually pinpoint the site for penetrating ulceration. Magnetic resonance imaging (MRI) (Fig. 14–3) may be superior to CT in differentiating the acute intramural hematoma from atherosclerotic plaque and chronic intraluminal thrombus. The effectiveness of MRI in diagnosing penetrating ulcers is just beginning to be realized.[3]

AORTIC ATHEROSCLEROTIC ULCERS

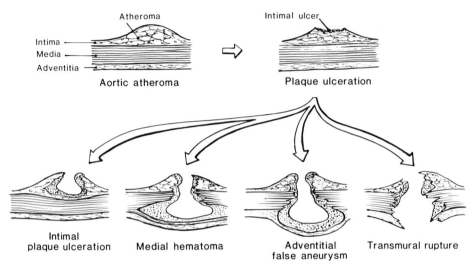

Figure 14–2. Potential fate of penetrating aortic atherosclerotic ulcers. An intimal tear into the atheroma results in an ulcerated tract that often becomes lined by thrombus. Extension of the ulcer may produce an incomplete rupture (if confined to the intima, media, or adventitia) or a complete transmural aortic rupture. The ulcer craters in incomplete ruptures commonly are filled with thrombus. As a result, the size of the remaining flask-shaped or nipple-shaped lumens may lead to an appreciable underestimation of the actual size of the involved aortic segment. In our surgical pathology series, medial dissection was the most commonly observed fate of penetrating ulcers. (From Stanson and colleagues,[1] by permission of Expansion Scientifique Francaise.)

COMMENT

There are several questions that should be addressed in reference to the penetrating aortic ulcer:

1. Is this a new entity?
2. What is its relationship to classic aortic dissection?
3. Has the natural history of this entity, as initially described, stood the test of time?
4. What are the implications of its natural history for treatment?

Questions 1 and 2 are intertwined with each other as are questions 3 and 4.

Although atheromatous ulcers are frequent in the carotids, infrarenal aorta, coronaries, and brachiocephalic arteries, there are few recorded instances in the literature of ulcers extending into the media of arteries.[4] The descending thoracic aorta has been an exception. As cited by Shennan[5], Virchow and some other early pathologists thought the cause of classic dissection was atheromatous ulceration with dissection through the edge of ulcer into the layers between intima and media or between media and adventitia. In contrast, Shennan[5] noted that of 218 recent dissections he reviewed, only 19 showed a relationship of atheroma to the primary

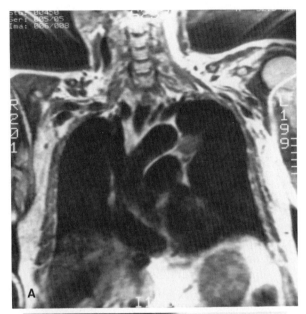

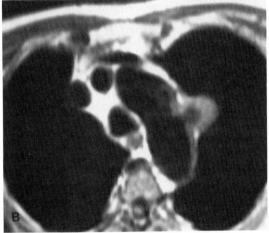

Figure 14–3. Magnetic resonance imaging scans of patient with penetrating aortic ulcer. Sagittal (*A*) and transverse (*B*) images reveal ulceration and penetration of proximal descending thoracic aorta, with thickening of wall at site of ulceration. (From Cooke and associates,[2] by permission of Mayo Foundation.)

rupture and dissection. In only four of his cases did the dissection actually begin in an atheromatous ulcer.[5] Hence, this is the exception and is uncommon. Atheromas are not common in relation to the spontaneous tears in the ascending aorta.[6] Larson and Edwards[7] noted extensive atheromatous plaquing in only 9% of dissections involving the ascending thoracic aorta in contrast to an 80% extensive atheromatous involvement in the lower thoracic aorta.

In a talk on aortic dissection published in 1941, Willius and Cragg[8] noted that some of the *primary* internal ruptures in their aortic cases involved the more distal thoracic aorta and many clearly appeared to be associated with "ulcerating atheromatous abscesses." Eyler and Clark,[9] as well as others, have described ulcerlike projections, similar in appearance to the gastric ulcers seen on barium examination on angiography of the aorta.[9,10] They thought these projections of contrast represented intimal defects leading to a clotted false channel. These ulcers were usually in the descending thoracic aorta and may represent penetrating ulcers, but pathologic confirmation is lacking. Tisnado and colleagues[11] have described ulcerlike projections of contrast from the true lumen into a false lumen in the ascending aorta. Their two cases identify the site of spontaneous intimal tear or lacerations and are examples of aorta dissection beginning in the ascending thoracic aorta, not associated with atherosclerotic plaque. The authors emphasized the importance of additional projections to clarify and expose the more typical appearance of classic type A dissection.

Hence, the entity under consideration is not new, nor is the angiographic appearance of ulcerlike projections new. The angiographic findings are not specific for penetrating atherosclerotic ulcers, when seen in the ascending aorta, but are strongly suggestive of same when seen in a descending thoracic aorta involved with extensive atherosclerosis. The entire symptom complex is sufficiently distinctive that it warrants differentiation from classic type A and B aortic dissections. That penetrating aortic ulcers in the descending thoracic aorta do represent localized aortic dissection in an unusual site and from an uncommon cause seems clear.

Our initial natural history data were based on our index case and a retrospective review of a small experience.[1] Since then, Hussain and colleagues[12] have noted that rupture of symptomatic ulcers may be less common than initially thought and that nonoperative management is appropriate as initial therapy, followed by serial evaluation with imaging and clinical follow-up. Further prospective data are needed to settle these issues. Our experience with penetrating aortic ulcers in patients with persistent or recurrent pain leads us to support surgical intervention for such patients, directed at graft replacement in the area of ulcer and intramural hematoma.[1,2]

SUMMARY

Penetrating atherosclerotic ulcers are part of a clinical entity with distinctive clinical, pathologic, angiogrpahic, and CT and MRI findings and should be differentiated from more classic aortic dissection and expanding aortic aneurysm.

REFERENCES

1. Stanson, AW, Kazmier, FJ, Holier, LH, et al: Penetrating atherosclerotic ulcers of the thoracic aorta: Natural history and clinical correlations. Ann Vasc Surg 1:15, 1986.
2. Cooke, JP, Kazmier, FJ, and Orszulak, TA: The penetrating aortic ulcer: Pathologic manifestations, diagnosis and management. Mayo Clin Proc 63:717, 1988.
3. Yucel, EK, Steinberg, FL, Egglin, TK, et al: Penetrating aortic ulcers: Diagnosis with MR imaging. Radiology 177:779, 1990.
4. Lord, RSA and Berry, NA: Atherosclerotic ulceration of the brachiocephalic artery. Aust NZ J Surg 44:370, 1974.
5. Shennan, T: Dissecting aneurysms. Special Report Series 193. Medical Research Council (Great Britain), 1933–1934, p 86.
6. Murray, CA and Edwards, JE: Spontaneous laceration of ascending aorta. Circulation 47:848, 1973.
7. Larson, EW and Edwards, WD: Risk factors for aortic dissection: A necropsy study of 161 cases. Am J Cardiol 53:849, 1984.
8. Willius, FA and Cragg, RW: Cardiac clinics LXXIX: A talk on dissecting aneurysm of the aorta. Mayo Clin Proc 16:41, 1941.
9. Eyler, WR and Clark, MD: Dissecting aneurysms of the aorta: Roentgen manifestations including a comparison with other types of aneurysms. Radiology 85:1047, 1965.

10. Stein, HL and Steinberg, I: Selective aortography, the definitive technique for diagnosis of dissecting aneurysm of the aorta. AJR 102:333, 1968.
11. Tisnado, J, Cho Shao-Ru, Beachley, MC, and Vines, FS: Ulcerlike projections: A precursor angiographic sign to thoracic aortic dissection. AJR 135:719, 1980.
12. Hussain, S, Glover, JL, Bree, R and Bendick, PJ: Penetrating atherosclerotic ulcers of the thoracic aorta. J Vasc Surg 9:710, 1989.

CHAPTER 15

Conservative Management of Occlusive Peripheral Arterial Disease

John A. Spittell, Jr., M.D.

For all persons with occlusive peripheral arterial disease, whether symptomatic or not, whether atherosclerotic or a less common type, whether involving the upper or the lower extremity or both, and whether acute or chronic, the management program should always include measures designed to protect the ischemic limb. In addition, there are conservative approaches to the management of patients with intermittent claudication. None of the conservative measures—protective or symptomatic—are as dramatic as the restoration of pulsatile flow, but their potential for benefit is every bit as great. Patient compliance can be a significant problem unless health care providers spend the time to emphasize the rationale, goals, and importance of each of the conservative measures.

CONTROLLABLE RISK FACTORS

When the occlusive peripheral arterial disease is due to atherosclerosis, the controllable risk factors—smoking, diabetes, hyperlipidemia, and hypertension—should be addressed in the hope of slowing progression of the atherosclerosis. Although some have advocated the use of fish oil or purified omega-3 fatty acids in atherosclerotic vascular disease, a reasonable alternative is replacement of foods containing large amounts of saturated fatty acids with fish in the diet.[1] If there are no contraindications to its use, aspirin in a daily dose of 325 mg is appropriate for the person with atherosclerotic vascular disease to lessen the risk of myocardial infarction and stroke[2]; antithrombotic therapy in the hope of modifying the natural history of atherosclerotic peripheral arterial disease is not indicated unless recurrent thrombotic arterial occlusion has occurred.

PROTECTION AGAINST VASOCONSTRICTION, INFECTION, AND TRAUMA

In the category of protective measures are those designed to avoid vasoconstriction, those to prevent infection, and those to lessen trauma to the ischemic

Table 15–1. Effect of Smoking on
Intermittent Claudication Outcome after
5 Years

	Continued, %	Stopped, %
Mortality	27	12
Major amputation	11	0
Claudication stable	40	56

Source: Modified from McDaniel and Cromwell Ann Vasc Surg 3:273, 1989.

part. The most important vasoconstrictive factor to address is the use of tobacco; care should be taken to explain that tobacco exerts its adverse effect by its vasoconstrictive effect on small arteries and arterioles, which are essential to develop and maintain good collateral circulation. Many persons can be influenced to stop their use of tobacco in all forms if the reported increased amputation rate in those who continue tobacco use (Table 15–1) is brought to their attention. It should be made clear, however, that the goal of stopping smoking is not symptomatic relief, lest failure to observe this admonition leads to the resumption of tobacco use. The patient with Buerger's disease (thromboangiitis obliterans) can be virtually assured, however, that the activity of the disease will be arrested when tobacco is stopped and just as certainly will restart if resumed.

Medications being taken for associated conditions—for example, hypertension, coronary artery disease or migraine—should be reviewed; alternatives to those agents that may induce vasoconstriction such as certain β-blockers,[3] clonidine, and ergot preparations should be utilized in the person with occlusive peripheral arterial disease if equivalent effect can be achieved. Using proper footwear to protect ischemic limbs from cold is likewise essential, but local heating of an ischemic limb should be avoided because it may burn the skin.

Because ischemic tissue tolerates infection poorly, instructing the patient in meticulous foot hygiene and the maintenance of skin integrity is essential. Feet should be washed carefully and gently with a mild soap and warm [not more than 32°C (90°F)] water. After thorough rinsing, drying is best done by blotting or patting with a soft clean towel—rubbing should be avoided since it may injure the skin. It is important to emphasize that the skin between the toes should be carefully dried. It is desirable to have the patient examine his or her ischemic foot (or hand) daily for any blisters, dryness, fissuring (Fig. 15–1) or infection and, following this examination, rub the skin of the feet gently with a lanolin preparation (or cocoa butter) to keep the skin soft. The patient should be cautioned to not leave an excess of the moisturizer between the toes. If the daily inspection reveals unusual discoloration, fissuring of the skin, or signs of infection in the foot (or hand), it should be reported promptly to his or her physician.

Most amputations in persons with occlusive peripheral arterial disease arise from some type of trauma—mechanical, chemical, or thermal—to the ischemic limb.[4] Because such trauma is often patient-induced, much of it can be prevented by patient education. Properly fitted shoes that do not bind or rub should be worn at all times. New shoes should be broken in gradually. Patients should be cautioned against going barefoot. Protection against cold injury with warm outer footwear is

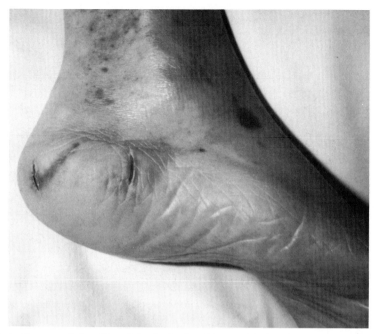

Figure 15-1. Fissures of the skin of the heel of a 46-year-old diabetic male with arteriosclerosis obliterans.

recommended in winter. Care never to place a hot object such as a heating pad on an ischemic limb or to expose the limb to water that is too hot should be emphasized. To avoid injuring the skin, strong ointments, corn cures, and antiseptics should be avoided by the person with occlusive peripheral arterial disease; minor injuries are better treated by gentle cleansing with warm [32°C (90°F) or less] water and soap, and bed rest; if prompt healing does not occur, the patient should contact his or her physician. Thickened or deformed toenails, calluses, corns, and bunions should not be cut or filed; these are best managed by a podiatrist who is aware of the impaired arterial circulation. Removal of ingrowing toenails from an ischemic toe can result in an ischemic ulcer (Fig. 15-2), so that such procedures, if necessary, are best carried out by physicians familiar with peripheral vascular disease.

In the patient with occlusive arterial disease in the hand secondary to chronic blunt trauma, occupational or otherwise, the source of the trauma should be identified (Table 15-2) and the affected hand protected from it by the appropriate use of tools or gloves or by a change in occupation.

The best approach to dermatophytosis is prevention by keeping the feet dry, wearing clean dry cotton or wool socks, and using one of the antifungal foot powders. If the blisters or cracks of dermatophytosis are noted between the toes, prompt treatment with an antifungal ointment is indicated. If there has been a delay in bringing the fungal infection to the physician's attention and secondary bacterial infection is present (Fig. 15-3), appropriate antibiotic therapy—administered systemically and not locally—is indicated. Although the usual bacterial organism causing lymphangitis and/or cellulitis as a complication of dermatophytosis is a streptococcus, culture and antibiotic sensitivities should be performed if there is an open sore or any drainage.

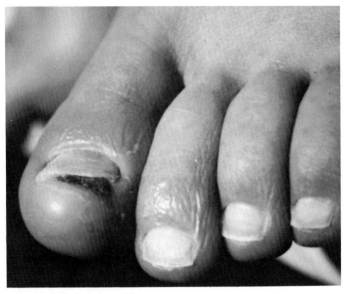

Figure 15–2. Ischemic ulcer at site of removal of ingrowing toenail of a 34-year-old male with arteriosclerosis obliterans.

INTERMITTENT CLAUDICATION

For the conservative management of intermittent claudication, there are several approaches that can be tried singly or in combination. In the obese person, weight reduction is an obvious initial approach. A regular walking program or other supervised dynamic leg exercise program (e.g., stationary bicycle, treadmill, or stair climbing) is associated with an improved pain-free and maximum walking distance in many persons with intermittent claudication.[5] It is important to advise the patient that the improvement is gradual and may not be maximal for up to 3

Table 15–2. Some Occupations with Potential for Chronic Blunt Trauma to the Hand

Occupation	Source of Trauma
Butcher	Hand tools
Carpenter	Hand tools
Creamery worker	"Hammerhand" to remove milk can lids
Dentist	Drills
Farmer	Tools and tractor steering wheel
Forestry worker	Chain saw
Laborer	Air hammer
Mechanic	Wrenches; "hammerhand"
Obstetrician	Outlet forceps
Packing house worker	"Hammerhand"
Pharmacist	Loosening bottle caps
Truck driver	Levers, steering wheel

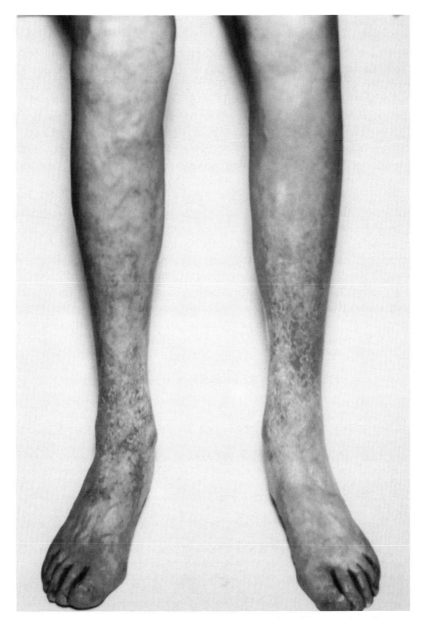

Figure 15-3. Acute cellulitis, a bacterial complication of dermatophytosis.

months, in order to maximize patient compliance. Although programs should be individualized, 30 minutes of dynamic leg exercise at least 5 days a week is reasonable for most persons; in the case of walking, when claudication symptoms occur, stopping for relief is advised. The basis for the improved walking distance with exercise programs is not clear; mechanisms proposed include improved oxidative metabolism in the limb,[6] increased blood flow due to improved hemorrheology,[7] and improved walking technique.[8]

Pharmacologic treatment of intermittent claudication is limited to pentoxifylline at present. None of the presently available oral vasodilators are effective for the management of intermittent claudication.[9] Pentoxifylline has been described as a "hemorrheologically active compound" that improves blood flow and tissue perfusion in the microcirculation[10] as a result of its effect on blood viscosity, erythrocyte flexibility, platelet aggregation, and plasma fibrinogen concentration.[11,12] Several studies have reported symptomatic improvement in 50% to 60% of persons receiving pentoxifylline,[13,14] whereas other investigators report no change in the walking distance.[15,16] One recent study may explain the controversial reports[17]; these investigators noted maximum benefit in persons who had intermittent claudication for more than one year and who had an ankle-to-arm systolic blood pressure index of 0.8 or less ("moderately severe occlusive arterial disease"). The recommended dose of pentoxifylline is 400 mg orally, three times a day, preferably taken with meals to lessen the most frequent side effects of nausea and indigestion. Blood counts should be monitored inasmuch as aplastic anemia has been reported in two persons receiving pentoxifylline.[18] In persons who are also receiving antihypertensive therapy or oral anticoagulants, frequent monitoring of the blood pressure or prothrombin time is recommended to detect any additive effect of pentoxifylline, though no interaction of pentoxifylline with commonly used cardiovascular drugs or antidiabetic agents has been noted. Because pentoxifylline is a methyl-xanthine derivative, the drug should not be employed in persons intolerant to this class of compounds (e.g., caffeine, theophylline, and theobromine).

REFERENCES

1. Goodnight, SH, Fisher, M, Fitzgerald, GA, and Levine, PH: Assessment of the therapeutic use of dietary fish oil in atherosclerotic vascular disease and thrombosis. Chest 95:195, 1989.
2. Clagett, GB, Genton, E, and Salzman, EW: Antithrombotic therapy in peripheral vascular disease. Chest 95:128S, 1989.
3. Roberts, DH, Tsao, Y, McLoughlin, GA, and Breckenridge, A: Placebo-controlled comparison of captopril, atenolol, labetolol, and pindolol in hypertension complicated by intermittent claudication. Lancet 2:650, 1987.
4. Weis AJ and Fairbairn, JF, II: Trauma, ischemic limbs and amputation. Postgrad Med 43:111–115, 1968.
5. Radack, K and Wyderski, RJ: Conservative management of intermittent claudication. Ann Intern Med 113:135, 1990.
6. Dahlof, AG, Bjorntorp, P, Holm, J and Schertsen, T: Metabolic activity of skeletal muscle in patients with peripheral arterial insufficiency. Eur J Clin Invest 4:9, 1974.
7. Ernst, EE and Matrai, A: Intermittent claudication, exercise, and blood rheology. Circulation 76:1110, 1987.
8. Schoop, W: Mechanism of beneficial action of daily walking training of patients with intermittent claudication. Scand J Clin Lab Invest 31 (Suppl 128):197, 1973.
9. Coffman, JD: Drug therapy: Vasodilator drugs in peripheral vascular disease. N Engl J Med 300:713, 1979.
10. Muller, R: Hemorrheology and peripheral vascular diseases: A new therapeutic approach. J Med 12:209, 1981.
11. Spittell, JA, Jr: Pentoxifylline and intermittent claudication. Ann Intern Med 102:126, 1985.
12. Angelcort, R, and Kresivetter, H: Influence of risk factors and coagulation phenomena on the fluidity of blood in chronic arterial occlusive disease. Scand J Clin Lab Invest 156(Suppl):185, 1981.
13. Porter, JM, Cutter, BS, Lee, BY, et al: Pentoxifylline efficacy in the treatment of intermittent claudication: Multi-center controlled double-blind trial with objective assessment of chronic occlusive arterial disease patients. Am Heart J 113:864, 1982.
14. Johnson, WC, Sentissi, JM, Baldwin, D, et al: Treatment of claudication with pentoxifylline: Are benefits related to improvement viscosity? J Vasc Surg 6:211, 1987.

15. Donaldson, DR, Hall, TJ, Kester, RC, et al: Does oxypentifylline ("Trental") have a place in the treatment of intermittent claudication? Curr Med Res Opin 9:35, 1984.
16. Gallus, AS, Gleadow, F, Dupont, P, et al: Intermittent claudication: A double blind crossover trial of pentoxifylline. Aust NZ J Med 15:402, 1985.
17. Lindgard, R, Bjorkman, H, Jelnes, R, et al: The evaluation of conservative drug treatment in patients with moderately severe peripheral vascular disease. Circulation 80:1549, 1989.
18. Mass, RD, Venook, AP, and Linker, CA: Pentoxifylline and aplastic anemia. Ann Intern Med 107:427, 1987.

CHAPTER 16

Nonsurgical Restoration of Pulsatile Arterial Flow

Robert A. Graor, M.D.
Bruce H. Gray, D.O.

Major changes in the treatment of cardiovascular disease have occurred in recent years. Technologic advances have fueled an intense renewed interest in interventional therapy for the treatment of peripheral arterial occlusive disease. Percutaneous techniques such as balloon angioplasty, thermal angioplasty, atherectomy, stent therapy, thrombolytic therapy, and ultrasound ablation methods have been employed with increasing frequency. These new and older procedures are often performed in coordination with surgical therapy and should be viewed as alternate options in patients with peripheral arterial occlusive disease.

These interventional techniques are also perceived as procedures with lower total patient treatment costs than surgical treatment. Although this perception is held by most, it has not yet been proved. Hospital stays and patient recoveries are clearly shorter, but whether or not this will translate to a lower cost in the long term is unclear. The interventional and surgical therapies palliate symptoms, and neither surgery nor interventional techniques treat the primary disease of atherosclerosis obliterans (ASO). Until biochemical means are developed to prevent the progession or the development of atherosclerosis, these palliative techniques will remain a critical part of patient treatment in a growing patient population with ASO.

HISTORIC DEVELOPMENT OF TRANSLUMINAL TREATMENTS

EVOLUTION OF CATHETER THERAPY

In 1964, Dotter and Judkins[1] reported an intra-arterial dilating technique using progressively larger arterial sounds to stretch the artery. With this report, the concept of catheter-directed therapy was born. In 1978, Gruntzig and Hopff[2] described balloon angioplasty. One year later, Gruntzig and Kumpe[3] introduced this technique in the United States.

These early reports were met with skepticism by the surgical community, and despite numerous reports involving hundreds of patients, there is still some uncertainty as to the long-term outcome of these interventional techniques.

DEVELOPMENT OF CATHETER TECHNOLOGY

Several generations of interventional catheters have evolved primarily by improving the profile, or diameter, of the balloon and its inflation characteristics. Compliance, profile, and trackability are the major characteristic features of modern-day catheters.

Compliance is the change in the balloon diameter per unit of pressure change ($\Delta D/\Delta P$). The trend is toward the development of less compliant catheters, and with this change, the evolution of polyethylene and polyurethane materials has become more common. An overstretching balloon or a noncompliant balloon resulted in the maldistribution of dilating forces, frequently resulting in balloon breaking, overdilation, and, less commonly, vessel rupture during angioplasty. The noncompliant balloons avoid the problem of increasing pressures resulting in overdistension.

Profile, another important characteristic, is best described as a cross-sectional diameter of a catheter, and in the case of balloon catheters, the balloon wrap must be tight to allow easy passage into the artery. The smaller the catheter and balloon wrap, or profile, the easier it is for the catheter to traverse tight areas of arterial narrowing, and this results in lower entry site complications. Low profile balloons are now as small as 2 mm in diameter and can follow a centrally placed guide wire easily.

Trackability refers to the tendency of a catheter to follow a wire placed in the desired position without disturbing the position or pulling back the wire. This characteristic depends on the axial components of the catheter and the technical capability of the operator. Positioning of the catheter precisely is important to avoid balloon dilatation in an area of nondiseased artery.

PATHOPHYSIOLOGY OF BALLOON ANGIOPLASTY

MECHANISM OF PTA (percutaneous transluminal angioplasty)

In the original description, the mechanism of balloon angioplasty was thought to be due to redistribution and compression of the atherosclerotic plaque.[3,4] Although this appeared to be logical, most atherosclerotic plaque in human arteries is composed of a dense fibrocollagenous tissue with varying degrees of calcific deposits and much smaller amounts of intercellular and extracellular lipid. Thus, it appears unlikely that plaque compression plays a major role in human artery angioplasty dilation.

Another mechanism of artery dilatation is the stretching of the plaque-free wall segments of eccentric atherosclerotic lesions.[5,6] Inflation of the balloon may extend or stretch the normal wall segment and produce little or no damage to the plaque. Stretching this plaque-free wall segment will result initially in an increase in arterial diameter, but the gradual relaxation over this overstretched segment reduces the lumen toward the predilation state within several weeks. This relaxation may be another explanation for early restenosis after an initially successful dilatation.

Table 16–1. Early and Late
Morphologic Changes
Associated with PTA

Early changes (<30 days)
1. Fracture of plaque
2. Intima and media splits or dissections
3. Lifting or separating of plaque from the surface
Late changes (>30 days)
1. No morphologic change
2. Intimal fibrous proliferation
3. Fibrocellular proliferation

A third possible mechanism for balloon angioplasty resulting in an increase in luminal dimensions is a combination of vessel stretching with minimal or mild plaque compression. An oversized angioplasty balloon may stretch the entire arterial segment that is concentrically narrowed by fibrocollagenous plaque. Although this overstretching technique has been highly successful, it has been plagued by two major problems at the angioplasty site: (1) early or abrupt closure and (2) late closure or restenosis.

Abrupt closure occurs at a peripheral arterial angioplasty site in fewer than 5% of patients treated with balloon angioplasty.[7] The obvious explanations for abrupt closure include spasm, localized thrombus formation, and dissection.[8,9] During overdilatation, if a large dissection occurs, the intimal flap can result in thrombus formation or simply result in mechanical occlusion of the arterial lumen. Abrupt closure may also be produced by relaxation of the overstretched, disease-free wall of an eccentric plaque.

Treatment, or prevention of abrupt closure, has consisted of repeated balloon angioplasty with prolonged inflation times, the infusion of thrombolytic agents, the use of intra-arterial stents, using thermal welding laser angioplasty, or employing an atherectomy device to remove large intimal flaps, thrombi, or other obstructing lesions.

The morphologic and histologic observations following balloon angioplasty are somewhat limited, but these data do provide clues as to the actual mechanism of action of balloon dilatation. The observations appear to be best divided into two categories: (1) early changes within 30 days after balloon angioplasty and (2) late changes beyond 30 days from the angioplasty (Table 16–1).

EARLY CHANGES AFTER PTA

The early morphologic changes in arteries have been described by several investigators. Block and associates[10] reported that in balloon-dilated coronary arteries, the fracturing of atherosclerotic plaque resulted in deep splits in the media. Mizuno and coworkers[11] described serially sectioned arteries at the site of balloon angioplasty and observed intimal and medial splitting that led to arterial dissection. Soward and colleagues[12] reported splitting, medial dissection, and lifting of the atherosclerotic plaque from the medial layer at the site of balloon angioplasty. These changes are all consistent with the initial injury produced by balloon dilatation.

LATE CHANGES AFTER PTA

Late morphologic changes observed in human arteries after PTA are divided into two major categories: (1) no morphologic evidence of previous angioplasty injury and (2) intimal fibrous proliferation. Waller[13] reported no morphologic or histologic changes at the site of angioplasty in three men who died suddenly after coronary angioplasty. Histologic assessment of the atherosclerotic plaque in the areas of previous angioplasty, compared with other areas of the atherosclerotic plaque in the same artery or in arteries in the same patient, disclosed no distinctive morphologic differences.

Essed and colleagues[14] were the first to report intimal fibrous proliferation at the site of coronary angioplasty. On cross sections of the dilated artery, they found evidence of previous disruption of the media with extensive proximal and distal dissection. After 5 months, fibrocellular proliferations surrounded portions of the atherosclerotic plaque, in addition to the area of previous plaque fracture, producing a severely narrowed artery. In all cases, the initial underlying atherosclerotic plaque was still clearly identified, and luminal channels created by angioplasty were filled with fibrocellular tissue that coated the denuded media.

Thus, at the angioplasty site, after angiographically successful balloon dilatation, a distinctive lesion or lesions may or may not be seen. Most commonly, a concentric fibrocellular proliferation is observed that is distinctly different from underlying atherosclerotic plaque. It is clear from these data that the healing process at the angioplasty site itself may increase or decrease the luminal size. An increase is the desired outcome, whereas a decrease is labeled "restenosis."

RESTENOSIS

The major problem with balloon angioplasty has been restenosis. The frequency of clinical restenosis ranges from 15% to 75%, depending on the size, location of the artery, and definition of restenosis. Multiple clinical, angiographic, technical, and pharmacologic factors have been analyzed to determine their role in promoting restenosis. Despite the large number of factors evaluated, studies diverge on the significance of many and concur on the significance of only a few.[15,16]

The most widely accepted theory for the development of restenosis is that fibrocellular intimal proliferation invokes responses from the damaged endothelium and media of the vessels.[17,18] The balloon angioplasty likely is the initial stimulus for the proliferation of the fibrocellular elements. The intimal proliferation may be precipitated by the release of thromboxane A_2, which leads to platelet deposition, the release of platelet-derived growth factors (PDGF), and fibroblast and endothelial growth factors.[19]

Other mechanisms implicated in late luminal narrowing or restenosis are the gradual elastic recoil from an overstretched, disease-free wall, the return to predilation state of an overstretched concentric lesion, and the progression of atherosclerotic disease. Plaque progression appears to be an unlikely cause in the 2 to 4 months after angioplasty, but it may be responsible for occurrences beyond this time interval.

ALTERNATE METHODS OF ANGIOPLASTY

THERMAL BALLOON ANGIOPLASTY

The use of thermal energy to produce plaque ablation or balloon angioplasty with thermal techniques is designed to decrease vessel elasticity at the dilatation site and remold the arterial segment to the size and the shape of the inflated balloon. In addition to the acute effects of remodeling, the thermal effects on the underlying media may destroy smooth muscle cells that may be involved in the late restenosis process.

Laser therapy to remove tissue has included hot-tipped probes and pulsed lasers of various energy spectra. Histologic studies of the vascular tissue after laser therapy show craters surrounded by concentric zones of protein denaturation and tissue vacuolization.[20] The resulting charred endothelial surface is not desirable and has led to high restenosis rates.[21-23]

Current laser research is concentrating on ablating tissue by limiting thermal injury. The two most common methods to achieve this goal are a modified tip for the delivery system of continuous wave lasers and the use of pulsed lasers. Other newer systems include employing fluorescence spectroscopy, which identifies tissue before laser treatment is delivered and thereby allows the energy to be delivered to the diseased tissue, sparing the normal arterial wall.

Although the current data reported on laser angioplasty has been disappointing, a future for laser therapy continues to be pursued with the development of further modified laser systems (Table 16–2).

ATHERECTOMY

New instruments to excise vascular obstructions have been promoted and are called atherectomy devices. The prototype of such instruments is the Simpson

Table 16–2. One-Year Results* of Laser-Assisted Balloon Angioplasty

Author	Lesion Location	Lesion Type	Lesion Length	Number Followed	Clinical Success at 1 Year
Diethrich[24]	Iliac	Stenosis		10	90%
		Occlusion		20	85%
	SFA†	Stenosis		28	93%
		Occlusion		69	90%
	Popliteal	Stenosis		5	80%
		Occlusion		8	63%
	Tibial	Stenosis		10	70%
		Occlusion		4	50%
Perler[25]	SFA/popliteal	Occlusion		22	35%
Sanborn[22]	SFA	Stenosis		21	95%
		Occlusion	1–3 cm	17	93%
			4–7 cm	26	76%
			>7 cm	35	58%

*Continuing clinical success in patients who were successfully treated initially.
†SFA = superficial femoral artery.

AtheroCath, an atherectomy instrument which consists of a circular cutting blade that can excise plaque when pressed against the diseased portion of the artery with an inflated balloon on the back side. Other atherectomy instruments use pulverization techniques to recanalize the artery. Only the Simpson device, however, retains tissue samples that can be removed from the catheter and examined microscopically, thereby providing a unique opportunity to evaluate removed tissue histologically.[26]

Atherectomy is an exciting new mechanical technique for the treatment of primary and restenotic lesions. A major concern of atherectomy is that the degree of tissue debulking may be an important concern in reducing the rate of restenosis. Exposure of large segments of medial smooth muscle may predispose atherectomy sites to intimal proliferation and restenosis. These concerns are currently under investigation. Improved guidance methods will likely be developed to more precisely remove tissue.

Published data accumulated at the Cleveland Clinic for directional atherectomy (Simpson AtheroCath) appear promising.[27] Calculations by the life table method demonstrate a 3-year patency for superficial femoral and popliteal artery treated lesions to be 82.4% for stenotic or short segment occlusions and 72.5% for long occlusions.

RESULTS OF BALLOON ANGIOPLASTY

Although early skepticism regarding PTA was voiced by the surgical community, it has become more widely accepted in recent years. Despite numerous reports involving hundreds of patients, there is still some uncertainty about the long-term outcome of PTA and about its role in the treatment of lesions of specific arterial segments in patients with different degrees of ischemia involving the lower extremity. This uncertainty is due, in part, to the lack of standardized reporting. As with any procedure, standardized reporting is critical for accurate evaluation and application of any technique.

The early reports of PTA appear to be comparable with those of surgery, but these reports often did not address the rate of acute failure, and these reports provided only a brief follow-up. More recent studies with observations from 1 to 5 years after the procedure have revealed less optimistic patency results in patients with severe ischemia. More optimistic patency has been observed in patients with lesser symptoms, that is, those with claudication alone.

An example of a trial comparing PTA and surgery in patients with milder disease was the prospective, randomized, cooperative trial that was reported by Wilson and associates.[28] In this study, PTA had a higher technical failure rate (immediate failure, 15.5%; technical failure, 7.8%; no mortality) compared with surgery (immediate failure, 7.1%; no technical failures; operative mortality, 0.8%), but the 3-year patency between the successful PTA group and the reconstruction surgery group is comparable. The patients in the PTA group probably were in a less advanced stage of the disease than patients in most surgical series because all lesions in both patient groups were correctable with angioplasty.

The results of PTA also vary according to the site of dilation and the extent and severity of the disease. Clinical variables proposed as predictors of good PTA results include the site of occlusion or stenosis (larger arteries yield better patency than smaller caliber arteries), the absence of diabetes, as well as several more con-

Table 16–3. Complications of PTA from Pooled Data

Type of Complication	Occurrence	% of Complications Requiring Surgery or Prolonged Hospital Stay
Angioplasty:		
Thrombosis	1–2%	50%
Guide wire dissection	1–2%	2–5%
Large angioplasty dissection	1–2%	5–10%
Embolus	0–3%	25%
Artery rupture	< 1%	100%
Puncture/entry site:		
Hematoma	5–15%	< 1%
Pseudoaneurysm	1–3%	90%
Thrombosis	1–2%	75%
Other:		
Contrast-induced renal failure	2–5%	10–20%
Fatal outcome	0–0.7%	

troversial variables such as the length of the lesion, runoff artery patency, indications for PTA, severity of the lesion (stenosis versus occlusion), and the degree of ischemia.[29–34]

Complications of PTA also have been inconsistently reported. Some studies reported all hematomas as complications, yielding complication rates as high as 20%, whereas others listed only complications requiring surgical intervention, yielding rates of 2% to 3%. Reporting of complications should be standardized and perhaps should include those that lengthen hospital stay or that require surgical correction or when excessive blood transfusion is required[35] (Table 16–3).

PTA FOR AORTIC LESIONS

Focal and concentric atherosclerotic stenosis of the distal aorta has been treated successfully with PTA. Although these lesions are unusual and the published experience is small, the technical success rate is high and complications appear to be low. The combined results of three published series revealed that 48 of 52 patients had technically successful PTAs with an 83% patency at a mean follow-up of 13 months.[36–38] Three patients had a second PTA during the follow-up period. Three major complications occurred: a distal embolus in one patient, a pseudoaneurysm in one patient, and thrombosis of a common femoral artery in one patient.

PTA FOR ILIAC LESIONS

For dilation of iliac artery stenosis, immediate success rates ranged from 79% to 93%, and from 70% to 80% of the treated vessels are patent at 2 to 3 years (Figs. 16–1 and 16–2).[29–32] The clinical indications for PTA in the iliac artery segments have ranged from claudication to limb salvage. More than 95% of all PTAs in this group are technically successful.

Due to the high technical and long-term success rates of PTA in the iliac artery

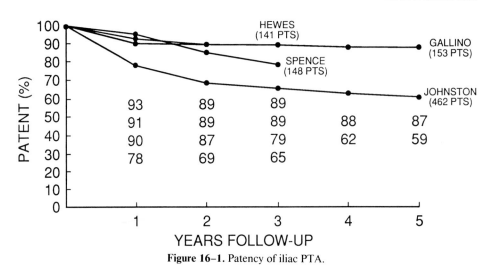

Figure 16–1. Patency of iliac PTA.

segments, it is the treatment of choice for patients with segmental stenosis involving these arterial segments. Alternative surgical therapy includes aortoiliac bypass surgery or aortoiliac endarterectomy, which is associated with a conservatively higher morbidity and mortality for the latter operation. In most series, serious complications during and following iliac PTA occur in less than 2% of patients treated.

Because PTA in the iliac region best serves those patients with segmental disease, that is, disease not extending into the aorta, suitable candidates for PTA represent less than 5% of patients encountered with lower extremity ischemia. One additional advantage of PTA compared with surgery for iliac disease is the cost savings associated with the low complication rates and short hospital stays (usually 1 to 2 days).

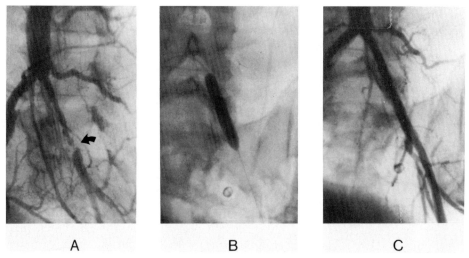

Figure 16–2 (*A*) Arteriogram of the abdominal aorta and iliac arteries demonstrating an occlusion of the left common iliac artery (*arrow*). (*B*) An 8-mm diameter balloon fully inflated at the site of the occlusion. (*C*) Completion arteriogram shows an excellent result without dissection of the arterial wall.

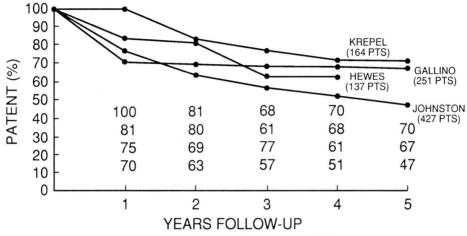

Figure 16–3. Patency of femoropopliteal PTA.

FEMOROPOPLITEAL PTA

Data from pooled studies reporting results of femoropopliteal PTA show an early mean patency of 89% in 979 patients.[29–31,33] The 5-year patency in this group was 61% (Figs. 16–3 and 16–4).

In a nonrandomized, prospective study, Martin and coworkers[39] evaluated PTA in the femoropopliteal system as compared with saphenous vein bypass grafting. Owing to the nonrandomized fashion in which the study was conducted, the lesions in both study groups would not necessarily be equivalent. With these study flaws in mind, the initial patency rates (76% for PTA and surgery groups) and 2-

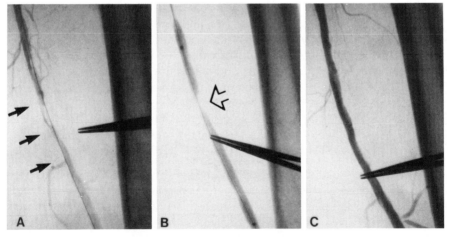

Figure 16–4 (A) Arteriogram of the left common, superficial (arrows), and profunda femoral arteries. (B) A 6-mm diameter balloon with a resistant "waist" (open arrow) that fully expanded with a higher pressure. (C) Completion arteriogram demonstrating resolution of the tight stenosis.

year patency rates (57% for PTA and 56% for bypass grafts) were the same. It should be noted that unusually low patency rates were observed in this study for saphenous vein bypass grafting. The majority of reported data regarding saphenous vein, femoropopliteal or femorotibial bypass grafting yields 70% to 80% 4-year patency.

Blair and colleagues[40] conducted a retrospective study comparing the results of PTA with those of infrainguinal bypass procedures in patients with *critical limb ischemia.* Thirty-nine of the fifty-four (72%) patients initially improved after PTA, but only 18% had improved Doppler studies at 2 years. Despite these poor results, limb salvage was 78%. In the surgical group, 2-year patency was 68% and limb salvage was 90%. Bypass grafts were statistically better ($p < 0.001$) than PTA results, but no significant difference was noted in limb salvage owing to the small number of patients in this study. In the PTA group, there were more subsequent procedures than in the surgery group ($p < 0.01$). These data support the contention that bypass grafting is more durable than PTA when limb salvage is the indication for the procedure. This is likely due to the more extensive disease encountered in the limb salvage patients. It may not be the expectation of the interventionist that PTA in this setting would be desirable.

Several individual studies are of interest. Zeitler[41] reported that in 437 patients with occluded superficial femoral arteries, 73% had initially good response to PTA and 60% remained patent at 2 years. Waltman and associates[42] reported succesful PTA outcome in 87% of stenoses and 76% of occlusions in an undisclosed follow-up. Johnston and coworkers[43] reported a 60% cumulative patency at 1 year for stenoses and a 40% patency rate for occlusions.[43]

Nonfatal complications associated with PTA in the femoropopliteal regions are believed to be less than 5%, and serious complications, less than 1%. The mortality rate has been reported to be 0.4%. This low mortality rate compares with a surgical mortality rate of 2% to 4% for femoropopliteal or femorotibial bypass grafting.

INFRAPOPLITEAL PTA

Recent studies published by Schwarten and Cutcliff[44] demonstrate that infrapopliteal PTA is commonly done in conjunction with proximal PTA or other more proximal inflow procedures. This study provides the most reliable data as a result of improvements in balloon catheters and adjunctive medications for angioplasty in this region. They reported 126 patients with an initial success rate of 94% and an undisclosed 2-year patency rate[44] (see Fig. 16–5).

OTHER SITES FOR ANGIOPLASTY

Owing to the broad scope of applied angioplasty, it is not possible to present detailed descriptions of renal or cerbrovascular balloon angioplasty in this text. In the area of renal angioplasty, successful application of angioplasty for fibromuscular disease has occurred. The results associated with atherosclerotic renal artery disease are highly dependent on the type of lesion and the location of that atherosclerotic lesion. In short, ostial lesions tend to restenose at a high rate and may be more amenable to treatment with future devices. A main renal artery stenosis can be

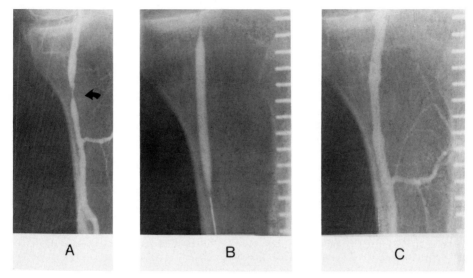

Figure 16–5 (*A*) Arteriogram of a left popliteal artery stenosis prior to balloon angioplasty (*arrow*). (*B*) A 4-mm diameter balloon was inflated to full expansion. (*C*) A higher magnification of mild post-angioplasty stenosis at the site of previous high-grade stenosis.

successfully dilated, and data support patency rates of 50% to 90% at relatively short follow-up periods.

Angioplasty for carotid, vertebral, and subclavian disease has also been reported with increasing frequency. More time and more data will be necessary to fully evaluate the application of this modality in these regions.

SUMMARY

Percutaneous transluminal angioplasty is an established method of revascularization in a variety of arterial stenotic conditions. When applied to specific morphologic and clinical indications, it can be very effective.

It appears to be the procedure of choice for focal stenotic lesions of the iliac and femoropopliteal system. Its role in infrapopliteal atherosclerotic disease is less certain, but more optimistic, with recent reports.

New methods for preventing restenosis and abrupt closure are currently being developed, and they appear to be promising as adjunctive therapy with mechanical catheter-directed intervention. The future of these adjunctive agents will likely improve the outcome and reduce the immediate failure rates of angioplasty. Other modalities, including thermal laser angioplasty and atherectomy, also appear to have a promising future. These methods, coupled with better endoluminal guidance, such as ultrasound, will help guide the interventional procedure more precisely and hopefully broaden the application and improve the outcome.

REFERENCES

1. Dotter, CT and Judkins, MP: Transluminal treatment of atherosclerotic obstruction: Description of a new technique and a preliminary report of its application. Circulation 30:654, 1964.
2. Gruntzig, A and Hopff, H: Percutane Rekanlisation chronisch arterieller Verschlusse mit einem neuen Dilatiionskatheter. Dtsch Med Wochenschr 99:2502, 1974.

3. Gruntzig, A and Kumpe, DA: Technique of percutaneous angioplasty with Gruntzig balloon catheter. AJR 132:547, 1979.
4. Zeitler, E, Schoop, W, and Zahnow, W: The treatment of occlusive arterial disease by transluminal catheter angioplasty. Radiology 99:19, 1971.
5. Waller, BF: Coronary luminal shape and the arc of disease-free wall: Morphologic observations and clinical relevance. J Am Coll Cardiol 6:1100, 1985.
6. Waller, BF: The eccentric coronary atherosclerotic plaque: Morphologic observations and clinical relevance. Clin Cardiol 12:14, 1989.
7. Caserella, WJ: Noncoronary angioplasty. Curr Prob Cardiol 11:138, 1986.
8. LeVeen, RF, Wolf, GL, and Biery, D: Angioplasty induced vasospasm in rabbit model: Mechanisms and treatment. Invest Radiol 20:938, 1985.
9. Sinclair, IN, McCabe, CH, Sipperly, ME, and Baim, DSA: Predictors, therapeutic options and long-term outcome of abrupt reclosure. Am J Cardiol 61:615, 1988.
10. Block, PC, Myler, RK, Stertzer, S, and Fallon, JT: Morphology after transluminal angioplasty in human beings. N Engl J Med 305:382, 1981
11. Mizuno, K, Jurita, A, and Imazeki N: Pathologic findings after percutaneous transluminal coronary angioplasty. Br Heart J 52:588, 1984.
12. Soward, AL, Essed, CE, and Serruys, PW: Coronary arterial findings after accidental death immediately after successful percutaneous transluminal coronary angioplasty. Am J Cardiol 56:794, 1985.
13. Waller, BF: Early and late morphologic changes in human coronary arteries after percutaneous transluminal coronary angioplasty. Clin Cardiol 6:363, 1983.
14. Essed, CD, Brand, MVD, and Becker, AE: Transluminal coronary angioplasty and early restenosis. Br Heart J 49:393, 1983
15. Myler, RM, Shaw, RE, Stertzer, SH, et al: Recurrence after coronary angioplasty. Cathet Cardiovasc Diagn 13:77, 1987
16. Zollikofer, CL, Redha, FH, Bruhlmann, WF, et al: Acute and long-term effects of massive balloon dilation on the aortic wall and vasa vasorum. Radiology 164:145, 1987.
17. Austin, GE, Norman, NB, Hollman, J, et al: Intimal proliferation of smooth muscle cells as an explanation for recurrent coronary artery stenosis after percutaneous transluminal coronary angioplasty. J Am Coll Cardiol 6:369, 1985.
18. Waller, BF, Gorfinkel, HJ, Rogers, FJ, et al: Early and late morphologic changes in major epicardial coronary arteries after percutaneous transluminal coronary angioplasty. Am J Cardiol 53:42C, 1984.
19. Fuster, V, Adams, PC, Badimon, JJ, and Chesebro, JH: Platelet-inhibitor drugs' role in coronary artery disease. Prog Cardiovasc Dis 29:325, 1987.
20. Sinclair, IN: Effect of laser balloon angioplasty on normal dog coronary arteries in vivo (abstr). J Am Coll Cardiol 11:108A, 1988.
21. Forrester, JS, Litvack, F, and Grundfest, W: Vaporization of atheroma in man: The role of lasers in the era of balloon angioplast. Int J Cardiol 20:1, 1988.
22. Sanborn, TA, Cumberland, DC, Greenfield, AJ, et al: Percutaneous laser thermal angioplasty: Initial results and 1-year follow-up in 129 femoropopliteal lesions. Radiology 168:121, 1988.
23. Cumberland, DC, Sanborn, TA, Taylor, DL, et al: Percutaneous laser thermal angioplasty; initial clinical results with a laser probe in a total peripheral artery occlusion. Lancet 1:457, 1986.
24. Diethrich, EB, Timbadia, E, and Bahadir, I: Applications and limitations of laser-assisted angioplasty. Eur J Vasc Surg 3:61, 1989
25. Perler, BA, Osterman, FA, White, RI, et al: Percutaneous laser probe femoropopliteal angioplasty: A preliminary experience. J Vasc Surg 10:351, 1989.
26. Simpson, JB, Selmon, JR, Robertson, GC, et al: Transluminal atherectomy for occlusive peripheral vascular disease. Am J Cardiol 61:965, 1988.
27. Graor, RA and Whitlow, P: Atherectomy for directional atherectomy for peripheral vascular disease: Two year patency and factors influencing patency (abstr). J Am Coll Cardiol 17:106A, 1991.
28. Wilson, SE, Wolf, GL, Cross, AP, et al: Percutaneous transluminal angioplasty versus operation for peripheral arteriosclerosis. J Vasc Surg 9:1, 1989.
29. Johnston, KW, Rae, M, Hoss-Johnston, SA, et al: Five year results of a prospective study of percutaneous transluminal angioplasty. Ann Surg 206(4):404, 1987.
30. Gallino, A, Mahler, F, Probst, P, and Nachbur, B: Percutaneous transluminal angioplasty of the arteries of the lower limbs: A 5-year follow up. Circulation 70:619, 1984

31. Hewes, RC, White, RI, Jr, Murray, RR, et al: Long-term results of superficial femoral artery angioplasty. AJR 146:1025, 1986.
32. Spence, R, Freiman, D, Gatenby, R, et al: Long-term results of transluminal angioplasty of the iliac and femoral arteries. Arch Surg 116:1377, 1981.
33. Krepel, VM, van Andel, GJ, van Erp, WFM, et al: Percutaneous transluminal angioplasty of the femoropopliteal artery: Initial and long-term results. Radiology 156:325, 1985.
34. Colapinto, RF, Harries-Jones, EP, and Johnston, KW: Percutaneous transluminal angioplasty of peripheral vascular disease: A two year experience. Cardiovasc Intervent Radiol 3:213–218, 1980.
35. Gardiner, GA, Jr, Meyerovitz, MF, Stokes, KR, et al: Complications of transluminal angioplasty. Radiology 159:201, 1986.
36. Heeney, D, Bookstein, J, Daniels, E, et al: Transluminal angioplasty of the abdominal aorta. Radiology 148:81, 1983.
37. Charlebois, N, Saint-Georges, G, and Hudon, G: Percutaneous transluminal angioplasty of the lower abdominal aorta. AJR 146:369, 1986.
38. Tegtmeyer, CJ, Kellum, DC, Kron, IL, and Mentzer, RM, Jr: Percutaneous transluminal angioplasty in the region of the aortic bifurcation: The two balloon technique with results and long term follow up study. Radiology 157:661, 1985.
39. Martin, EC, Fankuchen, EI, Karlson, KB, et al: Angioplasty for femoral artery occlusion: Comparison with surgery. AJR 137:915, 1981.
40. Blair, JM, Gewertz, BL, Moosa, H, et al: Percutaneous transluminal angioplasty versus surgery for limb-threatening ischemia. J Vasc Surg 9:698, 1989.
41. Zeitler, E: Result of percutaneous transluminal angioplasty. Radiology 146:57, 1983.
42. Waltman, AC, Greenfield, AJ, Noveline, RA, et al: Transluminal angioplasty of the iliac and femoropopliteal arteries: Current status. Arch Surg 117:1218, 1982.
43. Johnston, KW, Colapinto, RF, and Baird, RJ. Transluminal dilation: An alternative? Arch Surg 117:1604, 1982.
44. Schwarten, DE and Cutcliff, WB: Arterial occlusive disease below the knee: Treatment with percutaneous transluminal angioplasty performed with low profile catheters and steerable guide wires. Radiology 169:71, 1988.

Index

A "f" following a page number indicates a figure. A "t" following a page number indicates a table.